CW00495010

Rational Emotive Behavior Therapy in Sport and Exercise

Rational Emotive Behavior Therapy (REBT) is one of the most widely used counselling approaches in the world and is one of the original forms of Cognitive Behavior Therapy (CBT). *Rational Emotive Behavior Therapy in Sport and Exercise* is the first and only book to date to examine the use of REBT in sport and exercise.

It brings together leading international experts and practitioners to reflect on the use of REBT in sport and exercise, and examine the techniques used. Each chapter contains a case study, contextualising theory into practice, giving a rare and detailed insight into the use of REBT across a diverse range of issues. Some of the topics covered include:

- the theory and practice of REBT
- REBT intervention for competition anxiety
- the use of REBT interventions in Paralympic soccer
- the use of REBT in managing injury and loss
- using REBT to address symptoms of exercise dependence
- REBT intervention to improve low frustration tolerance.

Offering an invaluable insight into the practical application of REBT, this book is essential reading for undergraduates, postgraduates, trainee and qualified sport and exercise psychologists, and counsellors wishing to move into sport and exercise.

Martin Turner is a Chartered Psychologist and Associate Fellow of the British Psychological Society (BPS), is registered as a Sport and Exercise Psychologist with the Health and Care Professions Council, and is a Chartered Sport and Exercise Scientist with the British Association of Sport and Exercise Sciences. He is a prominent REBT Researcher and Speaker, and Senior Lecturer in Sport and Exercise Psychology at Staffordshire University, UK. His work using REBT in sport was featured in *The Psychologist*, the BPS's magazine. Martin was awarded the BPS Division of Sport and Exercise Psychology PhD of the year prize in 2013. He is currently Lead Psychologist for England Futsal with the FA. He has previously worked with Stoke City FC and Nottingham Forest FC, Staffordshire County Cricket and Nottingham County Cricket academies, and business organizations such as SONY.

Richard Bennett is a Chartered Psychologist and Associate Fellow of the British Psychological Society, is registered as a Clinical Psychologist with the Health and Care Professions Council, and is an accredited Cognitive Behavioral Psychotherapist with the British Association of Behavioural and Cognitive Psychotherapies. He has extensive knowledge and skill in the theory and practice of REBT after more than 20 years' experience working clinically within the NHS and private practice. In addition to his clinical experience, Richard has widespread experience of teaching and training in REBT. He is a Senior Academic Tutor in Cognitive Behavior Therapy (CBT) within the psychology department at the University of Birmingham, UK, where he is the lead for the Postgraduate Diploma in High Intensity Psychological Therapies, and Deputy Course Director of the Centre for REBT.

Routledge Psychology of Sport, Exercise and Physical Activity

This series offers a forum for original and cutting edge research exploring the latest ideas and issues in the psychology of sport, exercise and physical activity. Books within the series showcase the work of well-established and emerging scholars from around the world, offering an international perspective on topical and emerging areas of interest in the field. This series aims to drive forward academic debate and bridge the gap between theory and practice, encouraging critical thinking and reflection among students, academics and practitioners. The series is aimed at upper-level undergraduates, research students and academics, and contains both authored and edited collections.

Available in this series:

Rational Emotive Behavior Therapy in Sport and Exercise

Edited by Martin Turner
and Richard Bennett

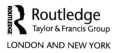
Routledge
Taylor & Francis Group

LONDON AND NEW YORK

First published 2018
by Routledge
2 Park Square, Milton Park, Abingdon, Oxon OX14 4RN

and by Routledge
711 Third Avenue, New York, NY 10017

Routledge is an imprint of the Taylor & Francis Group, an Informa business

© 2018 selection and editorial matter, Martin Turner and Richard Bennett; individual chapters, the contributors

The right of Martin Turner and Richard Bennett to be identified as the authors of the editorial material, and of the authors for their individual chapters, has been asserted in accordance with sections 77 and 78 of the Copyright, Designs and Patents Act 1988.

All rights reserved. No part of this book may be reprinted or reproduced or utilized in any form or by any electronic, mechanical, or other means, now known or hereafter invented, including photocopying and recording, or in any information storage or retrieval system, without permission in writing from the publishers.

Trademark notice: Product or corporate names may be trademarks or registered trademarks, and are used only for identification and explanation without intent to infringe.

British Library Cataloguing-in-Publication Data
A catalogue record for this book is available from the British Library

Library of Congress Cataloging-in-Publication Data
A catalog record for this book has been requested

ISBN: 978-1-138-68845-2 (hbk)
ISBN: 978-1-315-54180-8 (ebk)

Typeset in Goudy
by Apex CoVantage, LLC

Contents

Figures

Table

Contributors

Murat Artiran is the Director of the Affiliated Center of the Albert Ellis Institute-Turkey. He is an approved supervisor and trainer of Rational Emotive Behavior Therapy. After earning a bachelor's degree from Eastern Kentucky University he got his master's degree in a General Psychology program from the American APU University in West Virginia. He holds a doctoral degree in Clinical Psychology from Arel University.

Jamie Barker is Associate Professor of Applied Sport and Performance Psychology at Staffordshire University, with a research interest in the application of psychological techniques to maximize performance across a variety of domains. At the time of writing, Jamie is Chair for the British Psychological Society's Division of Sport and Exercise Psychology (DSEP).

Angela Breitmeyer is currently a licensed clinical psychologist in the state of Arizona and a faculty member at Midwestern University. Angela has consulted with sports teams and individual athletes, primarily at the university level. Designated as an Association for Applied Sport Psychology Certified Consultant (CC-AASP), she has been a member of the organization for ten years. In 2013 Angela became a member of the United States Olympic Committee's sport psychology registry.

Clare Churchman is dual registered with the Health Care Professions Council (HCPC) and works full time in the NHS as a clinical psychologist based in forensic services as well as offering REBT informed sport consultancy in an independent capacity. She is BASES Accredited and is a qualified Clinical Psychologist.

Rachel Cunningham currently works as a Professional Teaching Fellow at the University of Auckland (NZ) in Sport and Exercise Psychology. Rachel graduated with a Master of Science in Sport and Exercise Psychology from Staffordshire University. Historically, she has worked coaching adults and young people in sport, as well as training individuals as a fitness instructor.

Oana David is currently an Associate Professor within the Department of Clinical Psychology and Psychotherapy at Babeş-Bolyai University (BBU)

Cluj-Napoca, and a licensed clinical psychologist. She is the executive director of the International Coaching Institute and the European Coaching Center, services and research units of the Department at BBU. Oana is the founding president of the International Association of Cognitive Behavioral Coaching, dedicated towards the application of the cognitive-behavior theory in the coaching field.

Saqib Deen is studying for a PhD in the use of REBT to enhance resilience at Staffordshire University. Saqib is REBT-trained, has a passion for travel, fitness, and badminton, and is making the transition into being a sport psychologist after working in the finance sector. His enthusiasm has taken him to Malaysia to work as a research partner with the National Sports Institute (ISN) based in Kuala Lumpur.

Martin Eubank is the Subject Leader and Principal Lecturer in Sport Psychology at Liverpool John Moores University, Liverpool, England. He is a Registered Sport and Exercise Psychologist (Health and Care Professions Council) and British Psychological Society Chartered Psychologist, and is Chief Assessor for the BPS Stage 2 Qualification in Sport and Exercise Psychology. Martin has worked with numerous athletes and coaches across multiple sports, from local athletes to elite and Olympic performers.

Michelle Huggins is an Advanced Practitioner of the Albert Ellis Institute of REBT therapists and a Chartered Clinical and Sport and Exercise Psychologist. Michelle has a range of experience with athletes including those participating in team and individual sports. Her interest and enthusiasm for REBT is in the rationality of the model as a meaningful and person centred trans diagnostic approach.

Jonathan Katz is a Consultant Psychologist whose experience includes holding a wide variety of senior advisory and coaching positions in high performance sport and business environments. His roles have included National Lead for Psychology with the British Paralympic Association, National Governing Body Squad and Lead Psychologist across Olympic, Paralympic, and professional settings supporting all levels across high performance sport, and psychology support and coaching at four Paralympic Games.

Robert Morris is a Lecturer in Sport Social Science and Programme Leader for the BSc (Hons) Science and Football degree programme at Liverpool John Moores University, Liverpool, England. He is a Registered Sport and Exercise Psychologist (Health and Care Professions Council) and British Psychological Society Chartered Psychologist. Robert has worked with a number of athletes and coaches in the United Kingdom in a range of different sports including golf, football, and rugby.

Helen O'Connor is a Chartered Psychologist based in the United Kingdom. She has worked in the private, public, and charity sectors with a particular focus on health behavior change and emotional well-being. Helen first trained in and used REBT whilst working at a residential weight loss camp for children and young people, and has continued to practice REBT whilst supporting clients in areas such as weight management, smoking cessation, problem drinking, and substance misuse.

Leon Outar is a Trainee Sports and Exercise Psychologist studying for a PhD in the use of REBT in exercise settings at Staffordshire University. He is an REBT practitioner receiving his training from the Centre for REBT based at the University of Birmingham. His main interests include aesthetic manipulation and the role of body image upon psychological well-being. Moreover, he is a fitness model competitor competing previously in Miami Pro.

Aaron Phelps-Naqvi is a BPS Chartered Sport and Exercise Psychologist with extensive experience of working within high performance sport settings with a range of different sports and demographics in the United Kingdom. With qualifications and experience of delivering REBT education in sport and academia, Aaron has worked with groups and individuals to enhance understanding, performance, and well-being in addition to providing a counselling support network.

Gangyan Si is an Associate Professor at the Education University of Hong Kong and the President of the International Society of Sport Psychology (ISSP). Over the past 20 years, Dr. Si has worked directly with a variety of Chinese national teams and Hong Kong teams providing sport psychology services and has frequently provided on-site psychology support at big Games, such as the 2002, 2006, and 2010 Asian Games and the 2004, 2008, and 2012 Olympic Games.

David Tod is a Senior Lecturer in Sport Psychology at Liverpool John Moores University, Liverpool, England. He is a British Psychological Society Chartered Psychologist. David has worked with numerous athletes and coaches across multiple sports in New Zealand, Australia, and the United Kingdom, from weekend warriors to elite and professional performers.

Evangelos Vertopoulos is trained in REBT, which is the approach he uses in his work with athletes. He received his master's in Sport and Exercise Psychology from Staffordshire University. His practice in sport psychology counselling is influenced by his sports background both as a modern pentathlon and fencing athlete, and as a fencing coach.

Andrew Wood is Lecturer in Sport and Exercise Psychology and is completing a PhD investigating the effects of REBT as an intervention to enhance performance within the context of elite sport. As a consultant Andrew has worked with a wide variety of athletes, teams, and coaches, providing psychological support to develop sporting excellence and personal well-being. Andrew is currently the Lead Psychologist for the England Blind Football Team.

Charlotte Woodcock is a Chartered Psychologist with the British Psychological Society (CPsychol) and is an accredited Sport and Exercise Scientist with the

British Association of Sport and Exercise Sciences (BASES). Charlotte has ten years' experience working with a variety of performers from racing drivers to ballet dancers, and during this time collaborated with Elmhurst School for Dance, the English National Ballet School, and Scottish Rugby Union.

Chun-Qing Zhang is a Research Assistant Professor at Hong Kong Baptist University. Before obtaining his doctoral degree, he had been working for almost four years as a Sport Psychology Consultant at the Shenzhen Sport Training Center, China, and as a Research Assistant at the Hong Kong Sports Institute.

Acknowledgements

Martin

My sincerest gratitude goes to colleagues with whom I have collaborated over the years, especially those at Staffordshire University. I also extend my thanks to those who read and engage with my work examining REBT in sport, exercise, and occupational settings, from those who email me with questions and comments, to those who have attended my workshops and talks. I also thank Richard Bennett for joining me on this project; his expertise has been invaluable, and I learn more about REBT each time we speak.

But most of all, I thank my wife Jayne for her continued and unwavering love and support.

Richard

I am indebted to the wonderful community of people who have shaped my career in the fields of psychology and psychotherapy. You know who you are. In terms of the REBT community, I wish to extend my heartfelt thanks for the personal and professional influence of Jason Jones, Peter Trower, and Windy Dryden. Most of what I know about REBT I learned from you. I am also very thankful to Martin Turner for the invitation to co-edit this book. Your unswerving dedication to your work is an inspiration.

To my family and friends, and especially to Ingrid – you constantly work to hold me to a higher standard than the one to which I hold myself. I am forever grateful.

Both

We both want to extend our heartfelt thanks to the authors of the chapters in this book. Each author generously gave their time and effort to writing chapters that reflect the breadth, depth, and quality of the REBT work that is being done in sport and exercise settings across a range of contexts and issues. Special thanks go to William Bailey and Rebecca Connor at Routledge for their assistance in preparing this book.

1 The use of Rational Emotive Behavior Therapy (REBT) in sport and exercise

An introduction

Martin Turner and Richard Bennett

This book marks a significant development in studying the application of REBT within sport and exercise settings. Enclosed, across sixteen chapters, practitioners generously share their work using, and in many cases adapting, REBT within challenging but rewarding sport and exercise domains. The chapters that comprise *Rational Emotive Behavior Therapy in Sport and Exercise* demonstrate authors working across many psychological and performance related issues, across a variety of ages, abilities, and cultures, within an assortment of sport and exercise settings. As readers will discover, using REBT within sport and exercise environments has various challenges, some of which are predictable, and others that are unforeseen. Using REBT flexibly in these environments is paramount, because most practitioners do not have 50–60 minutes for a one-to-one session, and in most cases do not have the luxury of a private and dedicated consulting room. However, many practitioners do have the advantage of being able to consult with clients in the actual performance setting in which their clients toil, which, alongside many challenges, presents unique opportunities to apply and integrate REBT into a performer's environment more effectively.

Rational Emotive Behavior Therapy in Sport and Exercise was conceived due to the lack of published reports of the use of REBT in sport and exercise settings. Whilst practitioners probably quite frequently use REBT in sport and exercise settings, the presence of literature describing this usage is sparse. This presents a number of problems, such as lack of awareness about the utility of REBT, lack of evidence for the use of REBT in sport and exercise, and also a lack of guidelines for how REBT can be integrated into sport and exercise environments. In other words, how can practitioners use REBT in these contexts, and how might the mechanics of REBT be adapted to fit the unpredictable, constantly changing, and dynamic milieu of sport and exercise? This book aims to answer these important questions, whilst meeting a need within sport and exercise psychology literature for more reports of REBT being applied with athletes and exercisers.

The fact that there is a dearth of literature on the use of REBT in sport and exercise is curious, because REBT is not novel. We will comment in some detail on what REBT is (and what REBT is not) in the next chapter, but it is important to realize that REBT was conceived by Dr. Albert Ellis in the 1950s, with the publication of "Rational psychotherapy and individual psychology" in 1957

(Ellis, 1957). Therefore, REBT (or RT as it was first called) is 60+ years old. As such, REBT is not a new discovery, and furthermore even in sport and exercise, the use of REBT is not new. Although the use of REBT in sport and exercise has only recently begun to garner *significant* research interest, the first reported use of REBT in sport occurred in a book chapter by Professor Michael Bernard in 1985. In his chapter, Bernard describes his application of an REBT program with professional Australian Rules Football players. After the work, Bernard reports that the athletes were better able to control their thoughts to directly influence performance. Bernard's chapter had a major influence in the development of this volume, as it was essentially a detailed case study that captured the mechanics of using REBT in sport; a chief aim of *Rational Emotive Behavior Therapy in Sport and Exercise*.

The reader can engage with the extant literature that reports the use of REBT in sport and exercise independently, as a full review is not the focus of this introduction. Since Bernard (1985), around twenty papers have been published. Much of the research is covered in Turner (2016), but new research is emerging frequently. Notably, in most research papers, due to publication restrictions and the understandable focus on contribution to length, the intricate details of REBT interventions are often omitted from research articles. The current book addresses this omission by permitting authors to go into greater detail about how they applied REBT with their clients, including facets of the work that might be less glamorous or more difficult, contributing to an on-going narrative about how REBT can and "should" be used. In other words, the authors of the chapters in this book have been encouraged to take a balanced view of what they did, in the interest of self-reflection and transparency.

One notable consequence of REBT being written about and talked about in sport and exercise domains is the increased number of sport and exercise psychology practitioners and trainee practitioners becoming trained in REBT. Similarly, those who are already trained in REBT, and who typically work in clinical environments, are becoming more interested in how their skills may apply to athletes and exercisers. This represents a fascinating cross-pollination of skills and ideas across very different domains that can only serve to enhance our understanding of REBT, and more broadly, the psychological health and well-being of athletes and exercisers. With the current book, we hope to further engage and interest practitioners across domains, and hope to encourage those using REBT in sport and exercise to write about and publish their experiences.

Considering this brief introduction, it can be seen that REBT in sport and exercise is gaining research interest, is becoming more popular with practitioners, and is beginning to inspire performance-specific developments (e.g., the measurement of irrational performance beliefs). This book builds on the research to date by offering sixteen diverse, and in many cases pioneering, chapters that illustrate how, and importantly why, REBT has been applied in the sport or exercise setting the practitioner found themselves in. For the first time, a book brings together the expertise and experiences of practitioners applying REBT in sport and exercise settings from around the world. This book will appeal to established REBT practitioners who are curious about the various applications of REBT in sport and exercise, and sport and exercise psychologists who are curious about REBT. This book will appeal to neophyte and experienced practitioners, researchers and academics, athletes, and students who wish to understand more about REBT and how it can be used in sport and exercise settings.

References

Bernard, M. E. (1985). A rational-emotive mental training program for professional athletes. In A. Ellis & M. E. Bernard (Eds.), *Clinical applications of rational-emotive therapy* (pp. 227–309). New York, NY: Plenum.

Ellis, A. (1957). Rational psychotherapy and individual psychology. *Journal of Individual Psychology, 13*, 38–44.

Turner, M. J. (2016). Rational Emotive Behavior Therapy (REBT), irrational and rational beliefs, and the mental health of athletes. *Frontiers: Movement Science and Sport Psychology*, doi: 10.3389/fpsyg.2016.01423.

2 The theory and practice of Rational Emotive Behavior Therapy (REBT)

Richard Bennett and Martin Turner

This chapter outlines the philosophical and theoretical underpinnings of Rational Emotive Behavior Therapy (REBT) and places it in a historical context with other models within the cognitive behavioral tradition. The distinctive features of REBT as a model for understanding human psychological function and dysfunction will be outlined and Albert Ellis's ABC model will be described in detail. In defining the central tenets of REBT theory, the chapter will describe the primary role that rational and irrational beliefs, formed in response to real or perceived stimuli, play in predicting emotional, cognitive, behavioral, and physiological consequences. The chapter will describe how the ABC model can assist sport and exercise psychologists and others working in the field of performance management in the development of assessment, formulation, and intervention strategies.

REBT in context

Cognitive Behavioral Therapy (CBT) holds a dominant position within the field of psychological therapies. This is due to the significant evidence base that it has amassed for its efficacy across a range of different presentations and domains. Despite its often-reified status, it is important to establish at the outset that CBT is not a unitary 'thing'. Rather, it is a psychotherapeutic tradition, within which several different models have flourished, notably Cognitive Therapy (CT: Beck, 1976), REBT (Ellis, 1962), and more latterly Acceptance and Commitment Therapy (ACT: Hayes, et al., 1999).

The philosophical and conceptual foundations of CBT were initially established by Albert Ellis in the 1960s and many of the ideas and concepts central to REBT practice can be found in later variants of CBT, although Ellis's influence is not always acknowledged or credited (Velten, 2007). Ellis's (1962) pivotal text, "Reason and emotion in psychotherapy", presented his now familiar ABC model, although the roots of this model can be found in Ellis's writings further back (e.g., Ellis, 1958). Ellis was influenced by his love of philosophy, including the writings of Lao Tzu, Buddha, Epictetus, and Marcus Aurelius. With respect to these latter Stoic philosophers, Ellis was the first to apply a central tenet of their teachings to psychotherapy. This notion, that an individual's psychological disturbance is not wholly determined by events, but rather it is influenced by the beliefs that the individual holds about those events, has become a dominant feature of all models within the CBT tradition. Thus, Ellis paved the way for a sea change in the world of psychotherapy, in that formative experiences or parental attachments have been given less emphasis in pursuing an understanding of emotional distress, in favour of a more present-focused exploration of the way an individual's beliefs shape his or her emotions and associated behaviors. This 'here and now' focus has given rise to a more elegant form of psychological intervention; much more suited to today's healthcare economy. These characteristics also seem helpful within a sport and exercise context, given that practitioners are likely to be working under various constraints and that many athletes will not have the time or inclination to 'lie on a couch and talk about their mother' in the manner of the older psychoanalytic tradition. REBT is a short-term, structured, active, and collaborative therapy well-suited to the immediate and busy pace of many sport and exercise contexts.

There is a current trend within the CBT tradition for isolating the active ingredients of the model, such that it can be applied in much wider contexts, including for people with mental and physical health diagnoses, and in areas outside of the clinical realm, such as occupational and performance settings. To this end, there is a search for 'transdiagnostic' processes (Harvey, et al., 2004; Ellard, et al., 2010) and models of CBT with broad applicability. In this context, it is useful to be reminded that REBT was designed not as a means of diagnosing and treating 'mental illness', but as a means of understanding human function and dysfunction. It offers a perspective on human cognitive, emotional, and behavioral function that is equally applicable to an individual in a hospital ward diagnosed with paranoid schizophrenia (e.g., Bennett & Pearson, 2015) as it is to an athlete striving to maintain peak performance (e.g., Turner, 2016).

There is an extensive literature, including meta-analytic data, on the application of REBT to common mental health problems (Lyons & Woods, 1991; Engels, et al., 1993; Gonzalez, et al., 2004; Haddock, et al., 2015). REBT is also one of the interventions featured in the guideline for the treatment of depression by the National Institute of Health and Clinical Excellence in the UK (NICE, 2009). However, its application within the field of sport and exercise is in its relative infancy. The flexibility of REBT as a model that can help both explain and ameliorate distress and associated dysfunction irrespective of diagnosis or the form of that distress makes it well placed to address the many and varied issues that the sport and exercise context presents.

When one is delivering psychological interventions within a sport and exercise setting, there are certain advantages to adopting a theoretical model that can be flexibly applied across a range of cognitive, emotional, and behavioral issues. To illustrate with one example, it is possible that performance in a sporting competition might be viewed as a behavioral correlate of underlying emotional distress, such as anxiety or low mood. At a cognitive level, poor performance might also be a consequence of unhelpful beliefs around a demand for perfection, or global and negative self-evaluation when results do not go as desired. The ABC model of REBT is designed to elegantly account for this variation and allows the practitioner to apply the same assessment, formulation, and intervention template, irrespective of the precise content. Amongst the advantages of such a model is that it can be used as the basis for individual and/or group intervention without having to state narrow inclusion or exclusion criteria.

At the level of technique, there are a number of similarities between REBT and other forms of CBT. For example, REBT and CT have many similarities in both theory and practice, although there are some key points of divergence (for a review see Hyland & Boduszek, 2012). Notable amongst these differences is REBT's philosophical focus, in comparison to the more medical disorder-driven focus of CT. There have been few studies directly comparing REBT with CT, although in one study into the treatment of depression, Szentagotai, et al., (2008) found that whilst REBT, CT, and medication showed equal effectiveness post-intervention, REBT performed better at reducing irrational beliefs at six-month follow-up. This indicates that its impact may be longer lasting. When the underlying predictions of the different theoretical models have been explored using structural equation modelling, greater support has been found for REBT and the primary role of demandingness beliefs in the development of distress symptoms (Hyland, et al., 2014).

It is important for any model that is chosen to inform psychological intervention in sport and exercise to be able to explain the relationship between cognitions, emotions, and behavior. Poor performance is not an island and there are other influencing and interacting factors *within* an individual's experience, as well as in the interface *between* that individual and their environment. How often do we hear assertions such as, "Losing is so depressing" or, "That referee makes me so angry"? Whilst both beliefs might be associated with poorer sporting performance, the common interpretation here is that an external event has *caused* an emotional response, and that this leads directly to an undesirable behavioral consequence.

Such an interpretation, in REBT terms, represents an unhelpful 'A-C' model of thinking, in which an individual is powerless to resist the impact of external events, and where losing (A) makes him depressed (C), or refereeing decisions (A) make her angry (C). If this were really the case, and individuals were merely victims of circumstance, and there would be no role for a sport and exercise psychologist . . . but, what if the individual could learn to exert some influence between (A) and (C)? What if (C) were not dependent on (A)? What if the beliefs (B) that one holds about (A) were really what mattered? This book is about applying an ABC model to the issues relevant to sport and exercise psychology, in which an individual's beliefs about their situation are the driver for the emotion and behavior that follow.

REBT and the ABC model

Figure 2.1 illustrates the difference between an A-C model and an ABC model, the latter being consistent with REBT theory.

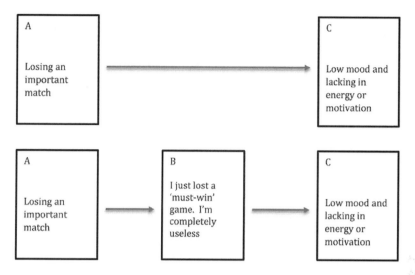

Figure 2.1 Comparing an A-C model and an ABC model

An individual who asserts that their emotions and behaviors are a direct result of external events (as in the A-C example) surrenders their agency in terms of influencing their own response. If someone takes the view that losing the match *made* them depressed, the only way to influence the depression is not to have lost the match in the first place, which is clearly impossible after the fact. This is a powerless position. If, however, one recognizes that the depressed feeling is largely determined by the beliefs that are held about losing the match, one is empowered to influence the depressed feeling and any associated patterns of behavior, since beliefs are amenable to change.

In the manner outlined previously, Ellis's ABC model established the principle, common to all CBTs, that beliefs about events are central in determining the range of responses one might have following any given event. Whilst common discourse is full of A-C language ("You make me so angry!" or "Airplanes terrify me!") and many people do not always recognize the power they have in terms of managing their own beliefs, REBT offers practitioners a tool for helping others to harness this power. One of the most striking things about the way the human mind works is how easily cognitions exert a regulatory function over behaviors. Most of what human adults do is done because their minds tell them to do it. Whilst most adults have acquired an enormously wide behavioral repertoire, this repertoire tends to become narrowed over time, for no other reason than one's mind takes control. An adult might decide that she is not the sort of person who dances or attends fancy dress parties, although it is highly probable that in her learning history she will have engaged in these behaviors, if only as a child. The important point here is that such behaviors will not have dropped out of her repertoire; rather, she simply chooses not to perform them. It is her beliefs that control these choices. In this example, her beliefs might be entirely rational, exemplified by flexible preferences, such as, "I don't really like dressing up and I don't have to go if I don't want to". However, on many occasions, the beliefs that limit our behavioral repertoire are not rational, and include rigid demands and condemnations, such as, "I don't really like dressing up and there-fore I must avoid it at all costs. I would look stupid and I could not tolerate that. Going to that party would be awful". This distinction is important, since the psychological experience of *freely choosing* not to attend the party is likely to be quite different from feeling that she *cannot* go. The ABC model is a tool for helping people identify when and where their irrational beliefs are impinging on the choices they make and giving rise to unhelpful emotional and behavioral consequences. At a philosophical level, the model implicitly values the common human drives for survival and enjoyment (DiGuiseppe, et al., 2013). It promotes the idea that if individuals can be enabled to think more flexibly and rationally, they will maximize their chances of living their lives in a manner that is consist-ent with a desire for a long and meaningful life in which emotional distress and self-defeating behavior are decreased.

Figure 2.2 illustrates the ABC model of REBT. This formulation of REBT prin-ciples has remained the dominant way in which the theory is expressed, although there have been variations suggested, due to debate amongst theorists around the relationship between different aspects of our belief systems (Hyland & Boduszek, 2012). The theory as advanced by mainstream REBT (Ellis & MacLaren, 2005) will be adopted in this volume. This model provides clarity to the practitioner around the distinctions between Activating Events or Adversities (A), Irrational

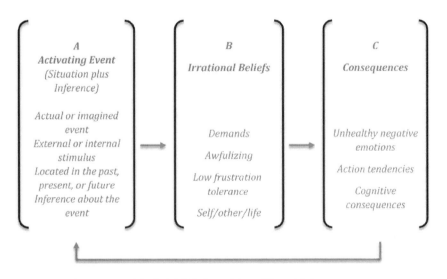

Figure 2.2 The ABC model of REBT (adapted from Ellis, 1994)

Beliefs (B), and Consequences (C). Each of these aspects of the model will be discussed in turn.

Activating events

An activating event (A in the REBT model) is any event which, when perceived, activates beliefs, which in turn prompt emotional, behavioral, cognitive, or physiological consequences. These activating events may be real or imagined, internal or external phenomena, and may be located in the individual's past, present, or future. Within the model, A has two components, consisting of the stimulus *plus* the inference made about the stimulus. Thus, in an exercise example, A might consist of feeling pain in a muscle and the inference, "I can't go on any longer". From the REBT practitioner's perspective, what is important to know about activating events is twofold:

1   What happened in the event being perceived? (situational A)
2   What inference did the individual make about the event? (inferential A, also sometimes referred to as the 'adversity')

Thus, in any exploration of activating events, the practitioner will elicit information both about the situation and the inferences made about it. It is important to take a flexible approach to eliciting this information, since anything can be an activating event. For example, the situational A could be:

1   An actual event (e.g., acquiring an injury)
2   An imagined event (e.g., assuming that the coach prefers another player in your position)
3   A past event (e.g., remembering a previous defeat against an opponent)
4   A present event (e.g., struggling to concentrate mid-game)
5   A future event (e.g., worrying that the team will be relegated)
6   An internal event (e.g., feeling pain in a hamstring)
7   An external event (e.g., being shouted at by a teammate)

The inferential A is any thought about the situational A. However, what is most useful is to ask the individual to identify which thought about the situational A seems to provoke the most disturbance. In the first example from the list, the most disturbing thought about acquiring an injury might be, "My career will be over". In this way, the practitioner can begin to track the train of cognitions that have led the individual from perceiving an event to feeling distressed and behaving in an unhelpful manner.

Conversations designed to elicit activating events are most helpful if they are clearly focused on specific events and distressing inferences about those events. Effective therapeutic interactions can quickly digress into unproductive areas if individuals are given the opportunity to discuss events in too much detail, or in vague and over-general terms, or in a way that leads them to give numerous examples of the same basic issue. Once the practitioner has a clear sense of the kinds of events in which the individual's disturbance manifests, it is helpful for both parties to agree on one specific example of the situational and inferential A and move on to the other aspects of the model. Dryden and Branch (2008) provide a clear and comprehensive overview of navigating the ABC model for anyone interested in learning the techniques described herein.

Consequences

Since they represent B in the model, the reader might reasonably expect 'beliefs' to be discussed next. However, experience of using REBT suggests that individuals seek therapeutic interactions either because they believe that their distress has been caused by some event (A), or because their feelings or behaviors are in some way problematic (C) (DiGuiseppe et al., 2013). Thus, it is often the case that as soon as an individual begins to discuss their presenting issue, the A or the C starts to be revealed. Once either is elicited, the practitioner can move on to the other. For example, assuming the individual describes having acquired an injury (A), the practitioner can start to explore the consequences (C).

Consequences in REBT comprise the emotional, behavioral, and cognitive aspects of the individual's response to the A. They are referred to as consequences because they are the result of the individual holding a particular set of beliefs about the A. These might be helpful and functional or unhelpful and dysfunctional. It is the dysfunctional consequences that are likely to be of most interest to the practitioner. Continuing with the previous example about injury, the following pattern might emerge:

Situational A	Getting injured
Inferential A	"My career might be over"
Emotional C	Anxiety
Cognitive C	Repeatedly worrying about the future
Behavioral C	Seeking excessive reassurance from peers

Since they follow the activating event so closely, it is often assumed that these consequences (C) are caused by the A. As has been stated previously, it is common in everyday parlance to hear A-C language, and the athlete in this example might draw the conclusion that the injury is making her anxious. However, the ABC model proposes that this is not a direct relationship, and the nature of a person's response at C is determined by the content of their evaluative beliefs (B) about A.

In practice, it is helpful to spend significant time on eliciting the C and there are several reasons for this. Firstly, the practitioner needs to know whether or not the consequences are functional. Ellis (1962) made a distinction between healthy and unhealthy negative emotions. Healthy negative emotions, such as sadness, tend to be associated with a tendency towards taking helpful or constructive actions. Indeed, whilst it might feel unpleasant, sadness is a wholly understandable and appropriate response to certain adverse experiences, such as loss. On the other hand, unhealthy negative emotions, such as depression, tend to be associated with unhelpful behaviors, including social isolation. Before offering a psychological intervention to an individual it is important to establish whether they really need it. Thus, the distinction between healthy and unhealthy negative emotions is useful in helping to determine whether intervention is required. The approach taken within REBT, and within this book, is that intervention tends to be indicated in the presence of unhealthy negative emotions and associated dysfunctional patterns of behavior, and not where healthy negative emotions and constructive behaviors are present. Put simply, concern and sadness are not reason enough to see a psychologist. Figure 2.3 (adapted from Dryden, 2008) provides an overview of the distinctions between common healthy and unhealthy negative emotions. It is important to stress that REBT is not about 'thinking positively' or being seduced by the idea of eternal happiness. If an emotional C about getting injured is anxiety, the more helpful alternative is not happiness. Who would be happy about being injured? The realistic emotional goal here would be healthy concern, rather than happiness. With respect to Figure 2.3, disturbed emotions and their more functional alternatives are considered together (e.g., anxiety-concern, depression-sadness, and so on).

Another reason for spending time clarifying the C is that for individuals to find the motivation to engage in the challenging task that psychological intervention often represents, they need to recognize that their current situation is clearly not helping them to pursue the life that they want. Whilst spending time worrying and seeking reassurance about an injury might seem like a good solution for the anxiety that surrounds it (it might actually help one feel less anxious in the short-term), it is more likely to contribute to the maintenance or worsening of anxiety in the long-term and is unlikely to prompt committed action towards recovery. Thus, whilst it can be difficult and stressful, clearly identifying the ways in which an individual's emotional, behavioral, and cognitive Cs are manifestly obstructing them from pursuing their values and goals is an important part of the therapeutic process.

Beliefs

In REBT theory, inferences about events (A) are not seen as responsible for emotional, behavioral, or cognitive consequences. For example, one might sustain an injury and infer, "My career is over". Whilst this is highly likely to be an uncomfortable thought, the ABC model asserts that this thought is not sufficient to result in significant emotional disturbance and dysfunction on its own. It is only the process of *evaluating* this inference negatively that will achieve that. Imagine an athlete who was coming to the end of their sporting career, and who was beginning to look with great interest at other business options. If, after an injury, they experienced the exact same inference ("My career is over"), they might not evaluate it negatively at all. The inference might be met with acceptance, perhaps even leading to excitement in the knowledge that this turn of events

Emotional (C)	Healthy or Unhealthy	Associated Cognitive (C)	Associated Behavioral (C)
Concern	Healthy	Viewing the threat realistically	Approach the threat in a constructive manner
Anxiety	Unhealthy	Overestimating negative features of the threat	Avoidance of the threat Reassurance-seeking
Sadness	Healthy	Seeing positive and negative aspects of a loss or failure	To express feelings about the loss or failure To seek out opportunities for reinforcement
Depression	Unhealthy	Seeing only the negative aspects of a loss or failure	Withdrawal and isolation Cutting oneself off from opportunities for reinforcement
Healthy anger	Healthy	Taking a realistic view of others' actions and motives	Asserting self with others Requesting that others change
Unhealthy anger	Unhealthy	Overestimating the extent to which others' actions and motives are malicious	Violence and aggression towards people or property Plotting revenge
Remorse	Healthy	Assuming an appropriate amount of personal responsibility for transgressions	Confronting the healthy pain that arises from acknowledging one's transgressions Asking for forgiveness
Guilt	Unhealthy	Assuming that one has 'sinned' and is wholly to blame for transgressions	Escaping or avoiding the healthy pain that arises from acknowledging one's transgressions Punishing oneself
Embarrassment	Healthy	Realistic about the extent to which others might be judgemental	Continuing to engage in social interaction Responding constructively to others' attempts to be compassionate
Shame	Unhealthy	Believing that something terrible has been revealed about oneself to others and assuming harsh judgement	Isolating self from the 'gaze' of others Defending one's self-esteem in self-defeating ways (e.g., by attacking others)
Sorrow	Healthy	Perceiving another's action towards one as bad, but not necessarily malicious, uncaring, or indifferent	Communicating one's feelings to the other Requesting fairer and more considerate treatment
Hurt	Unhealthy	Perceiving another's actions as deliberately malicious, uncaring, or indifferent	Closing down communication with the other Criticizing the other without disclosing why one feels hurt

Figure 2.3 Healthy and unhealthy negative emotions

might herald a new opportunity. REBT distinguishes between inferences (A) and evaluative beliefs (B) for this reason, taking the view that inferences need not be challenged or changed, since they are not in themselves intrinsically problematic. Evaluative beliefs *are* challenged, if only when they lead to unhealthy consequences, such as depression and withdrawal.

Ellis's ABC is a model of both function and dysfunction. Healthy or adaptive consequences are determined by rational beliefs, whereas unhealthy or dysfunctional consequences are determined by irrational beliefs. Rational beliefs are those that are flexible, preferential, and pragmatic in the sense that they facilitate outcomes that are consistent with an individual's goals. They also tend to have a quality of logic and a clear consistency with what is known about the way the world works. In contrast, irrational beliefs tend to be rigid, self-defeating, logically incoherent, and inconsistent with empirical reality (Dryden, 2008; Ellis, et al., 2010; DiGuiseppe et al, 2013). The model suggests that even if a person encounters a significantly adverse event, like a career-threatening injury, this is not sufficient on its own to *cause* an unhealthy emotional response. Should such a response develop, the determining factor is holding irrational beliefs about the adversity, rather than the adversity itself.

It is noted that when encountering this concept, many people react negatively to the term 'irrational beliefs', since it might appear to confer a pejorative judgement upon someone. There are two points to be made in respect of this. Firstly, by using the term 'irrational beliefs', Ellis implied that in the context of an individual's goals and valued directions, irrational beliefs are irrational because they are self-defeating and unlikely to facilitate progress in the desired direction. However, because of the potential for negative reactions, it is common for many therapists to avoid using the term 'irrational' with clients, in favour of other terms, such as 'unhelpful'. Secondly, care is always taken to be clear that it is the belief, and not the person, that is irrational. Where beliefs are challenged, the individual will know anything that is said is not a personal attack, but rather it is an attack on a belief system that is working against them moving towards a life characterized by meaning and purpose.

REBT helps individuals to recognize the role of beliefs in shaping their response to the adversities they experience. It clearly places irrational beliefs at the heart of emotional disturbance, emphasizing teaching the importance of a B-C connection, rather than a reliance on A-C thinking. Ellis identified four types of irrational belief: demandingness, awfulizing, low frustration tolerance, and depreciation (Ellis, 1994). The combination of these beliefs is largely responsible for the cognitive, behavioral, physiological, and emotional problems that are associated with a variety of forms of psychopathology. The organization of the components within REBT theory has received empirical support through the use of factor and meditational analysis (Fulop, 2007; DiLorenzo, et al., 2007; Turner et al., in press). Figure 2.4 comprises an ABC form template (Trower, et al., 2015) and extends the aforementioned injury example and illustrates a full range of irrational beliefs, alongside rational alternatives.

Activating Event (A)

Situation (A^1): Getting injured

Adversity (A^2): "My career might be over"

Irrational Beliefs (iB)	Rational Beliefs (rB)
Demand: I really want my career to continue and therefore it absolutely must not end now	**Preference:** I really want my career to continue, but it does not absolutely have to
Awfulizing: It would be awful if this were the end	**Anti-Awfulizing:** It would be bad if this is the end, but it would not be the worst thing in the world
Low Frustration Tolerance: I would not be able to stand having to give up	**High Frustration Tolerance:** Although it would be tough to stand, I could stand it. The difficulties associated with it would be worth standing, in the service of me making the best out of my future
Self-Depreciation: I am nothing without this sport	**Unconditional Self-Acceptance:** It would be a blow to have to give up but it would not prove that I am nothing. It would prove that I am fallible and not always able to do everything that I want to do, when I want to do it

Unhelpful Consequences (C)	Helpful Consequences (C)
Emotional Consequences:	**Emotional Consequences:**
Anxiety	Healthy concern
Behavioral consequences	Behavioral consequences
Seeking excessive reassurance from peers	Seeking appropriate help with rehabilitation
Cognitive Consequences:	**Cognitive Consequences:**
Repeatedly worrying about the future	Thinking constructively about the way forward

---

Figure 2.4 A complete ABC analysis

Demands

The REBT model proposes that demandingness is the primary irrational belief implicated in the development of psychopathology, and that the others are derivative beliefs that are similarly extreme in nature. Humans tend to escalate their preference for the things that they want and desire into rigid and absolute demands, characterized by expressions such as 'have to', 'need', 'must', 'should', 'ought', etc. Such dogmatic beliefs are problematic because they are largely inflexible, illogical, inconsistent with reality, and they interfere with an individual pursuing their values and goals. In eliciting demanding beliefs, skilled REBT practitioners will also elicit the preference that precedes it as a means of clearly illustrating how the preference has been escalated into a demand. In Figure 2.4, there is a preference for wanting the career to continue, followed by a demand that it absolutely must. The rational alternative to a demanding belief is known as a 'Full Preference', in which the preference is re-asserted, and the demand negated ("I really want my career to continue, but it does not absolutely have to").

Awfulizing

Awfulizing is the process of evaluating an activating event as being the worst that it could possibly be. It often follows quite naturally from an individual not getting what they believe they must have. It represents a belief state where an individual extrapolates consequences and arrives at some catastrophic interpretation of how bad something is. Dryden (2008) describes awfulizing as being on a continuum of badness from 101% to infinity. In truth, much of what people describe as awful is simply undesirable, and various REBT intervention techniques can help the individual to see this more clearly.

Low frustration tolerance

Also referred to in the literature as 'frustration intolerance' or LFT, this concept refers to the belief that one is incapable of tolerating the conditions presented by the adversity. Individuals often unhelpfully tell themselves, "I can't stand it", when they do not get that which they believe is essential, as if not getting it will cause them to somehow disintegrate or bring about a state where they will never experience happiness again. This is an unhelpful belief since it exaggerates the discomfort one naturally feels when thwarted and prevents contact with the notion that experiencing discomfort is an inevitable part of having values and pursuing goals. With reference to sport, it seems reasonable to assert that no great victory was ever won without a degree of emotional or physical discomfort somewhere along the way. In the pursuit of success or other valued goals, this discomfort is bearable and is worth bearing.

Depreciation

Depreciation beliefs are global and negative evaluations that are applied to oneself, another person, present conditions, or life in general. Thus, one will hear REBT practitioners describe 'self-, other-, or life-depreciation'. These beliefs involve a process of attributing blame when an individual does not get what they demand they must have. Depreciation beliefs are problematic because they tend to establish equivalence between a whole person and an aspect of their situation in a way that becomes self-defeating (e.g., "I failed, therefore I am a failure"). A more rational philosophy asserts that experiences such as failure or defeat can only ever provide evidence of fallibility, as opposed to a complete lack of worth. Losing a match is evidence that an individual or a team is capable of losing, and not evidence that he/she/they are total losers. Their history will also probably indicate that they are capable of drawing and winning as well. It can be useful to draw attention to the logic used in these global negative evaluations, since people rarely conclude that they are 'total winners' on the back of a single victory, although the logic is essentially the same.

Change methods in REBT

In moving through the REBT process, after eliciting an ABC that describes the current situation, as illustrated in the left-hand column of Figure 2.4, an REBT practitioner attempts to reinforce the B-C connection, helping the individual to understand the central role of their irrational beliefs in mediating their current disturbance. They would then elicit a more functional goal, defined by its emotional, behavioral, and cognitive components. This is primarily achieved by asking how the individual would like to think, feel, and behave if it were not possible to change the A. The individual would be encouraged to consider what beliefs they would need to hold to facilitate such a functional goal, as opposed to holding the current beliefs, which are leading to unhelpful consequences. Once a more workable set of alternative beliefs and their consequences has been elicited, the focus moves to strengthening conviction in the rational alternatives and weakening conviction in the irrational beliefs. The purpose of this is that the individual can begin to see that the irrational beliefs lead to emotional distress and other unhelpful consequences (Dryden, 2006) and that a more functional outcome is possible. Different REBT practitioners vary the precise order of the process, although one view is that it is helpful to establish a clear ABC sequence with irrational beliefs (left-hand side of Figure 2.4) and a clear ABC sequence with rational alternatives (right-hand side of Figure 2.4) before moving on to any change method. This is because it helps the individual to clearly understand that from the same A, different Cs are possible, and that the key to determining which outcome they will get is their belief system. One might simply ask the individual to look at a completed ABC form and consider that if they were to undertake further work with the practitioner, would they want that work to help them get better at achieving the outcomes on the left-hand side or the right.

Common to many approaches within the CBT tradition, REBT emphasizes cognitive change as a central ingredient of the change mechanism. REBT therapists use a technique called 'disputing', which is a specific method of questioning the beliefs that have been contributing to distress and self-defeating behaviors. Disputing aims to effect change in a person's belief system such that they adopt an effective new philosophy that will serve to reduce their disturbance. The 'D' in disputing and the 'E' in effective new philosophy have led some authors to refer to an ABCDE model of REBT, which perhaps more fully describes the whole assessment, formulation, and intervention process.

REBT challenges irrational beliefs using a wide range of strategies, and examples of these can be found throughout the subsequent chapters. One distinctive feature of REBT is this focus on evaluative beliefs at B, rather than focusing on challenging inferences at A, which might be seen in CT and other models. Our view in this book is that this approach confers a number of advantages in the sport and exercise context. Firstly, a practitioner challenging an individual's interpretation of actual events (as in, "This doesn't mean your career is *over*") may pose a potential threat to the therapeutic relationship. Thus, the practitioner and the individual being helped can become distanced in their understanding, and in a worst-case scenario, the challenge can feel invalidating, as if the practitioner lacks empathy into how significant the event is. Secondly, without addressing the beliefs about the inference, the individual may not generalize any gains that are made. Inferential change can be unstable, meaning that when the individual makes similarly dramatic inferences in the context of other injuries or setbacks, s/he may rehearse the same pattern of self-defeating beliefs and experience the same consequences. Thirdly, and perhaps most importantly, the inference may be true, and challenging a realistic inference has no utility whatsoever. The athlete's career may be over, but that does not mean that distress and dysfunction inevitably follow. By focusing on challenging evaluative beliefs rather than inferences, REBT paves the way for philosophical change that better equips individuals to deal more effectively with adversities of all kinds in a range of different contexts. It teaches a generalizable set of skills, to which the following chapters are testament.

The main disputing techniques involve empirical, logical, and pragmatic challenges delivered using a Socratic style of dialogue. With a completed ABC form in front of the practitioner and the person being helped, attention can be drawn to the irrational and rational belief pairs (e.g., demand – preference, awfulizing – anti-awfulizing, low frustration tolerance – high frustration tolerance, depreciation – acceptance) and both can be subjected to the same scrutiny. With reference to Figure 2.4, the different disputing techniques might be summarized as follows:

Empirical: "Which of these beliefs (rational or irrational) seems most consistent with reality – the idea that because you don't want your career to end, it therefore must not end, or the idea that even though you don't want it to end, it is still possible that it could?"

Logical: "Which of these beliefs makes most sense – the idea that your career ending would mean you are nothing, or the idea that your career ending would mean you are simply fallible?"

Pragmatic: "Which of these beliefs will help you most going forward – the idea that the end of your career is completely unbearable, or the idea that the end of your career is an adversity that you can survive and learn something useful from?"

Each of the three disputing methods can be applied to each pair of beliefs, giving the practitioner numerous options for intervention. Disputation is a process that requires practice and perseverance and the idea of working to strengthen conviction in rational beliefs is encouraged via the use of between-session practice tasks. Behavioral methods, such as graded exposure or deliberately widening one's behavioral repertoire to confront previously avoided situations or emotions, may also be employed to facilitate the process of more functional change. Another commonly used technique is rational emotive imagery, in which guided imagery exercises are used to facilitate the practice of identifying disturbed emotions and seeing if they can be changed to more healthy variants. Subsequent chapters of this book illustrate a wide range of change methods in a number of different contexts, attesting to the technical flexibility that is possible whilst maintaining theoretical integrity with the ABC model.

Conclusion

The editors of this book take the view that when working in a sport and exercise context there is a need for an established and evidence-based approach that addresses emotional distress and dysfunctional behavior without necessarily promoting a medical model. REBT allows both parties to construct explanations of distress and dysfunction that are non-stigmatizing, acceptable, accessible, and draw from common experience outside of notions of mental illness. REBT is a well-established and much-researched approach to psychological intervention that mixes elegance with a great potential for power and precision. This chapter has provided an overview of the theoretical foundations of the REBT model, and the remainder of the book provides numerous examples of its application. For those interested in pursuing the use of this model in their work, this volume is a useful starting point. As with any psychotherapeutic approach, novice and more experienced practitioners require on-going training and supervision from competent practitioners to ensure safe and ethical practice. Using REBT in practice will provoke questions and raise challenges that are beyond the scope of this book, although we hope the reader will find enough here to be stimulated to find out more.

References

Beck, A. T. (1976). *Cognitive therapy and the emotional disorders*. London: Penguin.

Bennett, R., & Pearson, L. (2015). Group rational emotive behavior therapy for paranoia. In Meaden, A. & A. Fox (Eds.), *Innovations in psychosocial interventions for psychosis: Working with the hard to reach* (pp 167–183). Hove: Routledge.

DiGuiseppe, R., Doyle, K. A., Dryden, W., & Backx, W. (2013). *A practitioner's guide to rational emotive behavior therapy* (3rd Ed.). Oxford: Oxford University Press.

DiLorenzo, T. A., David, D., & Montgomery, G.H. (2007). The interrelations between irrational cognitive processes and distress in stressful academic settings. *Personality and Individual Differences, 42*, 765–777.

Dryden, W. (2006). *Helping yourself with REBT: First steps for clients*. New York, NY: Albert Ellis Institute.

Dryden, W. (2008). *Rational emotive behavior therapy: Distinctive features*. Hove: Routledge.

Dryden, W., & Branch, R. (2008). *Fundamentals of rational emotive behavior therapy: A training handbook*. Chichester: Wiley-Blackwell.

Ellard, K. K., Fairholme, C. P., Boisseau, C. L., Farchione, T., & Barlow, D. H. (2010). Unified protocol for the transdiagnostic treatment of emotional disorders: Protocol development and initial outcome data. *Cognitive and Behavioral Practice, 17*, (1), 88–101.

Ellis, A. (1958). Rational psychotherapy. *Journal of General Psychology*, 59, 35–49.

Ellis, A. (1962). *Reason and emotion in psychotherapy*. New York, NY: Lyle Stuart.

Ellis, A. (1994). *Reason and emotion in psychotherapy (Revised and Updated)*. New York, NY: Birch Lane Press.

Ellis, A., David, D., & Lynn, S. J. (2010). A historical and conceptual perspective. In David, D., Lynn, S. J., and A. Ellis (Eds.), *Rational and irrational beliefs: Research, theory, and clinical practice* (pp 3–22). Oxford University Press, Oxford.

Ellis, A., & MacLaren, C. (2005). *Rational emotive behavior therapy: A clinician's guide*. San Luis Obispo: Impact Publishers.

Engels, G. I., Garnefski, N., & Diekstra, R. F. W. (1993). Efficacy of Rational Emotive Therapy: A quantitative analysis. *Journal of Consulting and Clinical Psychology*, 61, 1083–1090.

Fulop, I. E. (2007). A confirmatory factor analysis of the attitude and belief scale 2. *Journal of Cognitive and Behavioral Psychotherapies*, 7, 159–170.

Gonzalez, J. E., Nelson, J. R., Gutkin, T. B., Sauders, A., Galloway, A., & Shwery, C. S. (2004). Rational Emotive Therapy with children and adolescents: A meta-analysis. *Journal of Rational and Behavioural Disorders*, 12, 222–235.

Haddock, E., Bennett, R., & Jones, C. (2015). A meta-analysis of rational emotive behaviour therapy as an intervention for emotional distress (under review).

Harvey, A., Watkins, E., Mansell, W., & Shafran, R. (2004). *Cognitive behavioural processes across psychological disorders: A transdiagnostic approach to research and treatment*. Oxford, Oxford University Press.

Hayes, S. C., Strosahl, K. D., & Wilson, K. G. (1999). *Acceptance and commitment therapy: An experiential approach to behaviour change*. New York, NY: Guilford Press.

Hyland, P., & Boduszek, D. (2012). Resolving a difference between cognitive therapy and Rational Emotive Behaviour Therapy: Towards the development of an integrated CBT model of psychopathology. *Mental Health Review Journal*, 17, (2), 104–116.

Hyland, P., Shevlin, M., Adamson, G., & Boduszek, D. (2014). The organisation of irrational beliefs in posttraumatic stress symptomology: Testing the predictions of REBT theory using structural equation modelling. *Journal of Clinical Psychology*, 70, (1), 48–59.

Lyons, L. C., & Woods, P. J. (1991) The efficacy of Rational Emotive Therapy: A quantitative review of the outcome research. *Clinical Psychology Review*, 11, 357–369.

National Institute of Health and Care Excellence (NICE) (2009). *Depression the nice guideline on the treatment and management of depression in adults (Updated Edition)*. www.nice.org.uk/nicemedia/live/12329/45896/45896.pdf. Accessed 29/09/2013.

Szentagotai, A., David, D., Lupu, V., & Cosman, D. (2008). Rational-Emotive Behaviour Therapy versus cognitive therapy versus medication in the treatment of major depressive disorder: Mechanisms of change analysis. *Psychotherapy Theory, Research, Practice*, 4, 523–538.

Trower, P., Jones, J., & Dryden, W. (2015). *Cognitive behavioural counselling in action* (3rd Ed), London: Sage.

Turner, M. J. (2016). Rational Emotive Behavior Therapy (REBT), irrational and rational beliefs, and the mental health of athletes. *Frontiers in Psychology*, 7, 1423.

Turner, M. J., Carrington, S., & Miller, A. (in press). Psychological distress across sport participation groups: The mediating effects of secondary irrational beliefs on the relationship between primary irrational beliefs and symptoms of anxiety, anger, and depression. *Journal of Clinical Sport Psychology*, accepted August 2017.

Velten, E. (Ed). (2007). *Under the influence: Reflections of Albert Ellis in the work of others*. Tucson: Sharp Press.

3 A short-term Rational Emotive Behavior Therapy (REBT) intervention for competition anxiety with a trampoline gymnast

Michelle Huggins

Context

Cara (pseudonym) was a 26-year-old female trampoline gymnast who had been performing at a National level for several years. She had referred herself for psychological support following many competitions where she had felt disappointed that her performance had not equalled or surpassed what she knew herself to be capable of, based on her training sessions. Her coach had suggested seeking support and so she made contact with the sport psychology service via e-mail expressing an interest in attending sessions.

The service was based in a building that was predominantly used to support people with clinical difficulties such as depression and anxiety. The building housed a waiting room with refreshments, a receptionist, and a suite of well-resourced consulting rooms. Typically sport psychology consultations would take place in the athlete's environment, an educational establishment, or a sporting context; however, the environment described here is the place that I had access to through my work as a Clinical Psychologist.

Cara was offered an initial assessment session of 90-minutes followed by a course of six 50-minute sessions, totalling seven contacts over eight weeks. Two months after the final session, there was a follow-up contact via e-mail. As a Clinical Psychologist, I would usually meet with outpatients for an initial 90-minute assessment followed by subsequent weekly sessions of 50-minutes duration. I find this way of working helpful for maintaining therapeutic boundaries and planning my workload and so I have transferred this way of working to how I work with athletes.

Within the National trampolining competition structure, there are around five competitions available to attend each year. Cara explained that when competing there is usually a 30-minute warm-up period followed by the completion of a qualifying round consisting of two routines. Each routine has ten elements and lasts around 1-minute in duration. The first routine in the qualifying round is often a compulsory routine set out for the competition. The second routine is completely voluntary and Cara reported that she would choose to perform a harder routine at this time. As long as both of these routines had been completed and she had scored within the top eight places then she could perform in the final round. The final round is another voluntary routine where Cara reported that she would repeat her second routine.

Presenting issues

Cara's e-mail correspondence highlighted that her main issue was being unable to consistently transfer her training performance to the competition environment. During the 12 months prior to the referral there had been three occasions where she did not complete her final routine, which was more often than her usual performance at competitions. Cara identified that over the past year she had increased the pressure on herself to achieve more and this had led to worrying thoughts such as, "I should have been able to do it" that were difficult to manage during competitions. In addition, her competition performance had been less consistent than her performance during training.

Needs analysis

Multiple methods were used to conduct the initial assessment, including a semi-structured interview, the use of a psychometric assessment (Sport Anxiety Scale-2; SAS-2; Smith, Smoll, Cumming & Grossbard, 2006), and the application of a Multilevel Classification System for Sport Psychology (MCS-SP; Gardner & Moore, 2006). Using multiple assessment methods assisted with gathering a broad range of information to enhance my understanding of Cara's presenting issues.

Psychometric assessment

The use of psychometric assessments in sport psychology can provide additional information by focusing on a specific area of concern or interest. In this case Cara had reported concern with her competition performance, rather than her training performance. An assumption was made that anxiety may be having an impact on the performance during competitions, and so the SAS-2 was administered. The SAS-2 is a 15-item self-report questionnaire that asks about how the athlete usually feels before competing in their sport. The SAS-2 takes approximately 5-minutes to administer and the athlete is instructed to provide answers on a 4-point Likert-scale from 1 (*not at all*) to 4 (*very much*). High scores indicate more cognitive and somatic anxiety related symptoms. The SAS-2 has good psychometric properties (Smith et al., 2006), has been applied in a range of sports settings (e.g., Schwebel, et al., 2016; Scott-Hamilton, et al., 2016; Papadopoulos et al., 2014), and has been used to examine the effectiveness of REBT in past research (Turner & Barker, 2013).

Multilevel Classification System for Sport Psychology

The Multilevel Classification System for Sport Psychology (MCS-SP; Gardner & Moore, 2006) is a framework that can be applied to the information gathered about athletes during a sport psychology consultation. It enables the practitioner to readily identify which area of need is most prevalent for formulation and intervention. There are four classification levels that can be applied to the identified issues: Performance Development (PD); Performance Dysfunction (PDy); Performance Impairment (PI); and Performance Termination (PT). Each classification is further divided into two levels to capture different elements of each category. The framework considers a broad range of information to assist the classification process including the athlete's environmental, interpersonal, intrapersonal, behavioral, and performance history and expectations (Gardner & Moore, 2006).

During the assessment I reviewed each of the classification levels one at a time using the information obtained. The Performance Development category best fit the information obtained. A PD-I classification can be applied to an athlete who needs to enhance the physical skills for peak performance. This did not apply to Cara because she had the physical skills to perform well and did so during her training routines. The PD-II classification can be applied to an athlete who has adequately developed the physical skills required for high performance and requires support with mental skill development to benefit from the consistent execution of optimal performance. The assessment information indicated that this category could be applied to Cara.

Formulation

Prior to deciding on an intervention plan, it is important to develop a formulation with the athlete. A formulation is a collaborative understanding of the psychological processes involved in the development and maintenance of the presenting problem. It is important that this understanding is shared between the athlete and the sport psychologist and that both are encouraged to collaborate on its development. Using the athlete's own words directly from the assessment can enhance therapeutic rapport and further develop a shared understanding of the problems. During the initial session, a preliminary ABC was identified and is shown in Figure 3.1.

Cara's main difficulty was the experience of impaired performance during a competition relative to the performance during training sessions. The impaired performance was hypothesized to be a behavioral consequence of an increase in anxiety that was experienced both cognitively (with worrying thoughts/catastrophizing/black and white thinking) and physically (changes in body sensations, feeling tense, shaky). Predisposing this experience was the presence of irrational beliefs, where Cara demanded that she 'should' perform well and 'must not' fail. These beliefs were elicited when her self-expectations were high, which was during the competition environment. Cara held the belief that if she failed at her sport then she herself would be a failure, which predisposed her to experience anxiety.

Each time there was a competition Cara would demand that she perform well, which precipitated anticipatory anxiety (also described by her as panic) regarding the possibility of not performing well or failing. Furthermore, the experience was perpetuated by cognitive distortions that are typical of people experiencing anxiety: an internal focus on physiological experiences immediately prior to and

Situation

During a competition routine the performance is not as smooth as the routine in training
Adversity – I am not in control, I am going to fail

Irrational Beliefs

I should always be able to remain in control and complete the routine; I've done it before
I must not fail
If I fail I am a complete failure

Consequences

Thoughts:

I should have been able to recover from the fourth move
I feel out of control
This is awful
Oh my gosh I'm really close to the edge
I need to get my balance
I'm going to fail
I need to do something, what shall I do?

Emotions:

Panic, worry, out of control, tension

Body Changes:

Stiff, erratic, tense, not flowing easily, moves are slower, shaky

Behavior:

Feeling rushed, having difficulty completing the routine, the timing and tempo of the
  routine is faster, I end up on the side of the mat

Figure 3.1 Preliminary ABC form

during the competition routine, and noticing feelings of tension and panic that
distracted her and prevented her from concentrating fully on the skill execution required to perform well. Cara was further distracted by having a negative
focus on her performance, and being very aware in the moment of each error
that occurred. When errors did occur, she paid special attention to them and
attempted to analyze them during the routine.

There were several factors that were protective and provided optimism for successful change. These included that she was motivated and curious to learn about
her experiences, and she had a supportive coach who had encouraged her to seek
support. Cara experienced difficulties under certain conditions yet performed well
at other times, suggesting that her belief structure was not experienced globally
and that she had an alternative set of rational performance-enhancing beliefs,
accessible to her on certain occasions.

Goals for REBT

Goal setting is an important aspect of any psychological intervention because
it provides a marker for assessing progress. Cara's goals were to improve her

competition performance and we agreed to do this by making the following cognitive, emotional, and behavioral changes:

- Changing irrational beliefs to rational alternatives
- Reducing the experience of anxiety and panic during competitions
- Consistently completing the three competition routines

The primary outcome measures were: changes in irrational beliefs as measured using conviction in belief ratings; changes in anxiety as measured using the SAS-2 scores; and performance measured by the successful completion of the three competition routines.

REBT intervention

Cara was introduced to the ABC model of REBT. In this model A is the activating event or situation; B represents the beliefs held about the activating event; and C describes the thoughts, feelings, body changes, and behaviors which occur as a consequence of holding certain beliefs (B) about the situation (A). During this introduction, the emphasis was on teaching that the beliefs about the situation lead to the consequences (B-C link), as opposed to the situation leading directly to the consequences (A-C link).

When intervening with REBT, I used a formulation table that highlighted the ABC process (Figure 3.2). This table had been adapted from the Advanced Practicum training course that was delivered at the Centre for REBT, University of Birmingham, UK. I wrote the table onto the white board so that it could be viewed and worked on collaboratively during the session. Figure 3.2 outlines the ABC formulation that was completed using the following seven steps:

1   Identify and describe the situation.
2   Highlight the critical activating event that occurred at the time of the situation.
3   Identify the current cognitive, emotional, and behavioral consequences that are problematic.
4   Identify a more helpful set of cognitive, emotional, and behavioral consequences; how the athlete would rather think, feel, and behave in the same situation.
5   Identify the irrational beliefs held about the situation and rate the conviction with which they are held by the athlete.
6   Identify the healthy, rational alternatives to the irrational beliefs and rate the conviction with which these are held.
7   Question the rationality of the beliefs held with logical, empirical, and pragmatic disputations and re-rate the conviction in the belief.

At the end of the session photographs were taken of the work and printed as a handout for the following session and later given to the athlete for out of session work. Steps 1–5 were completed during session 2 and then steps 6 and 7 were

Situation

Description – During a competition routine the first three moves went okay but by the fourth move I was off balance and near the end of the mat. I panicked into the fifth move and ended up on the side mat and was unable to progress further with the routine.

Adversity – I am not in control; I am going to fail

Irrational Beliefs	Rational Beliefs
Demand: I must always be able to remain in control and complete the routine, I've done it before	**Preference:** I'd really, really like to be in control every time, I know I've got the skill, I've done it before, but just because I really want to do it, doesn't mean I always will do
Low Frustration Tolerance: If I can't remain in control and finish the routine, I can't tolerate it	**High Frustration Tolerance:** It is frustrating and difficult for me to accept if I don't stay in control but I can tolerate it and it is worth tolerating so that I can improve
Awfulizing: It is awful that I lost control and didn't finish the routine	**Non-Awfulizing:** If I lose control it is really disappointing for me, but it's not absolutely awful
Self-Depreciation: If I can't remain in control and finish the routine, it shows that I am completely rubbish at my sport and I am a failure	**Self-Acceptance:** If I lose control it shows that I have done so on this occasion, and not that I am completely rubbish at my sport; I am a dedicated athlete who makes mistakes at times – I am not a complete failure

Consequences	Consequences
Thoughts:	**Thoughts:**
I should have been able to recover from the fourth move	Stay strong, lift up into the fifth move
I feel out of control	
Oh my gosh I'm really close to the edge	
I need to get my balance	
I need to do something, what shall I do?	
Emotions:	**Emotions:**
Panic, worried, out of control	Calm, in control, slight concern
Body Changes:	**Body Changes:**
Stiff, erratic, not flowing easily, moves are slower	Body flows evenly, movements are familiar
Behavior	**Behavior:**
Feeling rushed, having difficulty completing the routine, the timing and tempo of the routine is faster, I end up on the side of the mat	Timing and tempo are controlled
	Focus on breathing and pace
	Acceptance – it has happened, now move on

Figure 3.2 Completed ABC form

completed the following week in session 3. The following sessions were used to reinforce the learning, to engage in rational emotive imagery exercises, and to re-formulate her beliefs.

Step 1: identify and describe the situation

It is important to focus on a single situation that is preferably a recent experience to enable the athlete to identify relevant and specific beliefs and consequences. The situation in this case was the athlete's performance during a recent competition. With prompts, Cara could describe in detail the moments leading to the start of her competition routine.

Step 2: highlight the activating event

It is necessary to highlight what part of that event led to the experience of adversity and this is the event that has activated the irrational belief system, and in turn, the unhealthy negative emotion. There will be factual elements of the event and then there will be inferences about the event that lead to the experience of adversity.

Step 3: identify the unhealthy consequences

Once a relevant and specific activating event had been agreed, I supported Cara to identify the unhealthy beliefs, feelings, and behaviors that occurred at the time. I asked her what she was thinking and feeling, and what she did. I also asked her to think about any changes in her body that she might have experienced at the time. During this step, I supported Cara to identify her major unhealthy negative emotion, which was anxiety. This was the most strongly experienced emotion and the one that was associated with the negative thoughts and behaviors (see Figure 3.2).

Step 4: identify the healthy consequences

Next I asked Cara to consider how she would prefer to experience this situation if it were to occur again, which facilitated the conversation about healthy consequences. The following transcript illustrates this dialogue:

Sport Psychologist (SP):   If you are in exactly the same situation again, how would you rather think, feel, and behave in that situation?

Athlete: I'd like to think about what I need to do next rather than what I've just done.

SP: And what would be an example of that type of thought?

Athlete: Erm, stay strong and lift up. To maintain tempo and timing I listen to my breathing and the sounds of the trampoline.

SP:	We try and have healthy alternatives to these consequences here. For anxiety, one alternative descriptive word we can use is 'concern'.
Athlete:	It's almost like accepting that it has happened and move on. On the practice comp I didn't accept it, I just panicked.

Once the form had been completed with the activating event and the two sets of consequences I introduced Cara to the links between situations (A), beliefs (B), and consequences (C). I highlighted that some people believe that there is a direct link between A and C; however, the link between A and C is moderated by B. Cara had originally thought that A did lead to C but was accepting of the suggestion that the A to C link was moderated by B. Using her own examples to illustrate this enabled her to accept this way of thinking.

Step 5: identify the irrational beliefs

The irrational beliefs were activated during competitions and contributed to her disturbance. I asked her what she believed about the situation (A) that was leading her to think, feel, and behave in the way that we had written down (C). I often find that people may struggle to identify their beliefs because they are less freely available to our conscious thinking than our automatic thoughts are. As such I offer hypotheses about the beliefs based on the assessment information. We started by identifying demands that Cara had about the situation before moving on to identify derivatives (low frustration tolerance, awfulizing, depreciation beliefs) of the demand. Cara said that she believed she must always be in control and complete her routines. This demand was added to the irrational belief box in Figure 3.2. Next, I explored whether she experienced any of the derivatives. The following transcript illustrates this dialogue:

SP: If you can't or don't [remain in control] can you tolerate that?
Athlete: That's where the acceptance comes in, I do in training, in competition I didn't.
SP: Can you tolerate the fact that you didn't do it as well as you could do?
Athlete: No, normally I can tolerate it but I don't feel like I did on that one.

Cara also reported that she felt awful when she failed to remain in control, and that she had beliefs that she was rubbish at her sport and a complete failure (see Figure 3.2). Cara reflected that she did not feel this way all the time, but she recognized it as a set of beliefs that she experienced during competitions. We reviewed the beliefs and added or removed anything that did not fit. We also changed any terminology that I may have inadvertently imposed on the original descriptions. Before moving on to discuss the rational beliefs, Cara rated the strength of conviction that she had in the irrational beliefs so that the ratings were not diluted by the introduction of a new belief structure. The following transcript illustrates this dialogue:

SP: On a scale of 0 to 10, where 0 is not at all true and 10 is completely true, how true is it that you should be able to remain in control if you've done it before?
Athlete: 10.
SP: How true is it that if you don't remain in control you can't tolerate it?
Athlete: Maybe, 2.
SP: And how true is it that it is awful if you don't remain in control?
Athlete: Am I talking about just in the competition or in general?
SP: Keep it specific to the situation.
Athlete: Erm, maybe a 5.
SP: The belief, "If I don't get this right, I am rubbish".
Athlete: At the time, I felt it about a 7. . . . But now, I know it's not realistic.

This transcript shows that Cara had already started to reflect on her experience and recognize that her beliefs were not rational. The session ended at this point and time was available for questions. We agreed to finish the form the following week and at the next session we re-rated the beliefs without reminding her of the previous ratings. There was a change in the strength of the low frustration tolerance belief from 2 to 4 out of 10 indicating that this was experienced more strongly than previously reported. All the other ratings remained the same. I find it useful to re-rate beliefs if there is a break in contact, even if there has been no direct discussion about how rational these beliefs are. I often find that the athlete will report lower conviction in the irrational beliefs because people are generally not as aware of the beliefs they hold about their experiences and once these are identified they have some time to reflect on them.

Step 6: identify rational alternative beliefs

Once all the beliefs had been re-rated we looked again at the right-hand side of the form and reinforced the B-C link. I asked the athlete to explain to me what led to or caused the consequences to occur in the situation, which helped me to check for understanding before moving on. We outlined phrases like those captured by the irrational beliefs and wrote them in an empirically validated, logical, and pragmatic way. I used Cara's language and asked whether the final phrase was something that she could imagine saying to herself to ensure that it was personally meaningful. Cara then rated her strength of conviction in each of the alternative rational beliefs and they were all rated 10 out of 10, indicating that she believed them to be 100% true. We discussed that these are the beliefs that she experiences during training, and when she is in the competition environment it is the irrational beliefs that are uppermost. It is possible that this is why Cara had an inconsistent performance, because she held two sets of beliefs.

This would be supported by the MCS-SP assessment that found her to have the physical skills to perform well, yet requiring psychological support to do so. The reason that Cara had poorer performance during competitions was because she held the beliefs on the left-hand side of the ABC form (see Figure 3.2). The next step taught Cara that these beliefs were irrational and encouraged her to more fully adopt the rational beliefs.

Step 7: question the rationality of the beliefs held using disputation

The final step was to review the form and begin a conversation about the irrational beliefs using three philosophical arguments: empirical, logical, and pragmatic. This is called disputation (D) because Cara is disputing the irrational belief. When reviewing the ABC form in Figure 3.2, the demand reads, "I must always be able to remain in control and complete the routine". This is irrational because empirically there is no evidence that she must always remain in control. The very fact that she has not remained in control on this occasion refutes the notion that she must always remain in control (empirical argument). In addition, it is not logical for Cara to demand that she must always remain in control and finish the routine because she will not be able to do this each time, no matter how desirable it might be (logical argument). Finally, it is not helpful for Cara to hold this belief because it is something that she cannot consistently attain, and holding the belief hinders, rather than helps, her performance (pragmatic argument). In the following transcript, all three philosophical arguments are used in addition to Cara being asked to explain why it was not helpful for her to demand that she must always remain in control and asking her to re-rate the strength of conviction in the belief.

SP: Who says you must always complete the routine?
Athlete: Me.
SP: Okay, and do you always do it?
Athlete: Er, well no.
SP: Because this is an occasion when you didn't do it?
Athlete: Yeah.
SP: So where's the evidence that you absolutely must always be able to do it?
Athlete: Mmm, just in my head.
SP: Okay, you'd really, really like to be able to do it every time but who says that you absolutely must do it every time?
Athlete: Well nobody apart from me.
SP: Okay, is it helpful for you to demand that of yourself?
Athlete: No.
SP: How come?
Athlete: Because it puts more pressure on myself to do it.
SP: And then what happens on the occasions when you don't achieve it?

Athlete:	I then get more disappointed with it, I panic about it.
SP:	So must you always be in control and finish the routines?
Athlete:	Erm, no.
SP:	You would really, really like to?
Athlete:	Mmm hmm.
SP:	So how true is it that you must always remain in control?
Athlete:	Like, 1 out of 10.
SP:	What's keeping the score from being zero?
Athlete:	Nothing, zero.
SP:	Are you happy with a zero?
Athlete:	Yeah.
SP:	Tell me again why, why this statement is not true.
Athlete:	Because it puts more pressure on me, if I say I have to do it all the time.
SP:	In reality, is this true that you absolutely must be able to do it all of the time?
Athlete:	No.
SP:	No, have you always done it [remained in control and finished the routine] every single time that you've tried it?
Athlete:	No.
SP:	So it's never been the case that this has been true?
Athlete:	No.

Cara was curious about this type of conversation and intrigued to learn more. She was surprised that her beliefs were irrational and bewildered that she had held them with such conviction. Next, we had a similar conversation about the low frustration tolerance belief and Cara re-rated her conviction in this belief as 0 out of 10. During the disputing of this belief she was asked to think about what she would be doing if she were unable to tolerate a situation and she said she would be annoyed, cry, and give up. On reflection, Cara acknowledged that she did not do these things, and that she was able to tolerate the frustration of losing control. We then discussed the awfulizing belief and I highlighted that REBT conceptualizes awful as being 101% bad. Together we disputed whether or not this applied to her situation.

SP:	When we talk about awful we are talking about the worst thing ever, 101% bad. Is it 101% bad?
Athlete:	Erm, no.
SP:	What would be worse?
Athlete:	I don't know, dying.
SP:	Yeah, how in this situation might you end up dying?
Athlete:	Unless I did something really, really, really awful then it's unlikely that I would die.
SP:	Sure, but I guess you could die?
Athlete:	Yeah.

SP:	And would that be the worst thing ever?
Athlete:	Yeah.
SP:	Would that be worse than if you fell off the trampoline, injured some-one else, and then died?
Athlete:	No.
SP:	Okay, so things can always get worse, now I don't want you going round and jumping off the trampoline injuring people, and please try not to die too!
Both:	Laughing.
SP:	When we use the term 'awful' we experience a heart sink response, like, "Oh gosh it's awful", a sinking down feeling and we tell ourselves that it's 101% bad. It's hard for us to experience 101% bad. So when you do the routine and you make a mistake, is it awful?
Athlete:	No.
SP:	Okay, so how true is it on a scale of 0–10 that it is awful when you lose control and don't finish the routine?
Athlete:	Zero.

During the disputing conversation about the self-depreciating belief Cara acknowledged that she had no empirical evidence that she was rubbish on the trampoline and a complete failure; that logically it did not make sense to believe she was rubbish because she knew this was not true; and pragmatically it was not helpful for her to tell herself this. Cara re-rated the strength of her conviction in this belief as 0. Cara could dispute all the irrational beliefs and change the strength with which she held them to zero acknowledging that they were not true, logical, or helpful. However, she reflected that she was not sure whether she could hold on to these thoughts in the moment and fully experience them during competition. As such, I introduced her to an exercise of rational emotive imagery (REI) to help her to build confidence in her ability to do this.

REI is a skill used to support people to experience a rational thought when they experience the unhealthy negative emotion linked to an activating event. During this exercise, Cara was encouraged to bring the irrational belief to mind and notice her experience of panic and worry. After a short time with this emotion, she was instructed to bring the alternative rational belief to mind and to monitor how her emotions changed.

SP:	The main feelings from the first belief were panic, worry, and being out of control. The matching healthy emotion was concern. Okay, so in a moment, I would like you to bring this situation to mind where you're at the competition and you're telling yourself that you must be able to do it. I want you to tell yourself this over and over again until you start to feel a sense of panic, worry, and feeling out of control. Exactly like you did at the time so you really need to put yourself back in this situa-tion. Worry yourself about the situation.

SP: Once you get the emotion, sit with this for a few seconds and notice how uncomfortable it is and then I want you to think this thought, "I'd really like to be able to do it but sometimes I won't". Keep telling yourself this until you notice the emotions change and you feel more of a sense of concern. Okay?

Athlete: Mmm hmm, yeah.

This can be a difficult exercise for people to understand so I asked Cara to tell me what I had asked her to do so that I could check her understanding and provide an opportunity for any questions to be asked.

SP: Okay, so tell me what I've asked you to do?

Athlete: Erm, make myself feel panicked and worried.

SP: Okay, and how are you going to do that?

Athlete: By saying that I must be able to finish all the routines as if I were at the competition. And then make myself less worried by saying that I'd like to be able to but sometimes I won't.

SP: Okay, when you're ready I want you to have a go, take as long or as short a time as you want over it and you can have your eyes open or closed too. So, when you're ready make a start and when you're done, just turn to me and we'll have a chat.

I also find it important to get immediate feedback about how the exercise has been experienced. Here I am checking for understanding and exploring how they applied what we had discussed.

SP: How did you find that exercise?

Athlete: I wouldn't have thought that I would really like to change my belief to a preference because I always say, "I *must* finish the routine". I feel like the preference puts less pressure on me.

SP: Did you notice your emotions change at all?

Athlete: Yeah, I think because it's the fear of not finishing that gets me and that's why I don't adopt a preferential belief. But, when I actually do use a preference, it feels more accepting.

Cara had engaged well with this exercise and I set it as a between-session task to complete on at least a daily basis to further encourage her to reject the irrational beliefs in favour of the rational alternatives. Cara was asked to independently complete tasks outside of the session time to increase the efficacy of what was discussed. These included monitoring her thought content for examples of 'must' thoughts; practicing the REI exercises; noticing irrational beliefs and changing these to more rational alternatives. Cara was motivated to engage in all aspects of the work, seeking clarity where needed and bringing back examples and reflections of how her independent work had progressed.

Outcome analysis

Cara's goals were to improve the consistency of her competition performance. The primary outcome measures were: changes in irrational beliefs as measured using conviction in belief ratings; changes in anxiety as measured using the SAS-2 scores; and her performance during competition measured by the successful completion of three competition routines. Secondary outcome measures were anecdotal responses from Cara about changes that were experienced in her thoughts, feelings, and behavior.

Changes in the belief structure

During the intervention, Cara was supported to identify four irrational beliefs related to her competition performance. In addition, there were four rational alternative beliefs that were experienced during non-competitive performances. Cara had a strong conviction in these alternative beliefs from the moment that they were discussed, as they formed part of her existing belief structure (see Table 3.1). Initially, there was strong conviction in the demand that she must remain in control and complete her routines. However, following philosophical disputation, Cara accepted that it was an unhelpful, illogical, and unsubstantiated belief to hold.

Changes in the experience of anxiety and panic

Cara completed the SAS-2 at four different time points (see Figure 3.3). The total scores show a reduction in self-reported levels of sport related anxiety over time. This concurs with Cara's presentation during the sessions and her experience of competition anxiety whilst we were working together.

Changes in performance

As the intervention progressed, Cara reported that she had completed the three routines in full at each competition that took place. This was the main outcome

Table 3.1 Changes in the strength of conviction in beliefs

	Irrational Beliefs			Rational Alternative Beliefs
	Initial Rating	Interim Rating	Post-Disputation Rating	Rating Throughout
Demand	10	10	0	10
LFT	2	4	0	10
Awfulizing	5	5	0	10
Self-Depreciation	7	7	0	10

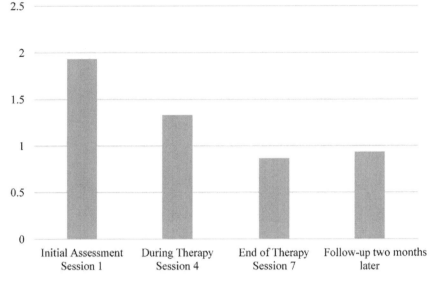

Figure 3.3 Change in mean SAS-2 scores

goal that she was hoping to achieve and it was encouraging that she had been able to succeed.

Anecdotal evaluation evidence

During the sessions there were a number of examples of change taking place that supported the end goal of a change in competition performance. These included:

- Recognizing 'I must' statements and when they are more likely to occur

  - "I notice the musts more when things aren't going very well"
  - "I'm a lot more aware of them"

- Noticing changes in her thinking

  - "I'm using less 'I must' statements and more 'I'd really like to' and I've noticed this is how I'm thinking much more now"
  - "I didn't have as many musts . . . I was able to continue training and although it took me a bit longer to achieve what I wanted to, I got there"

- Building skills and confidence using REI

  - "I practiced every day and it got easier the more I did it"
  - "Getting myself worried was the hardest part and changing it was easy and quick"

- "Doing it live, the worry was there quickly but less than it's felt before and the exercise helped keep it in control"
- Having more consistent performances during both training and competitions
  - "It was the consistency through all three routines that we were looking for, which I did"
  - "During these practice competitions the performance has been better and more consistent, like the training competitions"

Summary

In summary, the athlete worked well throughout the sessions and achieved the goals that she had set out to achieve. The change in her belief structure had occurred quickly, by session 3, and the following sessions were used to generalize the learning and reinforce the changes using REI. This case study demonstrates that REBT can be used successfully with athletes who are motivated to change and who engage meaningfully in the process of therapeutic intervention.

Critical reflections

This has been a positive short-term piece of work where Cara achieved her goals within the time set. The athlete factors that enabled this change included Cara's motivation to actively engage in the process, her ability to understand the concepts and framework of REBT, including asking questions if she was unsure about something, and her commitment to do the out of session work. Formally measuring Cara's readiness to change at the beginning of this process could have assisted me in understanding just how motivated she was. Social factors enabling the change included a supportive coach, a flexible employer (enabling attendance at psychology sessions), and a supportive social network.

Therapist factors included having a good technical knowledge of REBT to enable change; the ability to develop a therapeutic relationship to facilitate meaningful conversations; and being time-bounded and available via e-mail for between-session questions or concerns.

Environmental factors included having a quiet, reflective, and confidential space without distractions. It is possible that meeting with Cara at the sports centre where she trained and/or observing her during training or competitions would have added information to the assessment that was otherwise missed. It would have provided me as her therapist with a lived example of her environment, which I did not have. To overcome this, I asked Cara to explain things to me in a lot of detail and I also watched generic video footage of trampoline gymnasts training and in competition.

On reflection, it was useful to have identified how the goals could be measured and what the expectation was for a successful outcome. This made the direction of change clear throughout the work and the process for achieving these were shared between us. The goals that were set were not all SMART goals (Specific,

Measurable, Attainable, Realistic, and Timely). In the future I would encourage myself to support the athlete to set SMART goals to further enable this process of change. Overall, I have learned that motivated athletes are more readily engaged and experience change more quickly. When the enabling factors described previously are in place, REBT is an effective model to guide this change process.

References

Gardner, F., & Moore, Z. (2006). *Clinical sport psychology*. Champaign, IL: Human Kinetics.

Papadopoulos, E., Muir, C., Russell, C., Timmons, B. W., Falk, B., & Klentrou, P. (2014). Markers of biological stress and mucosal immunity during a week leading to competition in adolescent swimmers. *Journal of Immunology Research, 2014.*

Schwebel, F. J., Smith, R. E., & Smoll, F. L. (2016). Measurement of perceived parental success standards in sport and relations with athletes' self-esteem, performance anxiety, and achievement goal orientation: Comparing parental and coach influences. *Child Development Research*, 1–13.

Scott-Hamilton, J., Schutte, N. S., & Brown, R. F. (2016). Effects of a Mindfulness Intervention on Sport Anxiety, Pessimism, and Flow in Competitive Cyclists. *Health and Well-Being*, 8(1), 85–103.

Smith, R. E., Smoll, F. L., Cumming, S. P., & Grossbard, J. R. (2006). Measurement of multidimensional sport performance anxiety in children and adults: The sport anxiety scale-2. *Journal of Sport & Exercise Psychology*, 28, 479–501.

Turner, M. J., & Barker, J. B. (2013). Examining the efficacy of Rational-Emotive Behavior Therapy (REBT) on irrational beliefs and anxiety in elite youth cricketers. *Journal of Applied Sport Psychology*, 25(1), 131–147.

Editors' commentary on Chapter 3: "A short-term Rational Emotive Behavior Therapy (REBT) intervention for competition anxiety with a trampoline gymnast"

One of the really important aspects Michelle details in her chapter, which is often omitted from the research literature, is the belief conviction measurement. Here, Michelle asks Cara how *true* she feels her irrational beliefs are at key moments during the work. As the intervention progresses, Cara's conviction in her irrational beliefs wanes, as would be hoped. This is important because intellectual insight is an early step towards helping a client implement rational beliefs in their lives. Although in the early stages the client might understand that the beliefs they hold are irrational, they may still hold some conviction for them. As the work progresses, the practitioner works hard with the client to instil emotional insight, reflecting a full and deep understanding of irrationality and rationality. While intellectual insight is important, it is unlikely to lead to changes in behavior. Emotional insight is more likely to lead to changes in behavior, and thus is a marker of significant change (Dryden, 2009).

Those new to REBT will often search for and focus on the four core irrational beliefs *only*. One of the important details of Michelle's chapter is the recognition of cognitive distortions that follow irrational beliefs, typically associated with anxiety. Rumination, black and white thinking, distraction, paralysis by analysis, and an unconstructive focus on physical symptoms all contribute to Cara's performance issues. But crucially, through REBT these cognitive symptoms of anxiety resulting from irrational beliefs are not addressed directly; rather they are addressed *indirectly* by working with the root cause of the anxiety: namely irrational beliefs. This approach is one of the reasons that REBT is often described as 'elegant'; REBT addresses core beliefs, thus affecting a myriad of symptomology, rather than only addressing one symptom (such as rumination).

Reference

Dryden, W. (2009). *How to think and intervene like an REBT therapist*. London: Routledge, Taylor & Francis Group.

4 Anxiety, unhealthy jealousy, and exercise avoidance

A Rational Emotive Behavior Therapy (REBT) intervention

Helen O'Connor

Introduction

'Sarah', a 24-year-old woman, had struggled with her weight since puberty and at the start of our work together she weighed 203lb. Although the complete intervention also tackled issues of discomfort disturbance relating to healthier eating, this case study presents aspects of the REBT intervention which focused on ego disturbance issues underpinning Sarah's avoidance of exercise. As an example, when Sarah noticed attractive women she inferred that her partner would reject her by preferring these other women. By demanding that her partner must never find other women attractive, believing that it would be truly awful and unbearable if he did, and that his doing so would prove her to be worthless and unlovable, Sarah made herself distressed and anxious about being rejected. One consequence of this was avoidance of situations in which she might encounter attractive women, including exercise and fitness settings.

Sarah lost 20lb across the ten-session consultancy, which spanned six months. She had been making healthier dietary choices more consistently, and, instead of damning herself, she responded more constructively to the occasional slip. She also initiated and maintained a regular exercise routine. As Sarah developed a healthier rational philosophy (e.g., preferring, but not demanding, that her partner didn't find other women attractive, and preferring not to be judged by others), she experienced less distress to real or perceived adversities. For instance, she could feel concerned (rather than anxious) that her partner might notice other women, and healthy jealousy (rather than unhealthy jealousy) when he did, which supported her in overcoming some previous causes of exercise avoidance. This case study highlights the complexity of potential causes of exercise avoidance, some of which might extend beyond the exercise setting and affect a client's wider life and relationships.

Context

I am a chartered psychologist in the UK and have worked in the private, public, and charity sectors with a focus on health behavior change and addictions. I first trained in and used REBT whilst working at a residential weight loss camp. I have since used REBT interventions to support clients in weight management, as well as smoking cessation, problem drinking, and substance misuse. I am continuing my training at the Centre for REBT at the University of Birmingham.

I sit between a practitioner-led and client-led philosophy and approach to psychological intervention (Keegan, 2010). I believe people have a natural ability to change themselves and that REBT can facilitate this change through a more active, practitioner-led agenda due to its focus on specific aspects of a problem and its solution. I see the ABC formulation process of REBT as a method of "accurately describing the situation" and gaining a shared understanding of it with the client, as opposed to "uncovering and identifying the underlying cause of a clockwork problem" (Lindsay, et al., 2014; p. 47). I adopt a collaborative style where I bring the client into the decision-making process about what we hope to achieve and a roadmap for how we might get there. I also consider it to be important to foster a healthy working alliance in which the client and I are in agreement on the goals and tasks of the work, and that we share a warm, trusting bond (Flückiger, et al., 2012). The work described in this case study took place in my private practice over ten sessions at tapered intervals across six months because the client's financial situation limited the number and frequency of sessions.

Presenting issue

Sarah is a white British female, who was 24 at the time of this consultancy. At 203lb, she was overweight for her 5'8" frame and wanted to lose weight. She considered that she had overeaten and been overweight since the age of 13. Sarah had tried to lose weight numerous times following various plans. Typically, she would lose weight for a few weeks but was unable to maintain the changes for long enough to get close to a healthier weight. Sarah also frequently had intentions to exercise but struggled to initiate or maintain the exercise component of a weight loss plan. She felt self-conscious and ashamed about her "disgusting body" and felt unhappy being around other women who were slimmer than her.

Sarah's shame and thoughts about her shape and size had affected her sexual and romantic relationships. She considered that her past, current, and any future partners were (or would be) dissatisfied with her and be actively seeking to meet "someone better". Within her current relationship she experienced jealousy and hyper-vigilance in social situations. She would scan her environment for attractive women and point them out to, and seek reassurance from, her partner. Even when she was not with her partner and saw a woman who she considered to be "better" than herself, Sarah would imagine that her partner would prefer them, and feel anxious about the imagined rejection. Consequently, she tried to avoid situations where she would be around attractive women, including exercise settings.

In REBT parlance, Sarah was not particularly entrenched in A-C thinking (i.e., situation A causes my distress at C) and was aware that she was distressing herself and making herself feel more anxious because of her beliefs (B) about situations. Sarah's understanding of the influence of cognition on emotions helped me illustrate the REBT model as we collaborated on how it might be used to support her in taking necessary action towards reaching her goals. Her primary reason for working with me was to help her reach and maintain a healthy weight of 140–150lb through eating better and exercising more.

Needs analysis

I had been introduced to REBT on a residential work placement where the model was used to help overweight adolescents and young adults to tolerate the necessary discomfort of forgoing dietary pleasures and increasing their daily physical activity to lose weight. Having seen the positive effects of an REBT intervention in this setting, an REBT conceptualization shaped my assessment session with Sarah. Nothing in her initial presentation or information provided in the assessment suggested the presence of an eating disorder or other clinically significant mental health difficulty. Sarah admired "strong, toned and sporty" women and her goal weight and physique seemed healthy and appropriate.

In an REBT interpretation, overeating or avoiding physical activity (when one is overweight but would *prefer not to be*) can be viewed as a self-defeating action tendency in response to, or designed to avoid, a distressing unhealthy negative emotion (C). Sarah and I collaborated to understand what evaluative beliefs (B) were influencing some of her unwanted behaviors and distressing emotional consequences (C) in response to certain situations and inferences about those situations (A). The initial assessment suggested that Sarah was defeating herself in two ways: by holding irrational demanding beliefs (iBs) about her emotional and physical comfort (*discomfort disturbance*), which seemed to particularly influence her eating habits, and by holding demanding iBs about the self (*ego disturbance*), which seemed to particularly underpin her avoidance of exercise. When presented with a choice about what she wanted to prioritize in our sessions, Sarah considered that the distressing emotions around exercise were affecting her life most negatively.

We did identify additional issues relating to ego disturbance in terms of Sarah's diet (e.g., self-depreciation about lapses) and aspects of being physically active that related to discomfort disturbance (e.g., feeling sweaty, out of breath, sore). However, the remainder of this chapter focuses on the work we did relating to ego disturbance issues that were interfering with her goal of exercising regularly.

Ego disturbance

One of REBT's tacit absolutist demands is "I must do well and win the approval of others or else I am no good". A person who holds this demand places unrealistic expectations on themselves, is overly concerned with the opinions of other people, and conditionally bases their self-worth on their competence, achievements, and popularity ("If I do not do well/am not approved of, then I am worthless"). At an emotional level, an individual who holds these beliefs will experience ego anxiety if they perceive that their self or self-worth is threatened (Ellis, 1990). Behaviorally, they are more likely to avoid (uncomfortable) situations, which might give rise to disapproval or failure, and look to others for approval (Dryden, 2013).

The ego disturbance that Sarah experienced in exercise contexts contributed substantially to her avoidance of exercise. When she became aware of herself, for example, by noticing herself in a mirror, or realizing how much noise she was making on a piece of equipment (situational A), she would tell herself that people were noticing and judging her (inferential A). Beliefs about needing to avoid disapproval and not make mistakes, and labelling herself as "ridiculous" and "disgusting" (B), would create distressing feelings of shame (C). She would then want to flee from the shameful experience. Anxiety (another C) about the mere thought of this happening led to exercise avoidance.

Sarah also experienced distress from unhealthy jealousy and anxiety as a result of unfavourable comparisons with other women, which threatened her self-evaluative judgments. Taking a third-person 'male gaze' Sarah would evaluate other women in terms of how attractive they would be to men and particularly to her own partner. She would then engage in prediction, assuming her partner would prefer these attractive women, that he was dissatisfied with her (because her size made her unlovable), and would eventually leave her for someone more attractive. By demanding that her partner must never find other women attractive, whilst also indulging in imagining how truly awful and unbearable it would be if he did (and how this would prove her to be worthless and unlovable), Sarah felt anxious and "panicky" about being rejected which would include certain consequences:

- Physiological – feeling jittery, diarrhoea
- Cognitive – always worrying about being rejected
- Behavioral – hyper-vigilance to notice all the attractive women in her environment, and avoidance of situations in which she might encounter attractive women, including exercise

Despite these emotional responses in exercise settings, Sarah had tried to exercise before and one of her key goals was to feel more comfortable about going to the gym and taking classes.

It is essential in REBT to help the client emotionally access their distressing unhealthy negative emotions (UNEs), rather than simply intellectually describe a distressing situation. This allows the iBs that are behind the UNEs to be discovered, and is done by asking the client to reconnect with and re-tell a specific example of a distressing event. Sarah provided an example of a time when she had noticed a "stunning" woman in the gym and we worked together on the ABC formulation of this situation as presented in Figure 4.1.

Activating Event (A)

Situation (A¹): See a stunning woman in the gym.

Adversity (A²): She's so much better looking than me. My partner would notice her. He would prefer her looks to mine. That would be a rejection of me.

Irrational Beliefs (iB)	Rational Beliefs (rB)
Demand: I really don't want my boyfriend to ever fancy another woman. *And therefore he must never do so.*	**Preference:** I really, really want my boyfriend to only ever have eyes for me. *But unfortunately he doesn't absolutely have to.*
Awfulizing: It would be catastrophically awful if he found another woman attractive.	**Anti-Awfulizing:** Although it's unfortunate and I prefer it didn't happen – there are far worse things than him thinking someone else looks hot.
Low Frustration Tolerance: It would be totally unbearable if he found anyone else attractive.	**High Frustration Tolerance:** Although it would be tough to bear – I could bear it if he noticed someone else – and, in the service of my desire to exercise more, it would be worth it for me to bear it.
Self-/Other-Depreciation: It would prove how utterly and completely disgusting and unlovable I am (because of my size).	**Unconditional Self-Acceptance:** It would be bad if he noticed another woman, but his doing so doesn't make me disgusting or unlovable as a person. I am the same fallible human being whether he notices anyone else or not.

Unhelpful Consequences (C)	Helpful Consequences (C)
Emotional Consequences:	**Emotional Consequences:**
Unhealthy jealousy – at thought of partner finding others attractive.	Healthy jealousy – at thought of partner finding others attractive.
Panic/anxiety – about the idea of being rejected.	Concern – about the idea of being rejected.
Behavioral Consequences:	**Behavioral Consequences:**
Crying. Seeking reassurance. Hyper-vigilant – for attractive women. Escape from, or avoidance of, exercise.	Continue with exercise class/plans. Less checking for attractive women.
Cognitive Consequences:	**Cognitive Consequences:**
Catastrophizing – he's dissatisfied and will leave me for someone 'better'. Worrying about imagined rejection.	Use forceful coping statements.
Physiological Consequences:	
Jittery, diarrhoea ('flight'). 'Hollow' in pit of stomach.	

Figure 4.1 Example ABC conceptualization of Sarah's ego disturbance when exercising

The intervention

We explored what Sarah did, thought, and felt in this scenario, as well as how she would have preferred to have responded. This helped us identify what kind of healthy negative emotion (HNE) would have been more likely to lead to those preferential behaviors and cognitions, with a particular emphasis on engaging in, rather than avoiding, exercise. The UNE and corresponding HNE she selected to work on were, firstly, her anxiety (concern) at the imagined rejection by her partner, and second, her unhealthy jealousy (healthy jealousy) about the imagined scenario of him noticing the attractive woman. Later in the consultancy we worked through the process with UNEs relating to the adversity of being judged by others.

Within REBT theory there remains an unanswered question about whether dysfunctional UNEs and their corresponding functional HNEs differ mostly along a quantitative dimension (i.e., intensity), or whether they are qualitatively different, regardless of intensity. The latter idea of UNE and HNE being qualitatively different is original to REBT (David, 2015). What is most important is that experiencing a HNE in response to an adversity causes a person less distress, allowing them to respond in more self-supporting ways – for instance, assertively expressing how someone has disappointed them rather than being passive-aggressive or sulking.

Sarah and I spoke about REBT's model of HNE as we looked for how she would need to be feeling differently in order to respond differently (chiefly, to continue exercising) in the specific situation where she saw the attractive woman, *assuming that the adversity was accurate* (i.e., that had her partner been there, he would have noticed this woman and found her attractive). She found it reasonably easy to accept the idea that if she had felt concerned rather than anxious, then she would have experienced less distress and would not have felt an urgent need to flee the situation. For Sarah, concern was different to anxiety mostly in terms of intensity and a lack of physiological symptoms. Feeling concerned would also help her notice and express another HNE of wry annoyance about the very existence of this attractive person.

Sarah struggled more to accept healthy jealousy as unhealthy jealousy's functional twin, considering "any jealousy" to be an "ugly emotion". However, she settled on the idea that if she was healthily jealous she could relax more in environments where there were attractive women who her partner might notice, and would not constantly be on the look-out for these women, which would reduce the time she spent making herself "concerned". Later, Sarah was able to accept that feeling "ugly emotions" was just a sign of her human fallibility.

Beginning with the demand (absolutist musts) and then the derivatives (awfulizing beliefs, LFT beliefs, depreciation beliefs), we started to assess the iBs that connected to Sarah's emotional distress (anxiety, unhealthy jealousy). My preferred method of eliciting iBs is to ask direct questions derived from REBT theory (e.g., "What are you demanding about your boyfriend liking that other woman's appearance to make yourself feel so distressingly anxious?"; "What kind of person do you think it makes *you* if he did like her appearance?"). The benefit of having the client describe and vividly recall a specific situation and re-experience the UNE is that the client can also be asked to give the UNE a voice ("If that unhealthy jealousy could speak, what would it say?"). Some of Sarah's iBs that we identified, and which she understood were perpetuating her anxiety and unhealthy jealousy, are presented in Figure 4.1.

Having accepted the HNE goals of concern rather than anxiety, and healthy rather than unhealthy jealousy about her partner appreciating another woman's appearance, we worked through various disputation processes to develop rational beliefs (rBs) that would connect to her emotional goals.

Disputation

Pragmatic disputations such as, "How is evaluating other women's attractiveness helping you to exercise more and lose weight?" helped Sarah uncover possible benefits of thinking more rationally ("If I lost a pound in weight every time I saw an attractive woman it could make sense to keep looking out for them. But I don't lose any weight at all, in fact I just make myself unhappier and am even less likely to do anything about losing weight"). When we were talking about Sarah's demand that her partner "only have eyes" for her, an effective forceful disputation was, "Would you feel happy with your body and secure about your relationship if your partner was blind and unable to see other women?" Sarah found this amusing and we exaggerated the idea, wondering if it would be even more preferable if there were universal blindness, so that no-one could ever be judged or judge others by their appearance. Then we realized that people would simply start evaluating each other by 'feel' instead, and, being overweight, her problem would remain. Plus, she would have to tolerate being groped all the time! This particular disputation with dark humour seemed to helped Sarah see the futility and irrationality in insisting one person never notices other people or finds other people attractive. It also helped her to develop a more preferential belief about her partner noticing other women ("I really, really want my boyfriend to only ever have eyes for me. But unfortunately he doesn't absolutely have to") from which we were able to develop the rational derivative beliefs, including the notion that it would be worth it to Sarah to be able to bear the idea of this happening, as it would help her to exercise more and be more present in social settings (see rBs in Figure 4.1).

Sarah's self-depreciation and labelling of herself as "unlovable" because of how "disgusting" she was being forceful and caused her considerable distress. At the time of this case I weighed considerably more than Sarah's goal weight. I used a double-standard dispute to ask Sarah if she thought that I should believe that I was totally and utterly unworthy of anyone's love or approval because of my weight. I asked her if she was globally rating me as "disgusting" or "unlovable" because of my size and whether she thought that I should do so. Sarah intellectually understood that this would be illogical and unhelpful, but her conviction was weak. On this point I frequently reminded Sarah that weak convictions would not be sufficient to promote a robust lasting change, and stressed the importance of doing regular rational self-analysis and other between-session assignments (Dryden, et al., 2010). We also developed forceful rational coping statements to help address her entrenched thinking and depreciating self-talk.

Rational emotive imagery

Rational emotive imagery (REI) helps clients locate the HNEs in a particular problematic situation, and generate rBs and self-statements that could work for them in similar situations in future so that they disturb themselves less (Ellis, 1993). During session four, I asked Sarah to close her eyes and imagine a difficult situation (being in a class surrounded by attractive women) and label the strong UNE that the situation evoked (anxiety, unhealthy jealousy). Taking these emotions in turn, I asked her to try imagining the emotions being changed to the HNE we had previously discussed (concern, healthy jealousy). We explored how she was able to replace the UNE with the HNE (without changing any element of the situation at all) by thinking more flexibly about preferring for her partner to never find other women attractive, and using rational coping statements such as, "I wish there weren't any attractive women in this class – or even the world – and I do want to be slimmer, but it just doesn't help me if I allow someone else's attractiveness to affect my workout or happiness". We did this exercise twice (for anxiety and unhealthy jealousy), and I asked Sarah to practice it daily until our next session. When we met again she told me she had been doing the exercise about four times a week and had been feeling much less concerned about the presence of attractive women in general. However, although she was exercising regularly, she was staying in her 'least discomfort zone' and doing classes where she knew there would be fewer attractive women. That this avoidance was limiting Sarah's exercise options was less important than the fact that it revealed she was still vulnerable to distress in future situations where she couldn't avoid attractive women.

Behavioral assignments

Behavioral assignments are an effective way to help a client move from intellectual rational insight to emotional rational insight. These involve clients deliberately planning to enter situations that they would usually avoid and using coping strategies to manage themselves within those situations. This can help in a number of ways, including testing the validity of their inferences and beliefs – particularly strengthening their conviction in their rational beliefs, developing confidence in their ability to cope, and increasing their tolerance for things they find uncomfortable (Dryden, 1995; Froggatt, 2005).

In our second session I had asked Sarah to rate her exercise experiences from the least to most awful, uncomfortable, and distressing, and we explored her ratings. Top of the 'badness scale' were contexts in which she felt most self-conscious about her body and being looked at, and where there were slimmer and more attractive people (Body Pump™, yoga, Pilates). Sarah preferred classes (step, toning) with members who she felt more similar to in physique; with less chance of noticing attractive women she was less likely to upset herself with thoughts of who her partner might prefer. At that point, we agreed that to get her exercise plans underway and develop a habit of regular activity, she would start by attending the classes that provoked the least negative emotions.

By the middle of the consultancy, after Sarah had been exercising regularly but was still avoiding the 'more awful' classes, I explained that it would be useful if she considered attending a more emotionally distressing class as a way of developing a stronger conviction in her rational beliefs. I proposed a behavioral assignment that would help her to practice her developing rational outlook about situations where there were attractive women (including outside the gym setting). As this was something that continued to impact on her relationship, Sarah thought it was worthwhile and agreed to the between-session activity. We reviewed the list of exercise activities again and Sarah picked yoga. Not only would there be very attractive, stylish, competent, slim women in the class, she also felt ashamed that people behind her would see her backside in the poses and stretches and would be judging and laughing at her. To make the assignment more potentially shameful Sarah was to pick a spot that was somewhere between the front and the middle of the room. Sarah predicted that this would be about 75% awful in terms of feelings of shame and being upset by thoughts of rejection. We looked at coping strategies Sarah could use whilst she was in the class. She planned to remind herself of her rBs before the class, and during the class to use a forceful coping statement we had previously formulated as a form of mantra, going with the breath of the poses ("however much I weigh and whatever size and shape I am, I accept myself as a fallible human being").

In the following session we discussed this activity. Sarah rated the actual experience as 50% awful and had even done yoga again since, even though she did find it embarrassing to have her backside on show, and continued to be disappointed about her weight and shape. She had used her rational coping statement and thought about how she would laugh about the experience with me in our next session. Two women "might have been laughing" at her, but she had been able to feel annoyed about this (rather than angry, hurt, or ashamed). The key benefit to being annoyed was that she was able to remain focused on the class and what the teacher was saying, and did not withdraw by keeping her eyes down, but caught the eye and smiled at someone who had said hello to her and passed her a mat at the start of class. She did not have thoughts about any other woman's attractiveness or her partner, and felt she got a more complete experience of yoga because she had a "clearer mind". In this exercise, Sarah learnt to challenge the validity of her beliefs by discovering that the situation was not as bad in reality as it was in her imagination, and that she could, in fact, 'bear it'. She discovered that she had found an effective strategy to do so, and that it was more helpful and accurate to recognize that whilst some people might be judgmental, many are not. In terms of exercise avoidance, this expanded the range of activities Sarah had available to her.

Maintenance and relapse prevention

By the end of our sessions, the basis of Sarah's new rational philosophy for exercising could be summed up as:

> Feeling approved of and special is great, but not essential. In fact, the more I demand approval, the more I worry about not getting it or losing it. The more I demand I am special, the more I pity myself and get jealous when I am not. Demandingness takes me further away from my goals and a healthy happy life.

Byrne, et al. (2003) identified certain psychological factors that characterize people who gained weight after successfully losing weight, including: failure to achieve weight goals, dissatisfaction with the weight achieved, a black-and-white thinking style, a tendency to evaluate self-worth in terms of weight and shape, and to use eating to regulate mood. REBT can work on these issues directly, and many elements were present in the work with Sarah. Sarah considered that 'early warning signs' that she was at risk of abandoning her healthier lifestyle would include stopping planning and problem solving for high risk situations for food, starting to experience more emotional distress about attractive women, finding herself labelling herself disgusting, or indulging in catastrophizing thoughts about being rejected. She committed to doing her REBT exercises daily if she felt at risk of relapse or noticed she had started to slip, and understood that she needed to be consistent if she wanted to maintain and strengthen her healthy rational outlook.

Outcome analysis

We had agreed at the start of the consultancy that we would know the sessions were helping if Sarah was making healthier choices more of the time (as she tolerated the discomfort of resisting unhealthy choices and the frustration of slow weight loss better). A second indicator would be if she were exercising more regularly (because she was feeling less distressed whilst exercising or when imagining exercising). Effectiveness was determined through in-session observations and self-reported change. We also completed a client change interview (CCI) in our final session (Elliott, et al. 2006).

Sarah reported that she had lost weight every time we met, 20lb over the six months of our consultancy, and estimated that she had eaten healthily about 80% of the time. In the CCI, Sarah considered that the REBT intervention had helped her stick more consistently to her eating plans, stating that she hadn't lost more than 10lb on previous diets, none of which she had stuck to for longer than three months. The main shift was in her thoughts (unconditional self-acceptance) and feelings (disappointment) about her fallibility when she did make less value-congruent food choices, which led to more constructive and immediate responses to such occurrences. She felt less frustrated and self-pitying about the slow pace of change, which allowed her to focus on the less comfortable but longer-term and more worthwhile plan to consistently make healthy choices. Sarah found *Beating the comfort trap* (Dryden & Gordon, 1993), which I had lent her at the start of the work, particularly helpful in working through LFT issues around healthy eating. This sustained weight loss was a shift on a long-term problem for Sarah, and, given the amount of effort she needed to make between sessions to achieve it, demonstrated that she was 'getting better' rather than just 'feeling better' as a result of aspects of the intervention.

Sarah reported that she had kept to almost all of her physical activity plans during the consultancy, usually attending three classes a week. Sticking to these plans had also become a constructive action tendency in response to disappointments about occasional deviations from her eating plan. Sarah was experiencing less distress whilst exercising, even in classes further up her 'badness scale'. As her healthier rational philosophy contained more preferences than demands (e.g., preferring that her partner didn't find other women attractive, preferring not to be judged by others), she experienced healthier negative emotions, such as concern that her partner might find other women attractive, healthy jealousy when he did, and annoyance that the world contained lots of very attractive women. She had almost completely stopped predicting rejection by her partner, and considered that she spent far less time checking for attractive women in her environment or seeking reassurance from her partner. A key finding from the CCI was that Sarah had started to experience functional positive feelings (David, 2015) towards the step and toning classes she had been doing since we began our sessions. These included anticipation and enjoyment in taking part, a drive to make an effort, feeling a sense of belonging to the group, and pride in getting fitter and more competent. This was an unexpected change that Sarah did not think would have occurred without the intervention. She also considered this change to be very important as she saw it as the start of shifts on deeper issues such as her beliefs about her worth, both as a person and as a partner. Sarah found the REI exercise and between-session behavioral assignment helpful in feeling less distressed at the gym. More generally, she said that she benefitted from understanding more about "how the mind works" and "that it's OK to feel bad about things that we would rather weren't true".

The CCI also revealed changes which extended beyond the gym context, providing further evidence that Sarah was not only less disturbed about the issues she presented with, but also less disturb-able as a result of developing a more rational philosophy. For instance, she considered that her relationship with her boyfriend had improved because she was "more relaxed more of the time" and less avoidant or anxious about social events they went to together – a positive shift on a long-standing and important personal issue. She attributed this partly to the fact that she had lost weight, and also because she was "thinking differently".

Critical reflections

Despite Sarah's progress, some potentially important issues were left unexplored. The work concentrated on Sarah's evaluative beliefs about specific adversities and opportunities to look at her self-related beliefs (e.g., "to feel good about myself I must always be approved of and must avoid disapproval from any source") were missed. In REBT theory, the evaluative belief system is derived from an individual's core philosophy: if this continues to be unrealistic, inflexible, or not self-accepting, then an individual will still have vulnerabilities.

Although Sarah intellectually understood how it was causing her more distress to conditionally evaluate her own (and others') worth based on physical attributes, she did struggle to endorse this aspect of a healthy rational philosophy at an emotional level. She repeatedly returned to the idea that although it might not be pragmatic or logical, it was (according to her perception of "the way things are") reality-based and empirically true: the world, especially men, are shallow and don't care whether a woman has other positive qualities or not, as long as she is attractive and conforms to societal ideals. More forceful disputations, a didactic questioning style, or the use of examples and metaphors might have helped facilitate this head-gut shift. We might also have explored core irrational demands about how the world and others must be, think, and behave, with a view to developing unconditional life-acceptance and other-acceptance (e.g., of her partner as a fallible human being who might do things that hurt her feelings, such as take an interest in other women).

In REBT, humour and self-disclosure can be used both in the service of engagement, and as an aid to disputation, and humour is considered to be a desirable condition for therapeutic change (Dryden & Branch, 2008; Dryden, et al., 2010; Fryer, 2011). This was one of the first consultancies where I had felt comfortable using humour, possibly because Sarah and I were both, in our own perceptions, overweight and shared some of the struggles of trying to not be. Sport and exercise psychologists need to tread carefully when bringing humour and self-disclosure into the consultancy (Andersen & Peterson, 2005; Way & Vosloo, 2016) and some clients might not consider an 'overweight' psychologist to be the best person to help them lose weight. However, as Andersen and Peterson (2005) have noted, "when we talk in a matter-of-fact manner, with self-compassion and a touch of humor, about our struggles with how we look and how we have eaten, we model that it really is OK to talk about these things" (2005; p. 64). I consider that my self-disclosure and the use of humour modelled and supported cognitive shifts from irrational to rational beliefs that helped Sarah to experience healthier negative emotions, and consequently enact her diet and exercise plans more consistently.

When Taylor (1994) responded to Ellis's (1994) paper on REBT for exercise avoidance, one of his criticisms was that REBT does not place enough emphasis on "replacing irrational beliefs with more positive beliefs about the self and exercise/sport participation" (p. 264). Helping someone move towards a preferential view of exercise as an unpleasant, un-preferred, inconvenient necessity could seem sub-optimal, given what we know about the benefits and potential positive experiences that can arise from participating in physical activities. Yet, the "rational education" model of providing accurate and compelling information about the benefits of initiating and maintaining exercise has not been particularly effective in mobilizing people to be more active, because humans are frequently not rational decision-makers (Zenko, et al., 2016). Affective responses to exercise vary between individuals (Ekkekakis & Dafermos, 2012; Ekkekakis & Lind, 2006; Schutte, et al., 2016) and inferences about being judged and disapproved of in exercise contexts will sometimes be correct (Flint & Reale, 2016). So, it follows that some clients will experience exercise as more awful, uncomfortable, frustrating, and emotionally distressing than others.

It makes more practical sense to acknowledge that exercise might be a strongly un-preferred adversity for some individuals, and that people do not always make the 'rational' decision to exercise despite knowledge of its positive benefits. Only then can we develop effective interventions that help people be more physically active (Zenko, et al., 2016). Through REBT, people can learn to respond in less self-defeating ways to adversities, and it becomes more possible and more likely that they will make healthier choices, even if they still strongly prefer not to make those choices. REBT can help people put the 'awfulness' of exercise into perspective, become better at tolerating the discomfort of exercising, and practice unconditional self-acceptance about their size, shape, and exercise competence (even whilst preferring to be slimmer, healthier, or more competent). As Sarah discovered, reducing the emotional distress an individual experiences in exercise settings might, in time, help them discover positive experiences and emotions for themselves, which can reinforce and maintain regular physical activity.

References

Andersen, M. B., & Petersen, K. (2005) "I have a friend who": Group work on weight and body image. In M. B. Andersen (Ed.), *Sport psychology in practice* (pp. 61–74). Human Kinetics: Champaign, IL.

Byrne, S., Cooper, Z., & Fairburn, C. (2003). Weight maintenance and relapse in obesity: A qualitative study. *International Journal of Obesity, 27*(8), 955–962.

David, D. (2015). Rational emotive behavior therapy. In R. L. Cautin & S. O. Lilienfeld (Eds.), *Encyclopedia of Clinical Psychology*. Hoboken, NJ: Wiley-Blackwell.

Dryden, W. (1995). *Rational emotive behaviour therapy: A reader*. London: SAGE.

Dryden, W. (2013). *The ABCs of REBT revisited: Perspectives on conceptualization*. New York, NY: Springer.

Dryden, W., & Branch, R, (2008). *The fundamentals of rational emotive behaviour therapy*. Chichester: Wiley.

Dryden, W., Giuseppe, R., & Neenan, M. (2010). *A primer on rational emotive behaviour therapy* (3rd ed), Champaign, IL: Research Press.

Dryden, W., & Gordon, J. (1993). *Beating the comfort trap*. London: Sheldon Press.

Ekkekakis, P., & Dafermos, M. (2012). Exercise is a many-splendored thing but for some it does not feel so splendid: Staging a resurgence of hedonistic ideas in the quest to understand exercise behavior. In E.O. Acevedo (Ed.), *Oxford handbook of exercise psychology* (pp. 295–333). New York, NY: Oxford University Press.

Ekkekakis, P., & Lind, E. (2006). Exercise does not feel the same when you are overweight: The impact of self-selected and imposed intensity on affect and exertion. *International Journal of Obesity, 30*(4), 652–660.

Elliott, R., Mack, C., & Shapiro, D. A. (2006). *Client change interview*. Retrieved from http://peeft.blogspot.co.uk/2006/12/new-version-of-client-change-interview.html.

Ellis, A. (1990). Discomfort anxiety: A new cognitive behavioral construct. In W. Dryden (Ed.), *The essential Albert Ellis: Seminal writings on psychotherapy* (pp. 94–113). New York, NY: Springer.

Ellis, A. (1993). Rational-emotive imagery: RET version. In M. E. Bernard & J. L. Wolfe (Eds.), *The RET resource book for practitioners* (pp II-8–II-10). New York: Institute for Rational-Emotive Therapy.

Ellis, A. (1994). The sport of avoiding sports and exercise: A Rational Emotive Behavior Therapy perspective. *The Sport Psychologist*, 8(3), 248–261.

Flint, S. W., & Reale, S. (2016). Weight stigma in frequent exercisers: Overt, demeaning and condescending. *Journal of Health Psychology*. doi: 10.1177/1359105316656232.

Flückiger, C., Del Re, A. C., Wampold, B. E., Symonds, D., & Horvath, A. O. (2012). How central is the alliance in psychotherapy? A multilevel longitudinal meta-analysis. *Journal of Counselling Psychology*, 59(1), 10–17.

Froggatt, W. (2005). *A brief introduction to rational emotive behaviour therapy* (3rd ed.). Retrieved from www.rational.org.nz/prof-docs/Intro-REBT.pdf.

Fryer, D. (2011). Putting the fun back into dysfunctional: Is the use of humour in Rational Emotive Behaviour Therapy a desirable condition or an amusing aside? *The Rational Emotive Behaviour Therapist*, 14(1), 63–72.

Keegan, R. J. (2010). Teaching consulting philosophies to neophyte sport psychologists: Does it help, and how can we do it? *Journal of Sport Psychology in Action*, 1, 42–52.

Lindsay, P., Pitt, T., & Thomas, O. (2014). Bewitched by our words: Wittgenstein, language-games, and the pictures that hold sport psychology captive. *Sport and Exercise Psychology Review*, 10(1), 41–54.

Schutte, N. M., Nederend, I., Hudziak, J. J., Bartels, M., & de Geus, E. J. C. (2016). Heritability of the affective response to exercise and its correlation to exercise behaviour. *Psychology of Sport and Exercise*. doi: 10.1016/j-psychsport.2016.12.001

Taylor, J. (1994). On exercise and sport avoidance: A reply to Dr. Albert Ellis. *The Sport Psychologist*, 8(3), 262–270.

Way, W., & Vosloo, J. (2016). Practical considerations for self-disclosure in applied sport psychology. *Journal of Sport Psychology in Action*, 7(1), 23–32.

Zenko, A., Ekkekakis, P., & Kavestos, G. (2016). Changing minds: Bounded rationality and heuristic processes in exercise-related judgments and choices. *Sport, Exercise, and Performance Psychology*, 5(4), 337–351.

Editors' commentary on Chapter 4: "Anxiety, unhealthy jealousy, and exercise avoidance: a Rational Emotive Behavior Therapy (REBT) intervention"

This chapter raises the important issue of a careful assessment in line with the ABC model. Ostensibly, Sarah came to seek help with a goal of losing weight and maintaining an exercise regime. What Helen has demonstrated in her work is the importance of differentiating between *the goal as defined by the client* and *the goal as assessed by the therapist*.

The ABC model provides a way to frame Sarah's lack of adherence to a functional exercise regime as a behavioral consequence of her irrational beliefs. Thus, a clear B-C connection is established and *the goal as assessed by the therapist* is not losing weight per se, but working to strengthen Sarah's conviction in rational alternatives to the unhelpful beliefs that have thus far resulted in exercise avoidance. Without this attention to detail, a practitioner might find themselves offering healthy living advice or putting together exercise programmes, whilst failing to appreciate the precise nature of the beliefs that stop her acting in line with what she knows to be helpful.

One of the most striking things about human cognition is the way it exercises regulatory control over behavior. In this example, Sarah knew what to do to maintain a healthy weight – these behaviors were already in her repertoire. However, she was not doing these behaviors because her beliefs compelled her not to. Helen's careful examination of Sarah's beliefs in the context of attending the gym revealed the cognitive mechanism by which her behavior was being obstructed. In practicing REBT, it cannot be overstated how important it is to spend time on clarifying the ABCs of a situation before engaging in any intervention. As a wise supervisor once said, in a clever play on words, "Don't just do something, sit there!" It is important to resist the urge to provide a solution until one knows the precise nature of the problem.

5 "It will be the end of the world if we don't win this game"

Exploring the use of Rational Emotive Behavior Therapy (REBT) interventions in Paralympic soccer

Jamie Barker

Introduction

Cerebral Palsy (CP) is considered a neurological disorder caused by a non-progressive brain injury or malformation that occurs typically whilst the child's brain is under development. Whilst CP is a blanket term used to describe loss or impairment of motor function, CP is actually caused by brain damage. The brain damage is typically caused by brain injury or abnormal development of the brain that occurs whilst a child's brain is still developing – before birth, during birth or immediately after birth. However, CP can also be apparent in individuals following direct brain trauma, including a stroke or direct blow to the head. CP primarily affects body movement, muscle control, muscle co-ordination, muscle tone, reflex, posture and balance. It can also impact fine motor skills, gross motor skills and oral motor functioning. An individual with CP will likely show signs of physical impairment; however, the type of movement dysfunction, the location and the number of limbs involved, as well as the extent of impairment, will vary from one individual to another. CP affects muscles, and a person's ability to control them. Muscles can contract too much, too little or all at the same time. Limbs can be stiff and forced into painful, awkward positions. Fluctuating muscle contractions can make limbs tremble, shake or writhe (NHS, 2016).

Cerebral Palsy (CP) soccer

CP soccer is a seven-a-side a team sport played over 60-minutes. Whilst rules follow those developed by the Fédération Internationale de Football Association (FIFA) for mainstream soccer, some modifications have been included. These include: smaller pitch and goal posts, no off-side law and throw-ins being made by rolling the ball into the field of play using only one hand. Classification of disability provides a structure for competition. Athletes competing in CP soccer have Ataxia, Hypertonia or Athetosis – three impairment types that are most commonly associated with individuals having neurological impairment, with a motor control impairment of a cerebral nature, causing a permanent and verifiable Activity Limitation. Hypertonia is a condition marked by an abnormal increase in muscle tension and a reduced ability of a muscle to stretch. Ataxia is a neurological sign and symptom that consists of a lack of co-ordination of muscle movements and Athetosis is generally characterized by unbalanced, involuntary movements due to constant changes in muscle tone and a difficulty maintaining a symmetrical posture (International Federation of CP Football, 2015). On the field of play the teams consist of seven ambulant CP athletes ranging from classes 5 to 8 (5 being the most impaired to 8 being the least impaired). CP soccer is limited to classes 5, 6, 7 and 8. Presently, each team must field at least one class 5 or 6 player at all times, or the team will play with one less player. Each team may have one class 8 player on the field of play during a game. If the class 8 player is dismissed, a team is not allowed to replace a player in the field of play for a class 8 player (International Federation of CP Football, 2016). Due in part to the evaluative and somewhat subjective nature of the classification processes, classification remains an area of much stress for athletes and staff alike. Within the present context, the athletes are exposed to similar training loads, demands and expectations of those within mainstream soccer. To this end, they are regularly subjected to fitness tests with specific targets for aerobic fitness, body composition, power output and agility. Failure to maintain or improve on these aspects (along with poor soccer performance in training and competition) will typically result in transition or de-selection from the squad.

The context

In January 2014, the performance director (PD) of an international CP soccer team approached me about working with them to provide psychological support in the build up for a major international tournament. Until this point I had little experience of working in disability sport. Apparently, a colleague had recommended me to the PD as someone who may offer a different perspective (including REBT) to doing sport psychology and hence may be worth meeting with. REBT has been a fundamental component of my research and applied practice for a number of years (e.g., Turner & Barker, 2014). I favour the elegance and efficiency with which REBT techniques can challenge the beliefs and expectations of individuals to allow them to develop and maintain a rounded philosophical appreciation of themselves and the world around them (Ellis, 1957). In sport, as our research has illustrated, having skills to develop and maintain levels of perspective around beliefs and expectations is considered important for dealing with the turbulence of elite performance, along with having positive implications for well-being over the lifespan (see Turner, 2016).

From my initial meeting with the PD it was clear that whilst the team had many talented athletes, they had collectively underperformed in major championships, typically when faced with pressurized and adverse situations. During our initial conversations, the PD provided a very eloquent insight into CP soccer and the teams' performance environment. He also highlighted areas where he considered psychological intervention to be important (i.e., one-to-one support, working at a team level and working with the coaching staff). The PD explained that the aim for the team was to achieve a top six finish at a forthcoming international tournament to thus enable automatic entry for the 2016 Paralympics. During this meeting, I attempted to validate some of the observations offered by the PD using REBT principles (e.g., athletes and coaches creating unrealistic expectations and hence facilitating irrational beliefs) to highlight my approach should the PD wish me to begin work with the team. It was clear from this initial discussion that issues within this context appeared to relate to REBT principles. Upon being invited to work with the team, the PD and I agreed that a good starting point would be for me to attend a training camp in March 2014 to begin some initial observations and to further validate some of the PD's comments made in our initial meeting.

The athletes (aged between 18–29) were all presently amateur (although three had previously had professional contracts with teams within the UK) whilst most competed in regular high-level mainstream soccer. At training camps, the athletes were aided by a series of support staff including the PD, head coach, assistant coach, logistics manager, physiotherapist, medical doctor, strength and conditioning coach, sports therapist, performance analyst, kit manager and myself as the sport psychologist. The camps typically comprised physical testing, soccer training, team meetings (including performance analysis debriefs) and a match against fellow international CP teams or local professional soccer academies (aged 18 and below). Following my inclusion within the team, future camps would include one-to-one player and staff meetings, and team sport psychology sessions.

Needs analysis

During my conversations with the PD I had started to collect 'data' regarding the needs of the team and therefore to compile a thorough needs analysis. In the formulation of an appropriate intervention programme I followed a triangulation approach (see Barker, McCarthy, & Harwood, 2011) and thus during the training camps early in my appointment I collected a series of observational, interview and psychometric data.

My initial observations of training, pre-game, in-game and post-game situations yielded some interesting data. First, it was apparent that the language that coaches and senior athletes used to highlight expectations and provide instructions would more often than not be couched in terms consistent with irrational beliefs. To illustrate, demandingness and awfulizing were evident in pre-match instructions such as, "We must not give the ball away or concede an early goal", "We must win today" and "We must play to our potential or we may as well give up!" Further, language focused around demandingness and awfulizing was also prevalent within post-training and match reflection sessions. Second, at a behavioral level it was evident that some athletes and staff reacted to mistakes in unhelpful ways (including poor body language) and this appeared to highlight the prevalence of underlying individual irrational beliefs. Further, some athletes also demonstrably elicited low frustration tolerance (LFT), including petulant responses, and unhealthy anger (e.g., overzealous tackling) in situations where competence was questioned (i.e., a teammate played a poor pass to them and they gave possession away), and in situations where expectations of fairness were thwarted (i.e., poor refereeing decisions).

During the first camp, I also took the opportunity to interview key personnel within the team, including PD, coaches and senior athletes, to ascertain their thoughts around the typical psychological preparation and approach of the team, along with areas for development. In this phase, I asked open-ended questions around the aforementioned without focusing explicitly on irrational beliefs. These interviews typically lasted between 25–45-minutes and, overall, seven interviews took place. Information from the interviews highlighted several interesting areas including poor coping in relation to adversity (e.g., difficult training sessions and playing against tough opponents), poor emotional reactions (e.g., to mistakes, poor officiating, losing), tendencies to 'beat themselves up' following poor performances and inflated expectations (e.g., some athletes expecting perfection). Following the camp, I discussed this initial data during a peer-supervision session and thus settled on seeking to understand the observations and interviews through an REBT lens.

To finalize my conclusions about the needs of the team I collected psychometric data from all athletes and key members of the support staff regarding the prevalence of irrational beliefs during my second training camp. I used the Shortened General Attitudes and Belief Scale (SGABS; Lindner, et al., 1999), which up until this point had been a staple measure within our REBT in sport research (e.g., Turner & Barker, 2013).

Data was collected from 16 athletes and three support staff members (including two coaches and the PD). Analysis of individual data indicated a prevalence of irrational beliefs amongst eight athletes and two members of the support staff. In particular, high irrationality scores (above 2.5 on a 5-point Likert-scale) were observed for the following subscales: other depreciation ($M = 3.10$; $SD = .61$), need for achievement ($M = 3.18$; $SD = .63$), need for approval ($M = 2.74$; $SD = .66$) and demand for fairness ($M = 3.93$; $SD = .54$).

Through the triangulation of data during this needs analysis I developed an intervention plan, which focused on one-to-one REBT sessions for identified individuals, REBT psycho-education for the whole team and the development of a rational thinking training and performance environment. Whilst this needs analysis predominately focused on individuals and aspects in need of remedial work, it is worth highlighting that eight athletes displayed very good coping mechanisms and therefore these individuals were invited to take part in sessions which focused on strengths-based development aligned with postulations evident in positive psychology (Seligman, 2002). The following sections detail some examples of delivering REBT in this present context.

The intervention

Working one-to-one with REBT

In this case example, I will detail the application of a one-to-one REBT intervention with a player (aged 23 at the time of this work) who had had his professional soccer career terminated because of an acquired brain injury. Ben (pseudonym) had been around the team for 2 years following a period of rehabilitation after his brain injury. Prior to his injury he had been in a professional club environment since an early age, progressing through to obtaining a professional contract. Ben was clearly a talented player and because of this he had been given a pivotal role within the team. In my early observations of Ben in and around training and competition it was clear that he was experiencing a high level of anxiety prior to important situations and showing anger and frustration outbursts following individual or team mistakes and when receiving unfavourable refereeing decisions. Completion of the SGABS (Lindner et al., 1999) by Ben during the initial needs analysis highlighted high irrationality scores around the need for achievement (M = 3.48), and demand for fairness (M = 4.11).

Following a series of short meetings with Ben in order that we develop rapport, we began working together across six sessions (lasting between 45–60-minutes). Given Ben was an open, intelligent and articulate individual, he could describe and discuss his emotions in an eloquent manner. To illustrate, without prompting, in one of our initial meetings he spoke at length about the distress associated with his brain injury and how this had led to his professional career ending. It was clear that this life event had had a profound effect on his current thinking around himself and his soccer. As is typical in REBT practice (Dryden & Branch, 2008; Turner & Barker, 2014) I developed an intervention that was broken down into education, disputation and reinforcement phases (using the ABCDE model typical in REBT interventions); the length of each phase was dependent on Ben's understanding and progress.

The education phase lasted for two sessions. The main aim was to teach Ben the ABC model of REBT. Typically, in this phase I was interested in getting Ben to understand how his beliefs about situations caused him to feel certain emotions (i.e., the B-C connection) rather than him viewing the adversity (A) dictating how he responded (C) to situations. As we typically see in our work, athletes find this a very interesting insight and a liberating one. We are keen to emphasize that ultimately, individuals have volition and autonomy over their beliefs and emotions, and therefore working on changing their beliefs will allow them to deal more effectively with adverse situations. Due to Ben's self-awareness, we were quickly able to move onto the disputation aspect of the intervention. First, using the most poignant and recent challenging situation (a difficult international game) we collaboratively disputed (D) his irrational beliefs (see Figure 5.1) empirically (i.e., "Where is it written that the world must treat you fairly during a difficult game?"), logically (i.e., "Just because you want things to go your way does that mean they have to during a difficult game?") and pragmatically (i.e., "How helpful has it been for you to hold these beliefs about the world being fair during a difficult game?"). As expected, Ben demonstrated some resistance to my line of questioning and initially struggled to grasp the concept that things happen in the world which are unfair and that whilst playing soccer it was unhelpful to maintain beliefs that things will go as Ben would like. At this point I drew comparison to Ben's own life experience, to highlight how unfair things can happen, and to further develop his understanding of the disputation phase.

Activating Event (A)	
Situation: Playing and captaining the international team	
Adversity: "I'm not performing consistently"	

Irrational Beliefs (IB)	Rational Beliefs (RB)
Demand: "I want to succeed and play well all of the time and therefore I must"	**Preference:** "I want to succeed and play well all of the time, and it is not the end of the world if I do not"
Low Frustration Tolerance: "I can't stand it when I don't play well"	**High Frustration Tolerance:** "Not playing well can be hard to take but I can stand it and for the good of my career, it is worth standing"

Unhelpful Consequences (C)	Helpful Consequences (C)
Emotional Consequence: Pre-competitive anxiety	**Emotional Consequence:** Pre-competitive healthy concern
Behavioral Consequence: Disrupted sleep; confrontational and aggressive with teammates and match officials	**Behavioral Consequence:** More effective pre-game sleep patterns; protesting behavior to match officials; supportive reactions to teammates
Cognitive Consequence: Overthinking performance (pre-match)	**Cognitive Consequence:** Focus on controllable aspects of performance
Physiological Consequence: Increased heart rate	**Physiological Consequence:** Reduced heart rate

Figure 5.1 Example ABC analysis for one-to-one client

Over the course of the remaining four sessions (which were undertaken via Skype) we continued to dispute a series of irrational beliefs based around the need for achievement, and demand for fairness. Once the irrational beliefs were successfully disputed, in that Ben's conviction in them had weakened, we created a new set of rational beliefs (E), which we then disputed to validate their rationality (see Figure 5.1). This process helped to re-affirm and validate that the rational beliefs are true, logical and helpful. As the sessions progressed, Ben began to recognize the potential applications of the ABCDE model in helping him to deal with various challenging life and sport situations. The aim of this aspect of the intervention was to allow Ben to be autonomous in his ability to re-frame and regulate beliefs about future situations. To promote long-term change in relation to Ben's irrational beliefs we discussed various strategies to test out the ABCDE model and his newly created rational beliefs (Ellis & Dryden, 1997). First, we settled on Ben completing a diary, in which he would compile thoughts around daily events, notably, the challenging situations he encountered and the emotions that he and others expressed. This was to allow him to 'test' out his knowledge of the ABCDE model along with making some predictions about how he and others could have reacted more effectively had rational beliefs been adopted. When at camps I also encouraged him to converse with other athletes about what he had learnt from our work and the process he had gone through to change his beliefs. Finally, rational beliefs were collated from our sessions and compiled onto cue cards and info-graphics (which could be used as mobile phone and laptop screen savers). These reminders were designed to help Ben create a 'rational' culture for himself when at home or at the camps. Reading his new rational beliefs, along with re-affirming them with me pre-game, at half-time and post-game, would become a consistent routine for Ben and me.

Using REBT psycho-education

Based on data from the needs analysis (typically informed by observations from training and competition), I developed an REBT workshop for the athletes to increase awareness of the REBT principles, along with providing some initial skills to give the athletes an optional way of thinking and dealing with various situations. The use of workshops is a staple part of REBT practice and is an approach that has been used in past research with athletes (e.g., see Turner, 2016, for a review).

Consistent with previous research, the content of the workshop focused on exploring the prevalence and effect of demanding and awfulizing beliefs inside and outside of sport. Based explicitly on previous research in sport (see Turner, et al., 2014) the 90-minute workshop was delivered in three stages and used techniques widely advocated in REBT literature (e.g., Dryden, 2009; Ellis & Dryden, 1997): REBT education, recognizing and disputing demands (primary IBs), and recognizing and disputing awfulizing (secondary IBs). Typical to REBT workshop delivery in sport the athletes were educated in the ABC framework of REBT (Ellis & Dryden, 1997). I then asked athletes to write down their thoughts, feelings and behaviors in response to a series of scenarios they could face whilst being with the team. These included being deselected, suffering a long-term injury, making a series of critical mistakes in training and in competition, and approaching an important game. Athletes' responses were then collated on a flipchart and related to the ABC model. Next, athletes were asked whether their thoughts about the situations I had presented included: "I absolutely must play well today and it is awful if I do not", "I should not have made that mistake and I am an idiot for doing that", "Being deselected is awful" and "Getting injured and missing training is the end of the world". Using a show of hands, consensus formed specifically on "I absolutely must play well today and it is awful if I do not", "Being deselected is awful" and "Getting injured and missing training is the end of the world".

Many of the athletes had written down a demand to perform well (a consistent observation from our work in sport; Turner, 2014), so, consistent with the REBT disputation (D), I first focused on recognizing and disputing their primary irrational beliefs. Athletes were encouraged to dispute their primary irrational beliefs using empirical, logical and pragmatic questioning. To initiate the replacement of irrational beliefs with rational alternatives (E), athletes were asked what they could say to themselves instead of "I must" that would be more flexible, logical and helpful. Suggestions were encouraged that reflected preferences instead of demands.

For example, the rational belief, "I want to play well more than anything but I do not absolutely have to" reflects that a preference is not a weak belief and can in fact be very strongly asserted. Fluid discussions then took place about how athletes may want to play well more than anything, but it does not "have to" happen.

To help the athletes dispute beliefs relating to awfulizing, a badness scale was used which has been advocated for brief therapy (Ellis & Dryden, 1997). Broadly, the athletes placed a number of life events on sticky labels using a scale from 0–100%, with 0% representing *not at all bad* and 100% representing *worst thing possible*. Most athletes placed life events such as "being deselected" and "making a mistake in an important game" at around the 50% mark on the scale. Athletes were asked to challenge their thinking around how deselection or failure to perform well in important stations could be awful, if they did not place them anywhere near 100% on the badness scale? It was possible for the athletes to now understand that by using "awful" and "terrible" to describe what it would be like to underperform or be deselected, they were saying that these events were 101% bad, thus, potentially augmenting anxiety and an inability to be resilient in the face of adversity. The premise of such discussions is to assert that if underperforming and deselection are perceived as "awful", the prospect of failure becomes too threatening, and consequently, one feels too anxious to perform effectively.

Like replacing the demand (primary irrational beliefs), rational and preferential beliefs were encouraged for derivative irrational beliefs, such as, "It would be really bad to be deselected, but not the end of the world". This section of the workshop prompted some resistance and discussion amongst the athletes. To illustrate, several athletes struggled to grasp how making a mistake in an important game is not the end of the world in comparison to other life situations, particularly when playing soccer and wanting to be successful underpinned their motivation. Moreover, it was felt by some that by re-framing beliefs to include language, "it is not the end of the world" somehow reduces one's motivation and determination towards goal attainment. The discussion and disclosure in this aspect of the workshop further appeared to highlight the prevalence of some of the 'win at all costs' philosophies and ego-driven climates that athletes have been exposed to and have created (Harwood, 2008) along with the notion that winning is all that matters (Cockerill, 2002). Taken together, these philosophies and cultures have the potential to hamper athletes' resilience to adverse situations along with fuelling high expectations and demands, which in turn can perpetuate the prevalence of irrational beliefs in academy athletes (Turner, 2016). The session concluded with a summary of the salient points emanating from the workshop along with key reflections and take away messages for the athletes. From this session three athletes wished to follow-up the discussions on a one-to-one basis.

Creating a 'rational' performance environment

One-to-one work and psycho-education took place very much at the start of my work with the group. However, a longer-term aim was to use strategies that would foster rational beliefs and create a 'rational thinking' culture as we worked towards the international tournament and possible qualification for a major tournament in 2016. Accordingly, I planned to work with the coaches, senior athletes and performance analyst in fostering this culture.

A coach, through the development of a motivational climate (Ames, 1992), is fundamental to the generation and the fostering of rational and irrational beliefs in athletes as they are regarded as credible experts and role models. Coaches are key individuals in modelling for athletes, and in times of stress, are important sources of social support (Lu et al., 2016). Not only can coaches reinforce key tactical instructions but they can also foster the motivational climate and orientation of the group (Harwood, 2002). Accordingly, if coaches can develop their own awareness and psychosocial skills they are more likely to provide effective coaching to their athletes (including effective communication, behaviors and emotions) and foster effective performing environments (Mageau & Vallerand, 2003). Given that coaches have an important influence on the rational thinking and emotional well-being of their athletes, I was keen to work with this group to develop a rational thinking culture.

This work occurred primarily through the delivery of a 90-minute psycho-education workshop similar to that delivered to the athletes but with the inclusion of discussions and role-plays. The workshop was delivered to two coaches, a logistics manager and the PD. For this workshop, greater emphasis was placed on using scenarios and examples around beliefs associated with coaching instruction, philosophies, behavior(s) of athletes, underperformance and CP classification. Further, detailed discussions took place around how the coaches felt a constant need for approval (especially colleagues outside of the team environment) and how this affected their emotions and behaviors (during training, pre-match, in-match and post-match). Whilst the aims of this session were like those of the individual sessions, I was keen to explain and emphasize how the coaches' language and emotional reactions could facilitate irrational beliefs and rational beliefs in the team and the team's response to adversity (in games and during classification), along with some key areas for development. I was keen that this workshop would be the start of the development of our rational thinking culture therefore I wanted to allow the delegates to understand and recognize the application of the key principles in and around our performance environment. Throughout the session, I challenged the group to consider three aspects. First, for them to explore what they were saying to themselves about a situation and how these thoughts would influence their emotions and the emotions of others. Consistent with this, I also explored the notion of emotional contagion with the staff and the importance of this concept, especially in the dressing room prior to important games. Indeed, it has been argued that teams acquire a collective mood through team members responding similarly to shared events and also through the convergence of each member's mood (Totterdell, 2000). Moreover, team members may begin to mimic staff and fellow athletes' expressive displays and experience similar moods and emotions (Hatfield, et al., 1994) or compare their thoughts and feelings to others leading to moods becoming synchronized (Levenson & Gottman, 1983). Second, I wanted to challenge irrational language when they heard it in their own heads and from those around them to have effective strategies and conversations accordingly. To assist with this I created several role-play scenarios where I acted as an athlete and coach verbalizing irrational language. The staff were tasked with identifying this language and making assumptions about the possible effects of my beliefs, emotions and behaviors and their contagion to my colleagues. Finally, I wanted to help the coaches to develop training scenarios where athletes could create their own evidence to reject some of the irrational beliefs prevalent to the group (e.g., need for achievement, and demand for fairness). Therefore, I facilitated discussions about how best to operationalize this within the training environment. The session concluded with some key reflections being shared across the group, including the formulation of an action plan as to how to best integrate the salient points from the session within the team.

One of the action points was to work with the athletes on increasing their awareness in detecting and challenging irrational beliefs in and around the team and to develop effective pre-game, in-game and post-game messages to facilitate rational beliefs. To assist with this and the development of the rational thinking culture, I worked with the senior leadership group comprising four experienced athletes. Whilst this group served several other purposes, in this instance it provided a mechanism to filter and reinforce key rational thinking messages. We were interested in developing coherent and consistent rational thinking messages/mantras across the coaches, and senior athletes in and around the training and competition environments. Therefore, we outlined opportunities where effective conversations could take place to reinforce rational thinking in the dressing room, on the training ground and around the performance environment. To further help reinforce key rational thinking messages to the team I worked with the coaches at each training camp as they prepared their training sessions and content for their speeches to the athletes. In addition, rational thinking posters were created which included key rational messages and mantras, and the badness scale. Accordingly, posters were positioned around the dressing room, in the dining area(s) and in athletes' rooms along with being incorporated into pre-game tactical sessions and post-game review sessions. Athletes were also provided with information packs, distributed with their playing kit in the dressing rooms. The badness scale was used as a mechanism with which I could assist the team to regulate thoughts and feelings 'in the moment' prior to, during and post-game (Turner & Barker, 2014). Prior to pre-game tactical sessions, I worked with the performance analyst to draw on examples from our database of clips to emphasize behaviors we were looking for from the athletes along with incorporating salient rational beliefs messages (i.e., "We want to succeed more than anything in the world, but is not the end of the world if we don't"). Prior to the review sessions I also worked with the analyst to 'clip' instances of effective behavioral responses (e.g., accepting a poor refereeing decision and dealing effectively with mistakes) from the previous game along with reinforcing key rational beliefs messages.

The purpose of this aspect of the work was to increase awareness of REBT principles with key members of the team (including coaches and senior athletes) along with developing strategies, which could be used to create a rational thinking culture within the team. By incorporating the strategies outlined previously, I wanted to make sure that consistent messages were being delivered and received to enable effective coping (e.g., managing success and failure, or dealing with injury and classification decisions) across the group. Over time, I worked with key personnel (including the head coach and captain) on the integration of key REBT principles into their media interviews and public events (e.g., avoiding use of 'musts' and 'needs').

Critical reflections and outcome analysis

Working with this team has afforded me the opportunity to broaden my use of REBT into other aspects over and above typical one-to-one work. From the very start of my involvement, the team has been very open-minded to my ideas and rapport was established relatively early. Additionally, given that the head coach had a positive perception about sport psychology and a determination to develop his own skill set, this has helped me to be creative with my ideas and proposals. The acceptance I received from the group was in stark contrast to my previous experiences in soccer (e.g., Barker et al., 2011) and those of other sport psychologists working in soccer (Pain & Harwood, 2004), and undoubtedly made me feel at ease when around the group and delivering my work. With my value being clearly articulated by the PD and coaches early on in my work I feel this allowed me to relax and focus more on being effective rather than consistently looking to justify my role within the team. Unlike the case with my previous applied experiences, I focused more on my role as a sport psychologist and maximizing the psychological preparation of the entire group rather than adopting the immersion approach as a means of gaining entry and justifying my worth (Bull, 1995). I genuinely felt the group valued my 'expertise' and this gave me the confidence to drive a strategy I was comfortable with and one that was evidence-based. Throughout the work I was mindful of how I also needed to remain consistent with the rational thinking information I transmitted to the team whilst around the group. I therefore sought to reinforce key messages in team meetings and the dressing room whilst I also intervened and challenged 'irrational' language whenever I heard it. It was important that I remained authentic to REBT and the messages I was delivering to provide a role model for the athletes and to highlight the value of our work.

On reflection, I have recognized that whilst being formulaic, REBT is an extremely adaptable and flexible strategy that has applications above and beyond one-to-one work. To this end, the positive buy-in I had within this team allowed me to experiment in how REBT principles were integrated in and around the performance environment. As I move forward with the group we are exploring the use of rational thinking sessions for parents of athletes within the talent development programme(s) along with countrywide coach education.

During my work I have sought to determine my effectiveness in a systematic manner; however, working in such a fluid environment can make it difficult to consistently and objectively determine changes and effectiveness. I have relied predominantly on qualitative feedback from debrief meetings with athletes and staff, my own observations (including reflections) and discussions at peer supervision meetings to allow me to identify areas of effective and ineffective practice. Within the one-to-one work, this has afforded greater opportunity to collect quantitative data using some of the principles inherent in single-case research (Barker, et al., 2011). Therefore, I sought to collect pre- and post-intervention data (collected prior to the major international tournament) using the SGABS along with collating social validation data using principles outlined in the extant literature (Page & Thelwell, 2013). Overall, this data yielded positive changes over-time in specific irrational beliefs along with positive insights and feedback regarding my delivery of REBT. Specifically, data from the SGABS revealed notable reductions in four key irrational beliefs as highlighted as problematic by the needs analysis at the start of the work. To illustrate, changes in other depreciation (pre-M = 3.10; SD = .61; post-M = 2.70; SD = .64), need for achievement (pre-M = 3.18; SD = .63; post-M = 2.31; SD = .49), need for approval (pre-M = 2.74; SD = .66; post-M = 1.96; SD = .71) and demand for fairness (pre-M = 3.93; SD = .54; post-M = 2.45; SD = .51) were observed providing some insight into the effect(s) of the intervention programme on the beliefs of the athletes and key staff.

Regarding the challenges of using REBT within this context, one issue is the extent to which brain development and brain injury can affect an individual's ability to be rational. Indeed, neuroscience and developmental psychology would posit that the frontal lobe (typically associated with rational thinking) is one of the last areas to fully develop, with the greatest phase of development taking place during late adolescence (Wilson, 2014). With these principles in mind, consideration should perhaps be given to cognitive ability when using REBT with youth athletes, along with those who have suffered frontal lobe injuries. In the latter situation, interventions, which rely more heavily on behavioral principles, are possibly likely to be more appropriate and effective (Hill, 2001).

Within this chapter I have outlined the contextual demands of working in elite disability sport and how I used REBT in a range of applications to foster rational thinking strategies individually and collectively. I have identified areas of innovation along with stimulating thoughts for future practitioners and researchers. REBT is a fundamental component to my work and very much reflects my professional philosophy of improving psychological well-being and athletic performance. With those that I work with, I do not 'teach' REBT as a sticky-tape intervention to paper over the cracks, but as a life-skill that has numerous applications both in and outside of sport to enable humans to experience healthy emotions throughout life's many adversities (David, et al., 2010).

References

Ames, C. (1992). Achievement goals, motivational climate, and motivational processes. In G. Roberts (Ed.), *Motivation in sport and exercise* (pp. 161–176). Champaign, IL: Human Kinetics.

Barker, J. B., McCarthy, P. J., & Harwood, C. G. (2011). Reflections on consulting in elite youth male English cricket and soccer academies. *Sport & Exercise Psychology Review*, 7, 58–72.

Barker, J. B., McCarthy, P. J., Jones, M. V., & Moran, A. (2011). *Single-case research methods in sport and exercise psychology*. Hove: London.

Bull, S. J. (1995). Reflections on a 5-year consultancy program with the England women's cricket team. *The Sport Psychologist*, 9, 148–163.

Cockerill, I. (2002). In pursuit of the perfect performance. In I. Cockerill (Ed.), *Solutions in sport psychology* (pp. 74–88). London: Thomson.

David, D., Freeman, A., & DiGiuseppe, R. (2010). Social and cultural aspects of rational and irrational beliefs. A brief reconceptualisation. In D. David, S. J. Lynn, & A. Ellis (Eds.), *Rational and irrational beliefs: Research, theory, and clinical practice* (pp. 49–62). NY: Oxford University Press.

Dryden, W. (2009). *Rational emotive behaviour therapy: Distinctive features*. London: Routledge.

Dryden, W., & Branch, R. (2008). *The fundamentals of rational emotive behaviour therapy* (2nd ed.). Chichester: John Wiley & Sons, Ltd.

Ellis, A. (1957). Rational psychotherapy and individual psychology. *Journal of Individual Psychology*, 13, 38–44.

Ellis, A., & Dryden, W. (1997). *The practice of rational emotive behavior therapy*. New York, NY: Springer.

Ellis, A., Gordon, J., Neenan, M., & Palmer, S. (1998). *Stress counseling*. New York, NY: Springer.

Harwood, C. G. (2002). Assessing achievement goals in sport: Caveats for consultants and a case for contextualisation. *Journal of Applied Sport Psychology*, 14, 106–119.

Harwood, C. G. (2008). Developmental consulting in a professional soccer academy: The 5C's coaching efficacy program. *The Sport Psychologist*, 22, 109–133.

Hatfield, E., Cacioppo, J. T., & Rapson, R. L. (1994). *Emotional contagion*. Cambridge, England: Cambridge University Press.

Hill, K. L. (2001). *Frameworks for sport psychologists*. Champaign, IL: Human Kinetics.

International Federation of Cerebral Palsy Football (2015). *About classification*. Retrieved from www.ifcpf.com/about-classification

International Federation of Cerebral Palsy Football (2016). *What is CP football?* Retrieved from www.ifcpf.com/what-is-cp

Levenson, R. W., & Gottman, J. M. (1983). Marital interaction: Physiological linkage and affective exchange. *Journal of Personality and Social Psychology*, 45, 587–597.

Lindner, H., Kirkby, R., Wertheim, E., & Birch, P. (1999). A brief assessment of irrational thinking: The shortened general attitude and belief scale. *Cognitive Therapy and Research*, 23, 651–663.

Lu, F. J. H., Lee, W. P., Chang, Y. K., Chou, C. C., Hsu, Y. W., Lin, J. H., & Gill, D. L. (2016). Interaction of athletes' resilience and coaches' social support on the stress-burnout relationship: A conjunctive moderation perspective. *Psychology of Sport and Exercise*, 22, 202–209.

Mageau, G. A., & Vallerand, R. J. (2003). The coach athlete relationship: A motivational model. *Journal of Sports Sciences*, 21, 883–904.

National Health Service (2016). *Cerebral palsy*. Retrieved from www.nhs.uk/conditions/cerebral-palsy/Pages/Introduction.aspx.

Page, J., & Thelwell, R. (2013). The value of social validation in single case methods in sport and exercise psychology. *Journal of Applied Sport Psychology*, 25(1), 61–71.

Pain, M. A., & Harwood, C. G. (2004). Knowledge and perceptions of sport psychology within English soccer. *Journal of Sports Sciences, 22*, 813–826.

Seligman, M. E. P. (2002). *Authentic happiness: Using the new positive psychology to realize your potential for lasting fulfillment.* New York, NY: Free Press.

Totterdell, P. (2000). Catching moods and hitting runs: Mood linkage and subjective performance in professional sport teams. *Journal of Applied Psychology, 85*, 848–859.

Turner, M. J. (2014). Smarter thinking in sport. *The Psychologist, 27*(8), 596–599.

Turner, M. J. (2016). Rational Emotive Behavior Therapy (REBT), irrational and rational beliefs, and the mental health of athletes. *Frontiers: Movement Science and Sport Psychology,* doi: 10.3389/fpsyg.2016.01423

Turner, M. J., & Barker, J. B. (2013). Examining the efficacy of Rational-Emotive Behavior Therapy (REBT) on irrational beliefs and anxiety in elite youth cricketers. *Journal of Applied Sport Psychology, 25*, 131–147.

Turner, M. J., & Barker, J. B. (2014). Using Rational Emotive Behavior Therapy with athletes. *The Sport Psychologist, 28*(1), 75–90. http://doi.org/10.1123/tsp.2013-0012.

Turner, M. J., Slater, M. J. & Barker, J. B. (2014). Not the end of the world: The effects of Rational Emotive Behavior Therapy on the irrational beliefs of elite academy athletes. *Journal of Applied Sport Psychology, 26*(2), 144–156.

Wilson, R. Z. (2014). *Neuroscience for counsellors.* London: Jessica Kingsley.

Editors' commentary on Chapter 5: "It will be the end of the world if we don't win this game': exploring the use of Rational Emotive Behavior Therapy (REBT) interventions in Paralympic soccer"

One aspect that caught our attention in Jamie's chapter was the idea of a "rational culture". We share some of Jamie's observations concerning the language used in the context he worked in. That is, in our own work in sport we have also frequently observed the expression of "irrational language", or language that reflects irrational beliefs. One of us has spoken before about the propagation of irrational beliefs through language (Turner, 2016), and this chapter brings some of that into an applied environment for us all to see. To great effect, Jamie reflects on trying to change the language used around the athletes, and helps the team to develop a rational culture, with a view to deteriorating the spread of irrational language within the team.

But there is a broader issue. Irrational beliefs are evident in the language used in the daily sporting narrative by the media. It seems as though every other day commentators, coaches and athletes describe setbacks as awful, failure as "the end of the world", and dramatize "must win" matches. In fact, sport seems particularly endorsing of irrationality, where irrationality is openly promoted and often boasted about. This is important because language used to report on sport may play a role in not only reflecting irrational beliefs, but in developing and propagating irrational beliefs. Common cultural stereotypes in our language, our stories and our songs play a part in helping to develop rational and irrational beliefs (DiGiuseppe, et al., 2014). If the prevalence of irrational beliefs is in some part reflected in the utterances of athletes and coaches in the media, then a deeper analysis of this phenomenon is warranted.

References

DiGiuseppe, R. A., Doyle, C. A., Dryden, W., & Backx, W (2014). *A practitioner's guide to rational emotive behavior therapy* (3rd Ed.). New York, NY: Oxford University Press.

Turner, M. J. (2016). Rational Emotive Behavior Therapy (REBT), irrational and rational beliefs, and the mental health of athletes. *Frontiers: Movement Science and Sport Psychology.* doi: 10.3389/fpsyg.2016.01423.

6 Managing injury and loss

The use of Rational Emotive Behavior Therapy (REBT) with a collegiate football player

Angela Breitmeyer and Oana David

Brief introduction

I (first author) provided sport-focused counseling services at the counseling center at a National Collegiate Association of Athletics (NCAA) Division 1, American university. At that time, I served as the athletic department liaison for student-athlete counseling and sport performance referrals. In this capacity, I would typically obtain an average of one referral per month from various teams, and some athletes were self-referred. In addition, I formally served as the sport psychology consultant for the baseball team and consulted with the entire team on a weekly basis. I entered this role because I was the only counselor at the counseling center who had formalized education and training in sport psychology.

Context

My overall philosophy of practice is what I describe as the "3 Cs": Compassion, Clinical Knowledge, and Creativity. In my work with athletes and clients, I use clinical knowledge to inform my intervention style. Thus, I emphasize evidence-based practice, largely drawing from cognitive therapy, Rational Emotive Behavior Therapy (REBT), and mindfulness-based interventions, within the context of an empathic therapeutic relationship. When appropriate, I will also more formally incorporate creativity in my clinical intervention with clients. In my years of experience, I have noticed that both my clinical and sport clients are exceptionally hard on themselves, compromising their happiness and self-acceptance. Irrational beliefs or misperceptions tend to be at the forefront of their current dissatisfaction with life and/or sport performance. Such irrational beliefs also plagued Bill (pseudonym), who was referred by the Athletic Director (AD) of the university's athletic department. He was referred at the onset of the Fall Semester (beginning of September) and was seen for ten sessions over a two-and-a-half-month period.

The athlete's identified issues

Bill was referred to me after the AD identified concerns regarding his ability to effectively manage his anger. There had been an incident in which Bill had consumed alcohol and marijuana at an off-campus party, had become agitated, and had engaged in a physical altercation with another male university student. At the time of the referral, Bill had a pending legal charge of assault and was potentially in jeopardy of losing both his scholarship and his position on the football team (due to NCAA rules and regulations). After the physical altercation, he sustained a knee injury and was therefore medically red shirted. Although the original referral of this athlete was for anger management, upon further assessment during the intake interview, Bill disclosed ongoing grief secondary to the death of his father approximately two years previously. Thus, the focus of treatment was on grief and loss issues, not only due to his father's death, but also due to his recent knee injury. In collaborating with Bill, three primary issues were identified: grief and loss, transitional and adjustment issues, and emotional dysregulation.

As the intake progressed, Bill identified several losses for which he was grieving, namely the unexpected loss of his father two years ago to a heart attack. In addition, he experienced multiple losses secondary to his knee injury, including the inability to play football; impaired mobility, as he had to use crutches; and disruption of daily life tasks/activities. Bill also had two potential losses, including the potential loss of scholarship, as well as his status of student-athlete at the university, and potential loss of freedom if he were to be legally charged with assault and required to make restitution in jail. In addition to grieving these losses, Bill was also experiencing transitional and adjustment issues secondary to his move to college (approximately 90 miles from home), away from his family and friends. Simultaneously, he was making the adjustment from being a senior in high school to a freshman in college, including his adjustment to a new football team and new coaching staff. Finally, he had to adjust in his daily living skills post-injury. A final issue was Bill's emotional dysregulation due to a high level of acute life stressors. In addition to his athletic injury and pending legal charge, Bill experienced a high level of guilt for "abandoning" his mother and two younger brothers when they needed him most. I conceptualized his emotional response as grief that was displaced as anger.

When I met with Bill for the first time, during the review of the informed consent, I had to address a couple of unique ethical dilemmas in his treatment. First, since the AD was the referral source, I indicated that I would be providing updates regarding his attendance and participation in therapy. Bill acknowledged his understanding of this and agreed to consent to therapy. Second, since his trial was scheduled for the middle of December, and if he was found guilty of the assault charge and consequently dismissed from the team and-or university, I informed him that I would no longer be able to see him for counseling. Bill acknowledged his understanding of this. Given my philosophy of practice, it was important for me to be transparent with him regarding the course of therapy and potential barriers to providing therapy within the college counseling center. Knowing this going into the therapeutic relationship, I had mixed feelings about my ability to effectively clinically intervene. There were several "unknowns," and I realized regardless of the outcome, I was obliged to do the best I could with the time I had with him. During therapy, I really kept the focus on our therapeutic relationship and his goals for therapy instead of becoming frustrated with the parameters of the system.

Needs analysis

Typical for all counseling services provided at the university counseling center, I conducted a formal intake interview, in which behavioral observations, a mental status exam (MSE), self-reported information, and collateral sources (in this case, information provided by the AD) were consolidated to form a diagnostic impression and plan for intervention. The following is a synopsis of the behavioral observations and MSE.

Bill presented as an 18-year-old Caucasian male, who was casually dressed in athletic attire and well groomed. Given his status as a football player, he was taller than 6-foot and had a muscular, athletic build. His gait was impaired by his recent knee injury, and he used crutches to assist with walking. He appeared depressed with congruent flat affect and a downward gaze. He was attentive throughout the duration of the intake and did not appear to be easily distracted. Other than when exhibiting a downward gaze, he could maintain appropriate eye contact, and he was very cooperative during the intake, answering all questions in a forthright and appropriate manner. When asked about suicidal or homicidal ideation, he denied both, and expressed remorse regarding his recent physical altercation with the other student. He spoke at a soft volume, at a slower rate, and with little inflection. There was no evidence of psychotic symptoms. Bill was oriented to person, place, time, and situation. His intelligence was assessed to be average based upon his vocabulary, general fund of knowledge, and oral expression, with recent poor (impaired) judgment, but adequate insight. He did not appear to be under the influence of drugs or alcohol and denied use since the incident at the party approximately a month prior.

Activating Event (A)

Situation: Physical altercation with student
Adversity: "This other student is annoying me"

Irrational Beliefs (iB)	Rational Beliefs (rB)
Demand: "I don't like being annoyed by him and so he should not annoy me"	**Preference**: "I don't like being annoyed by him but he does not absolutely have to stop"
Low Frustration Tolerance: "I can't stand how this guy is annoying me"	**High Frustration Tolerance**: "While I don't like how he's annoying me, I can stand it"
Depreciation (other): "This guy is terrible"	**Acceptance (other)**: "We all are fallible at times"
Unhelpful Consequences (C)	**Helpful Consequences (C)**
Emotional Consequence: Unhealthy anger	**Emotional Consequence**: Annoyance
Behavioral Consequence: Aggression (punching the student in the face)	**Behavioral Consequence**: Assertion (ask him to stop annoying me)

Figure 6.1 ABC formulation for anger

In addition to the intake interview, as well as my behavioral observations, I instituted the AD as a collateral source. Per my initial conversation with the AD, he stated that Bill, "Had problems with substance abuse and anger management." When asked to elaborate, the AD shared details of the physical altercation that corroborated with Bill's story. After careful consideration of the details of Bill's case, REBT was arrived at as an appropriate intervention, within the context of a larger humanistic, existential framework. REBT was identified as particularly beneficial as Bill had a high level of guilt, self-blame, and irrational beliefs, particularly surrounding the death of his father. Moreover, there is empirical evidence to suggest that REBT is effective for grief and loss (Malkinson, 2010), adjustment difficulties (Calabro, 1997; Ellis, 1997), and emotional regulation (Banks, 2011). Bill's irrational beliefs are highlighted in Figure 6.1 within the context of various activating events.

Structure and content of REBT intervention

At the intake session and for the initial sessions, I directed most of my efforts on diagnostic assessment, rapport building, and treatment planning. It was important for me to establish myself as a "safe" person for Bill to speak to regarding his concerns. Throughout the course of therapy, and particularly during the intake, I displayed empathy, a non-judgmental attitude, and a high level of attending behaviors. As a result, despite the differences between Bill and me, particularly in terms of gender, age, and life experiences, I could establish rapport with Bill fairly easily. During an approximate two-and-a-half-month timeframe, I met with Bill for weekly sessions. Due to scheduling challenges, there were a couple of weeks in which I met with him twice. Below is a synopsis of the course of treatment:

Session 1:   Intake assessment, rapport building
Session 2:   Further exploration of psychosocial history, treatment planning
Session 3:   Active listening, continued rapport building, discussion of existential issues
Session 4:   REBT orientation/introduction
Session 5:   REBT working phase (target: physical altercation)
Session 6:   REBT working phase (target: injury/inability to play sport)
Session 7:   REBT working phase (target: guilt over leaving mother/brother)
Session 8:   REBT working phase (target: inadequacy about living up to father's expectations)
Session 9:   REBT working phase (target: upcoming court trial and fear of outcome)
Session 10:   Unanticipated termination session

Although REBT was provided within the context of a humanistic/existential framework, it served as the vast majority of intervention. Given the magnitude of Bill's losses, I emphasized exploring the meaning of such losses using existential themes, namely life, death, freedom, and responsibility. In my work with Bill,

I noticed that he exhibited a high level of negative self-depreciation. Examples of Bill's irrational beliefs include the following:

- "I am a complete disappointment to my father." (self-depreciation)
- "I am a terrible person." (self-depreciation)
- "I must be in control of my emotions at all times." (demand)
- "My life will be over if I can't play football again or if I lose my scholarship." (awfulizing)
- "I am a horrible person." (self-depreciation)

The intervention

In the orientation to REBT phase, I explained the overarching philosophy and the ABC model within the context of several of Bill's presenting concerns (Ellis, 1956; Ellis, 1991). For instance, when discussing the physical altercation with the other student, he explained that the activating event was how the student "annoyed" him. His emotional consequence was anger, and his behavioral consequence was aggression (punching the student in the face). Upon further exploration, Bill revealed his belief that the other student *should have* behaved the way Bill wanted him to behave. I assisted Bill in disputing the irrational belief by asking what evidence he had that people always behave the way we want them to. Bill acknowledged that we do not have control over how others behave. In the therapeutic dialogue, I indicated that although we do not control other people's behavior, we could influence it by our verbal, emotional, and behavioral responses. Bill also acknowledged the role of his choice to consume beer and marijuana, and that this subsequently influenced him in making a poor choice.

Furthermore, it became evident that Bill was interpreting this behavior as evidence that he was "a bad person" (self-depreciation). Therefore, I assisted him in distinguishing his poor choice and subsequent behavior from who he is as a person. I used disputation and Socratic questioning to assist him in coming to the conclusion that, "Even though I made a poor choice, this does not make me a bad person." Within the context of REBT theory, Bill was generalizing an isolated incident to his overall value as a person (Ellis & MacLaren, 1998). Thus, the objective of this intervention was to move Bill from a place of self-depreciating shame to self-accepting regret. I also explored the role of the loss of his father and its impact on his thought process and behavior at the time. He could acknowledge that he was "not thinking clearly" and that his head was "in a fog" at the time. In hindsight, Bill realized that he placed too much emphasis on the other student's behavior and he therefore reframed his belief about the student within a more logical/realistic framework. He was also able to display evidence of self-compassion and forgiveness, essentially internalizing the belief that he made a poor choice, but that choice did not define him as a person.

In my work with Bill, I applied cognitive disputation, a technique used to help clients evaluate the helpfulness and efficacy of their beliefs, in which clients can use empirical, functional, logical, and philosophical disputes to evaluate their beliefs. Disputing helps clients identify, debate, and replace self-defeating irrational beliefs with self-helping rational beliefs. It is important that clients practice disputing during non-stressful periods for maximum effectiveness when coping with stressful periods (Ellis & MacLaren, 1998). In my work with Bill, I employed cognitive disputation quite frequently. For instance, Bill maintained, "My life is worthless if I am not able to play football" (see Figure 6.2). Through cognitive disputation, he was able to refrain from awfulizing and identify that while he really values playing football and being a football player is a part of his identity, he is a resilient individual, and would make necessary adjustments post-injury. Bill also focused on the importance of rehabilitating his injury through physical therapy, and by focusing his efforts and energy on his recovery, he experienced less frustration and disappointment.

In addition to cognitive disputation, skills training, largely in the form of psycho-education, was provided to Bill. According to Ellis and MacLaren (1998), clients can be encouraged to pursue courses and workshops that provide information and training on specific skills such as communication skills, assertiveness skills, social skills, and anger management skills. Therapists can also work with clients on learning about and practicing such skills in the office (Ellis &MacLaren, 1998). Within the context of my therapeutic work with Bill, I specifically addressed communication skills and anger management skills, especially about his athletic injury and pending legal charges. For instance, the behavioral strategy of walking away when Bill notices his frustration tolerance began to wane. Within the context of REBT, I largely stressed the importance of developing more helpful emotional and behavioral consequences (C) when Bill encounters a potential activating event (A).

To enhance the benefits of cognitive disputation and skills training, I also utilized rational coping statements, particularly during and after forceful disputation based on Socratic questioning (DiGiuseppe, et al., 2014). For instance,

---

Activating Event (A)
Situation: Current inability to play football
Adversity: Perceived loss of life purpose (and a way to honor his father)

Irrational Beliefs (iB)	Rational Beliefs (rB)
Demand: "I want to honor my father through football and therefore I have to play"	**Preference:** "I want to honor my father through football but I don't have to play football to do that"
Depreciation (life): "My life is worthless if I am not able to play football"	**Acceptance:** "My life has worth, even if I cannot play football"
Unhelpful Consequences (C)	**Helpful Consequences (C)**
Emotional Consequence: Depression	**Emotional Consequence:** Sadness
Behavioral Consequence: Social withdrawal	**Behavioral Consequence:** Seeking social support

---

Figure 6.2 ABC formulation for depression

Bill maintained the belief, "I have abandoned my Mom and my younger brothers when they needed me most, and this means I am worthless." When I disputed this irrational belief with Bill (see Figure 6.3), he acknowledged that since moving away to college, he speaks with his mother and brothers daily (helpful behavioral consequence), and he reminded himself that he is only a short car ride away from his family (helpful cognitive consequence). In addition, I explored different ways in which Bill could be a source of emotional support for his family, even if not physically present. He acknowledged that phone calls, text messages, and e-mails would all be forms of supportive communication he could implement to show his care and concern for his family. Essentially, by exploring the ways in which he could show support for his mother and brothers, he was able to develop realistic, encouraging, self-helping statements to replace irrational beliefs, e.g., "I can accept myself even when I fail to be the son I want to be," "I can show my family I care, even though I'm not there," and "Deep down, my family knows I support and love them." Throughout the course of therapy, it was important that Bill practice these statements regularly to strengthen their impact. I recommended nightly between-session practice of these statements, as Bill acknowledged he experienced a high level of self-depreciation before going to sleep. In this case, rational coping statements were not just encouraging positive statements, but rather addressed self-defeating philosophies that Bill held (Ellis & MacLaren, 1998).

In addition to REBT techniques, modeling was also utilized, particularly in relation to Bill's father. For instance, Bill could identify that his father is a person

---

Activating Event (A)

Situation: Moved away from home to pursue athletic scholarship opportunity
Adversity: "I have abandoned my mother and younger brothers when they needed me the most"

Irrational Beliefs (iB)	Rational Beliefs (rB)
Demand: "I want to support my mom and brothers and I should have stayed back with them"	**Preference:** "I want to support my mom and brothers but I don't have to stay back with them to do that"
Depreciation (self): "I am a terrible person"	**Acceptance (self):** "Trying to balance my responsibilities does not make me a terrible person"

Unhelpful Consequences (C)	Helpful Consequences (C)
Emotional Consequence: Guilt	**Emotional Consequence:** Remorse
Behavioral Consequence: Avoid family	**Behavioral Consequence:** Call/visit his family when I can
Cognitive Consequence: Rumination of self-depreciating thoughts	**Cognitive Consequence:** More appreciative thoughts, e.g., "While I am not physically present, I am a good son and brother because I talk to my family on a regular basis"

Figure 6.3 ABC formulation for guilt

whom he admires and aspires to be more like. Bill identified specific qualities about his father and used him as a model to emulate making changes in his own life. Essentially, Bill made comparisons between his own way of thinking and that of his father (Ellis & MacLaren, 1998). More specifically, Bill acknowledged the level of love and respect he had for his father. In addition, both he and his father had a deep passion and love for football. When his father was younger, he played football, and as an adult, he coached football. Bill indicated that he and his father "bonded" over football, and he perceived playing football as means to honor his father. In the eighth session of therapy, Bill expressed a high level of disappointment in himself, stating, "I am worthless to my father." I assisted Bill in reframing this irrational belief and had Bill identify all the ways in which he made his father proud and honored his father's memory. This session was a highly emotional session, as Bill came to the realization that he never really grieved the loss of his father. He became tearful and vocalized an apology to his father for letting him down. As his therapist, I felt a high level of empathy and compassion for my client. I also believed this to be a "turning point" in therapy, in which he truly acknowledged the depth of the sadness, regret, and hurt he felt because his father was no longer here. I also realized the importance of my ability to remain present and tolerant of intense emotions displayed by my client, particularly as he wept and put his head in his hands.

Socratic questioning was a technique that was frequently implemented throughout the course of therapy with Bill. Through Socratic questioning, he also came to the realization that anger had become a secondary emotion for him, and at a core level, he was devastated and extremely hurt that his father died unexpectedly. Bill came to some profound realizations, particularly regarding freedom and responsibility within the context of his pending legal charge, an affirmation of his passion for football, the love he had for his father, and the value he placed on his athletic identity as a football player.

Throughout the course of therapy, both Bill and I acknowledged the potential of him being dismissed from the university, pending the outcome of his trial. His trial date was set for the beginning of December, which coincided with the end of the Fall Semester. His ninth session occurred before his court appearance, so most of the session focused on his fears surrounding the potential outcome of the trial. He expressed genuine remorse for having physically harmed the other student and acknowledged that he "was not thinking clearly at the time." Within the context of his worry of his pending trial, I implemented referenting (I had Bill identify the advantages and disadvantages of changing his irrational beliefs). For instance, he could identify that he felt less anger and guilt when he maintained more rational beliefs. He also acknowledged making better behavioral choices, e.g., calling his family, reaching out to a teammate. He acknowledged an understanding of the link between his beliefs (B) and subsequent emotional, behavioral, and cognitive consequences (C). The purpose was to help Bill keep track of why he wanted to change and to increase his motivation to change. He was encouraged to review this cost-benefit analysis regularly, especially when feeling discouraged (Ellis & MacLaren, 1998).

Regarding his upcoming trial, Bill acknowledged that a primary advantage of maintaining the irrational belief of, "My life is worthless if I can't play football again and if I lose my scholarship" (see Figure 6.2) is that "it's easier to think that way." Not surprisingly, the primary disadvantage that Bill identified about changing his irrational belief was that, "it's hard for me to imagine life without football." I assisted Bill in adopting a realistic perspective regarding the potential outcome of the trial. Bill came to the realization that although he was disappointed in himself for the choice he made, he was able to make better choices moving forward. He discussed the importance of owning how devastated he was at the loss of his father and how that impacted the choice he made at the time. This acknowledgement was crucial, as Bill largely avoided processing the grief over his loss, which consequently increased his potential for developing and maintaining irrational beliefs. In addition, Bill acknowledged a trust or belief that the outcome of the trial would assist him in making decisions moving forward. If the other student's parents pressed charges (as the other student was a minor), and he was found guilty, he would trust that the best outcome was to move back to his hometown to be with his mother and his brothers. Conversely, if the other student's parents opted not to press charges, he would trust that the best outcome for him was to stay at the university, continue to rehabilitate his injury, and plan to resume playing football next fall. Regarding his injury, Bill could acknowledge a sense of gratitude that his injury was not career-ending.

In discussing his injury further, Bill placed a high level of blame on himself for being careless. Throughout the course of therapy, he could acknowledge that he was emotionally preoccupied after the loss of his father and consequently not focused during football practice when he injured his knee. I implemented disputing quite frequently when Bill would make remarks such as, "I'm an idiot for not paying attention as I should at practice." For instance, I would ask him where holding this belief was getting him, and he was able to articulate that maintaining that belief was not helpful for him. This active approach assisted Bill in evaluating his irrational beliefs. Throughout the course of therapy, I implemented both didactic and Socratic styles of disputation. In the didactic style, which was used earlier on during therapy, I explained different terminology within the context of REBT, including the differences between rational and irrational beliefs. As therapy progressed, the Socratic style, which involved a series of leading questions, was incorporated more frequently (Ellis & MacLaren, 2005).

In addition, I also implemented forceful coping statements throughout therapy. To increase the strength of rational coping statements, it was useful to elicit an emotive element along with them. Practicing rational coping statements in a calm and unemotional manner may not adequately counteract the strongly held irrational beliefs. Bill could identify strongly held emotions regarding his recent series of losses. I worked with Bill to identify several rational coping statements, including, "While my judgment was clouded at the time, I can make better choices moving forward." Essentially, this belief refrains from global self-rating and instead recognizes his fallibility. Additional rational beliefs would include,

"While I prefer to be in control of my emotions all the time, I do not absolutely have to be" and, "I can accept myself when I am not in control and this could lead to me making better choices." After Bill developed rational statements, he was encouraged to practice them forcefully during and between sessions to increase their effectiveness. Bill appeared open to implementing between-session practice and acknowledged practicing the statements outside of session. Irrational beliefs tend to be held strongly and to weaken them, rational beliefs must be strengthened (Ellis & MacLaren, 1998).

A final REBT technique incorporated in therapy was reverse role-playing. Essentially, I adopted the role of Bill, and Bill adopted the role of the therapist. Toward the end of the therapeutic relationship, I adamantly verbalized Bill's irrational beliefs, and he was able to practice disputing and challenging them by using his newly developed rational beliefs. A specific example of this in therapy was when Bill stated the self-downing belief, "I am a complete failure to my father." In the reverse role-play, I stated this, and Bill disputed this statement with the self-acceptance belief, "While I sometimes fall short, I am never a complete failure to my father." Bill developed further insight in that because he cared so much about his father and what his father thought of him, he put added pressure on himself to do so well. He acknowledged, "What I did to myself caused me to break." By incorporating reverse role-playing, Bill's rational beliefs were strengthened and irrational beliefs were weakened. The primary objective of this exercise was for Bill to see how he sounds when defending irrational beliefs and to experience a live demonstration of active disputation (Ellis & MacLaren, 1998).

After the ninth session, I received a phone call from the AD who indicated that the other student's parents decided to press charges against Bill and consequently, he would be dismissed from the university and lose his scholarship. As his counselor, I knew this was a possibility from the outset, and I was prepared for the news. When Bill shared this news with me, I felt a high level of empathy for him, but also, like him, recognized there was a legal consequence for his action. The AD stated that I would be able to have one final session with Bill before his formal dismissal from the university. The AD thanked me for all I did to assist Bill, and the AD reiterated his sentiment from a previous phone call, "I don't know what you're doing with him, but whatever you're doing is working. I have noticed a positive shift in his attitude and his behavior. He has become less angry and calmer." I thanked the AD for his feedback and indicated that much of the work I did focused on getting Bill to change his perspective on things.

When Bill came in for his tenth and final session, he appeared to display a sense of relief. He briefly explained the course and outcome of the trial, stating that the 17-year-old student's parents decided to press assault charges against him. Rather than stating, "Life isn't fair," Bill was able to illustrate his recently formed effective new philosophy regarding the situation. He articulated a balanced perspective, acknowledging personal responsibility, but refraining from exhibiting a high level of self-blame and shaming statements. He acknowledged disappointment in himself, but recognized that he is not a complete and utter failure.

Within the context of these newly found realizations, I discussed the importance of Ellis's notion of unconditional self-acceptance (USA; Ellis, 2000). I reinforced the idea to Bill that a person cannot be judged by one aspect alone. Essentially, a person is not 100% bad because he or she has bad behavior. This philosophy allows a person to increase tolerance for being imperfect (Ellis & MacLaren, 1998). In the final session, Bill could acknowledge his development of a more balanced perspective of various aspects of his life, particularly regarding his sport participation, athletic injury, legal charge, sadness over his father's death, and sense of responsibility to his mother and his brother. He was able to acknowledge that deep down he had the sense that he needed to be there for his family and perhaps this was life's way of telling him that that is where he needed to be. Ultimately, he displayed compassion for himself and forgiveness for the poor choice he made.

In the termination session, Bill expressed his gratitude and appreciation of the work I did with him. He explained that he had a high level of skepticism and misperceptions regarding therapy and, "never really wanted to see a shrink." As a counselor, and especially within the context of sport, I have encountered this attitude quite frequently. However, I have come to the realization that much of the attitude is shaped by the coach's philosophy, particularly their perspective on the potential benefits of mental health counseling and sport psychology consultation. More specifically regarding Bill, he acknowledged that he experienced a high level of emotional pain, secondary to the loss of his father, and a high level of physical pain, secondary to his knee injury. However, he stated that he felt more equipped to handle the pressures and demands of life moving forward. When asked about his plans, Bill explained that he planned on moving back home to be with his mother and his brothers. He stated that he would continue to rehabilitate his knee injury and consider attending the local community college next fall. He acknowledged that he needed a break from school and would really like to have extra time to spend with his mother and his brothers.

A large theme that ran across the course of therapy was how he could live his life in a way that honors his father. Bill acknowledged that by playing football and identifying as a football player, he was honoring his father. He expressed that even though he may have fallen short at times, he ultimately knew that his father was still proud of him. Bill was also able to acknowledge the profound impact that losing his father had on him, especially since his father's heart attack was unexpected. He explained that the loss had been "eating away" at him and he was able to admit the role that alcohol and marijuana played in "numbing the pain." He and I spoke very candidly about the role of grief in compromising his judgment. He acknowledged his fallibility in that he had made some bad choices. In the end, my goal was to facilitate USA in Bill (Ellis & MacLaren, 2005). Throughout the course of treatment, I noticed identifiable shifts in his perspective, attitude, and behavior. Overall, he adopted a more realistic perspective about his life, particularly regarding the profound impact that his father had on him and his strong identification as a football player.

The efficacy of the work

Regarding the efficacy of the work, unfortunately, due to limited resources at the counseling center, formalized quantitative measures were not incorporated pre- and post-therapy. Thus, many of the insights gleaned regarding the effectiveness of therapy were largely anecdotal and through self-report. In terms of specific behavioral observations, I identified the following: visibly noted changes in affect and cognitions; punctual attendance at every session; active participation in sessions; increased eye contact after the third session (less of a downward gaze); and expressed gratitude toward the end of therapy. These changes were indicative of a marked improvement in Bill's initially depressed mood.

In addition to the changes in mood and behavior, I also received a phone call both mid-way through the course of therapy, as well as before the final session with Bill. In the initial phone call from the AD (just after the sixth session), he asked what I was doing with him, as his attitude and demeanor "completely shifted." In addition, he thanked me for helping Bill. In the second phone call (after the outcome of the court hearing), the AD expressed that he was initially skeptical that therapy could help someone like Bill. The AD explained that I "made a believer" out of him. My perception was that the AD maintained stereotypes and preconceived notions about psychotherapy and sport psychology work. I have found that coaches and ADs who have been in the sport world longer tend to have more skepticism than newer coaches and ADs who have likely been exposed to sport psychology in their sport experiences, education, and training.

Several months later, I received another phone call from the AD in which he indicated that Bill continued to undergo physiotherapy and had been successful at rehabilitating his leg. He was going to try out for the junior college football team for the upcoming Fall season. Bill endorsed being happy about his move home to be with his mother and two younger brothers and explained that, "things worked out the way they were supposed to."

Critical reflections

I noted several strengths and limitations regarding my implementation of REBT. Perhaps the most salient evidence for the effectiveness of the interventions was the reception of REBT from the AD: after speaking with the AD on several occasions, my perception was not specifically that the AD cared about the techniques that I was using, but rather that the interventions were working with Bill. Evidence for the success of the interventions included Bill's shift in perspective and a willingness to forgive himself for what he did, ultimately acknowledging that he was not a complete failure. Behaviorally, he exhibited increased eye contact, more positive affect, and was even able to laugh at appropriate times as therapy progressed. Moreover, I believed I handled the potential legal and ethical issues quite well and clarified my role at the onset. During the informed consent, I explained the limits of confidentiality and communicated that the AD may request general information regarding Bill's attendance and participation in therapy. I also addressed the potential issue of pre-mature termination, should the outcome of the court hearing lead to Bill's dismissal from the university. Also, I was careful and astute in my documentation of session notes, given the potential for sub-poena. While my notes were not ultimately requested, a general letter regarding attendance, participation, and progress was requested by the Court. Moreover, I prioritized grief/loss issues and the importance of Bill's athletic identity in my work with him. If I had the opportunity to continue with Bill in therapy, I would have continued to assist him in processing the grief secondary to his multiple losses, particularly the death of his father. I would have also continued to work on reinforcing the internalization of Bill's effective new philosophy, particularly his acceptance of himself as a fallible person.

The primary limitation of my work with Bill was my lack of standardized measures to quantify treatment gains. I relied solely on self-report, behavioral indicators, and the AD's report on noticed positive changes in Bill. In addition, while I used a majority of REBT interventions, because I did not adopt a purist REBT approach it was difficult to ascertain the role of REBT versus other aspects of the therapeutic relationship and process in Bill's treatment gains. Relatedly, I could have more consistently implemented the terminology of REBT with Bill, more effectively assisting Bill in self-identifying irrational beliefs regarding dogmatic demands, awfulizing, low frustration tolerance, and self/other rating (Ellis, 2000). In addition, another potential limitation was the context that influenced the way REBT was delivered. More specifically, it took place in a university counseling center where the students were on 15-week semesters, and Bill's eligibility for therapy ended once he was no longer a student at the university. Given both my personal investment and professional obligation to Bill, this harsh reality was difficult to accept, as I did not want Bill to perceive me as abandoning him. However, in our last session, Bill acknowledged his plan to follow up with counseling services in his hometown. He mentioned that he was still on his mother's insurance plan and would follow up with a provider within her insurance network.

In addition to overall strengths and limitations of my work with Bill, some general insights regarding the use of REBT can be gleaned. In my experience, the prevalence of irrational beliefs in exercisers/athletes is high. Not just in my work with Bill, but also in my work with other student-athletes, as well as recreational and competitive athletes, I have found the occurrence to be high. Arguably, all of the athletes with whom I worked have displayed at least one irrational belief per session, team meeting, practice, game, etc. However, I have found that sometimes athletes are not as consistent with between-session practice as psychotherapy clients. Thus, a suggested adaptation would be to make the work of REBT less scholarly and more active. I have found that the active disputation component of REBT is one that resonated with the athletes.

In addition, I have used components of REBT to assist myself in adopting a more realistic perspective in my work with clients and athletes. For instance, I previously held the irrational belief that I needed to be effective with all my clients all the time and that I should be the absolute best person to help every athlete/client/student with their issue. Through my 15 years of experience both in clinical and athletic settings, I have realized how irrational that belief is and have since adopted a more realistic, self-compassionate, and rational perspective.

Finally, regarding novel insights for using REBT in sport/exercise, the importance of a comprehensive assessment and case formulation was highlighted. For instance, in this case, Bill presented with more of a clinical issue, i.e., unresolved grief/loss. Therefore, traditional aspects of sport psychology related to performance enhancement were not a priority in this case. Instead, aspects related to the client's sense of loss on multiple levels were all addressed. Moreover, it was crucial for me to understand the importance of sport to Bill's life and attend to the expressed belief that his life would have been over if he could no longer participate in his chosen sport. This is one of the most challenging irrational beliefs to confront within an athlete.

In summary, Bill appeared to make significant changes to his beliefs, emotions, and behaviors over the course of therapy. As his counselor, I was proud of him for altering his irrational beliefs, developing more effective emotional regulation skills, and incorporating adaptive behavioral alternatives. Ironically, throughout the course of therapy, not only did Bill develop an effective new philosophy in his life as a football player, but also I developed an effective new philosophy in my life as a therapist.

References

Banks, T. (2011). Helping students manage emotions: REBT as a mental health educational curriculum. *Educational Psychology in Practice*, 27(4), 383–394. doi:10.1080/0266 7363.2011.624303

Calabro, L. E. (1997). 'First things first': Maslow's hierarchy as a framework for REBT in promoting disability adjustment during rehabilitation. *Journal of Rational-Emotive & Cognitive-Behavior Therapy*, 15(3), 193–213. doi:10.1023/A:1025039816806

DiGiuseppe, R., Doyle, K., Dryden, W., & Backx, W. (2014). *A practitioner's guide to rational emotive behavioral therapy* (3rd ed.). New York, NY: Oxford University Press.

Ellis, A. (1956). *The ABC model of rational emotive therapy*. Paper presented at the American Psychological Association (APA) Convention, Chicago, IL.

Ellis, A. (1991). The revised ABC's of Rational-Emotive Therapy (RET). *Journal of Rational-Emotive & Cognitive-Behavior Therapy*, 9(3), 139–172. doi:10.1007/BF01061227

Ellis, A. (1997). Using Rational Emotive Behavior Therapy techniques to cope with disability. *Professional Psychology: Research and Practice*, 28(1), 17–22.

Ellis, A. (2000). *REBT resource book for practitioners*. Albert Ellis Institute. Retrieved from www.rebt.org.

Ellis, A., & MacLaren, C. (1998). *Rational emotive behavioral therapy: A therapist's guide*. (1st ed.). Atascedero, CA: Impact.

Ellis, A., & MacLaren, C. (2005). *Rational emotive behavioral therapy: A therapist's guide*. (2nd ed.). Atascedero, CA: Impact.

Gee, C. J. (2010). How does sport psychology actually improve athletic performance? A framework to facilitate athletes' and coaches' understanding. *Behavior Modification*, 34(5), 386–402. doi: 10.1177/0145445510383525.

Malkinson, R. (2010). Cognitive-Behavioral Grief Therapy: The ABC Model of Rational-Emotion Behavior Therapy. *Psihologijske Teme/Psychological Topics*, 19(2), 289–305.

Editors' commentary on Chapter 6: "Managing injury and loss: the use of Rational Emotive Behavior Therapy (REBT) with a collegiate football player"

This chapter illustrates the flexible and 'transdiagnostic' nature of REBT as a psychotherapeutic model. While there was a clear rationale for the referral at the outset, namely, developing more effective skills for managing unhealthy anger, it quickly became apparent that there were other important issues at play. Having supervised hundreds of peer-counseling sessions on REBT training courses, I very clearly see how an apparently straightforward issue can spiral into something very complicated when one attempts to apply the ABC framework. This is often a surprise to the clients, who often apologize, saying that they thought this was going to be an easy issue for the trainee therapist to practice their skills with. Clearly, in the field of practice, issues are likely to be of even greater complexity than within a training environment.

In this chapter, once Bill began to talk about his anger, issues of loss revealed themselves, and as the therapist, Angela soon had to make choices about the direction of their work. She was faced with making sense of the relationship between the various issues, and formulating an intervention plan that was accessible and coherent. A frequent mistake observed in training is conflating two ABCs, either by trying to work on two different emotional problems at the same time, or mixing up two entirely different inferences about the same situation. What the different ABC forms illustrate in this chapter is the utility of keeping issues clearly defined and separate from each other. Unhealthy anger, guilt, and depression, while all being aspects of the presenting problem, are kept apart and formulated separately. This is a key decision in this case and is very helpful in maintaining clarity, both for the therapist and the client. Where the reader faces complex issues during assessment, we would endorse this strategy and encourage mindful awareness of which facets of the problem belong on which ABC form.

7   The use of Rational Emotive Behavior Therapy (REBT) to address symptoms of exercise dependence

Leon Outar

Contextual information

My practice was conducted in a local leisure centre, which advocated a passion for cultivating not only the client's physical well-being but also their mental well-being. Exercise dependence (greatly known as exercise addiction) is a rather new and taboo phenomenon, and since its emergence in mainstream exercise psychology it has been plagued with a myriad of definitions. Initially, exercise dependence held positive connotations, even being referred to as the "positive" addiction (Glasser, 1976). Such definitions grossly downplayed the deleterious effects it posed upon physical and psychological well-being. Exercise dependence is seldom mentioned in the fitness industry, with high-profile athletes advocating the importance of addiction in the pursuit of success, promoted through social media platforms via popular hash tags such as #exerciseaddict and #fitnessaddict. Corroborating this notion, previous literature demonstrates that those who are at risk of exercise dependence are unattuned to the adverse effects it can create (Johnston, et al., 2011). Finally, given the current climate, with health and well-being issues of inactive individuals, the push for physical activity has never been so robust. Therefore, leisure centres, fitness centres and gymnasiums spend masses of effort and time promoting the plethora of physical and psychological benefits of exercise. To this end, the notion of over-exercising appears somewhat paradoxical. Therefore, when presented with such notions, such establishments may be resistant to such beliefs due to goal conflict, consequently rupturing working alliances.

To steer clear of negative connotations associated with the word "therapy", whilst simultaneously being sensitive to the current misconceptions of exercise dependence, I conceived the programme "Intelligent Development". Intelligent Development (REBT) was a programme designed to bring greater awareness to current cognitive patterns, and to promote more "intelligent" beliefs toward exercise, therefore, beliefs that were healthy, flexible and helpful. Psychological benefits of the programme included improved psychological health and well-being, enhanced emotional and behavioral regulation, improved self-awareness and increased exercise enjoyment. The potential benefits proved favourable amongst staff and members and they were advised that this was achieved by teaching individuals psychological skills to assist them to identify, challenge and replace unhelpful beliefs (ABCDE model). It was during the delivery of this programme that I worked with many individuals, one of whom was Brian.

The case of Brian

Brian was an exuberant individual with a thirst for success and accomplishment. He exercised regularly and played Saturday League Soccer (sub-elite). Brian prided himself on being academically excellent, expressing aspirations of studying at one of the United Kingdom's most renowned Universities. His mindset was driven by success in all virtues of life, with failure being non-optional. With such drive and determination to reach success, Brian required means that would guarantee acquirement of success, accomplishment and accolades. Therefore, Brian implemented rigid structures, plans and routines within his life, and flexibility within such plans was non-negotiable. He viewed rigidity within his structure as key to his personal excellence, especially with regards to his exercise routine. In the screening process undertaken prior to my work with Brian, data showed that he displayed greater irrational beliefs and exercise dependence symptoms when compared with norms. I wondered whether his irrationality (i.e., his dogmatic view of success and achievement) could be responsible for his dependent exercise behavior. Ellis (1994) in his one published contribution to exercise psychology outlined the potential problem of exercise dependence (he referred to it as exercise overindulgence), postulating irrational beliefs as partly responsible for its occurrence and maintenance, chiefly low frustration tolerance. To this end, exercisers who possess greater irrationality may be more inclined to engage in excessive exercise due to dogmatic demands ("I need to exercise"), and perceived inability to cope without exercise ("I can't stand it when I miss the gym"). Therefore, Ellis conceived that through identification, challenging of irrational beliefs, and development and reinforcement of rational beliefs, healthier exercise beliefs and exercise behavior can be achieved.

As expressed earlier, exercise dependence is seldom mentioned within the fitness industry, however, the expression of irrational beliefs amongst exercisers is prominent. Being a keen exerciser myself, I was familiar with statements such as "I need to get bigger", "I need to go to the gym", "I need to be skinnier", "I need to lose this fat" and so forth. However, once I had undergone my REBT training, I began to identify consequences of such thought patterns. I realized that those who held such beliefs expressed feelings of guilt, anxiety and even depression when missing exercise bouts, and demonstrated dysfunctional behavior such as excessive exercise sessions, meticulous regimes, exercising whilst injured and failing to attend social events due to scheduling clashes with exercise sessions.

Although seldom mentioned, exercise dependence as a construct has been around for quite some time, but has been thwarted due to a myriad of terms and definitions, rendering clear definition difficult. However, progressive steps have been made and it is now recognized by the DSM-V, however, not as a stand alone disorder, rather as a symptom to another disorder (i.e., anorexia nervosa). To date, there is no clear and specific intervention to address symptoms of exercise dependence, however, due to the deleterious effects, tangible interventions are required.

Needs analysis

Initial conversations with Brian were informative, allowing my practitioner's ears to identify potential high irrationality, however, prior to any REBT work, it was important to assess the prevalence of irrational beliefs and symptoms of exercise dependence in Brian. Several measurement tools were deployed to ascertain Brian's level of irrational beliefs or presence of exercise dependence symptoms. The irrational Performance Beliefs Inventory (iPBI; Turner et al., 2016) was utilized to establish his irrational belief scores, and the exercise dependence questionnaire (ED-Q) was used to ascertain his risk of exercise dependence. Brian scored highly on the iPBI scoring 21.22 (out of 35), furthermore his ED-Q scores highlighted that Brian was categorized as non-dependent symptomatic (i.e., non-dependent yet showing symptoms of exercise dependence), which is achieved by scoring 3 or above.

Brian's results suggested that he held high irrational beliefs and that he suffered from symptoms of exercise dependence. The appropriateness of conducting REBT was largely anecdotal and based on an interpretation of the theory, and Ellis's notion of exercise overindulgence. To date, there have been no published articles on the use of REBT within exercise settings, however, promising use has been shown within sport (see Turner, 2016, for a review) so one would hope that such benefits could be transferred. It was conceived that identifying Brian's unhealthy, unrealistic, irrational beliefs, challenging them and replacing them with healthier, realistic rational beliefs, consequently would alleviate exercise dependence symptoms. This notion has been corroborated within other forms of addictions (e.g., to the Internet; Cardak, et al., 2009). Therefore, it was hoped that such results could be replicated within maladaptive exercise patterns.

The ABCDE of REBT

The structure of my work with Brian followed the traditional ABCDE model, however, presented quite differently. As mentioned prior, due to the context in which REBT was being carried out, Brian did not approach me with a problem he wished to circumvent; rather he wished to engage in self-development through Intelligent Development (REBT), and needs analysis had revealed symptomology of exercise dependence. Due to this, I believed that sessions were best to follow a didactic-Socratic approach, in which Brian was educated in REBT principles (via PowerPoint and diagrams) early in the work, followed by Socratic discussion as to how REBT principles were reflected in Brian's behavior and emotions. For example, session 2 involved educating Brian to differentiate between unhealthy negative emotions (UNEs) and healthy negative emotions (HNEs), analysis of As, Bs and Cs, and then Socratic discussion as to how his beliefs may influence his exercise behavior. Each of the six sessions lasted approximately 45 minutes and followed a session plan to optimize efficiency.

REBT follows a cognitive model of change; therefore a fundamental tenet of REBT is that clients rehearse what they have learnt to ensure that the effects become both meaningful and durable. This is achieved through homework assignments, which can take the form of cognitive (e.g., self-help worksheets), behavioral or emotive (e.g., facing the activating event with new rational beliefs) work. Homework can often hold negative connotations reflecting schoolwork or infancy, so it may be beneficial to refer to it as self-help work, rehearsal exercise or fieldwork. Each homework assignment was negotiated with the client, was specific, was consistent with the prior session, and was reviewed and administered systematically (reviewed at the start, and set at the end of each session).

Session 1

This session was all about setting the stage for the period of practice. It was driven by developing a therapeutic alliance, and establishing rapport to facilitate collaboration. I utilized this session to gain familiarity with Brian, which was achieved through an informal semi-structured interview. The purpose of this interview was twofold. First, it allowed rapport to develop as I began to know more about my client, and second, it allowed for discrete analysis of potential ABCs (activating events, irrational beliefs and emotional/behavior dysfunctionalities). The semi-structured interview included topics for discussion such as exercise initiation (i.e., why did he start exercising?), importance of exercise in Brian's life, implementation of exercise plans and consequences if they are not fulfilled, and finally motives for exercise (e.g., catharsis, body image, fitness, etc.). For example:

P: So, tell me why you exercise.
C: I train for strength for soccer as I play with adults so it helps my strength within my sport. I would also say that exercising regulates my mood, as when I do not exercise I can feel very irritated, as exercising is quite cathartic for me.
P: How important is exercise in your life?
C: Very important! I train six times a week for 12 hours and I can't imagine my life without it. I find it hard to comprehend why people do not train. We are here once so why be 40% body fat when you can be the best you can be?
P: Do you set dedicated time for exercise? If so what happens if this time is not adhered to?
C: I'm a very structured and planned person, so I set a plan and I have to execute it, for example, I'll go a minimum of four times; I feel irritated if I do not as I like my structure. If I wasn't to go the gym I would feel like I haven't fulfilled my daily plans.

Principles of REBT

The semi-structured interview preceded a short presentation of the fundamentals of REBT. This covered REBT history, irrational beliefs, rational beliefs, UNEs vs. HNEs and the ABC model. Content was expressed to Brian didactically, whilst allowing for pauses for clarity using analogies between slides. The slides provided real-life examples that helped Brian apply the content to his life. REBT was pre-sented this way, as it was believed that this would be more engaging for Brian, rather than long educational lecture-like speeches. For example, here is an anal-ogy (fruit basket) used to describe unconditional self-acceptance (USA):

P: So Brian, imagine that there is a basket of fruit. In the basket, there is a wide range of fruits, some good, normal, and some are bad. Can you label this fruit basket as either good or bad?
C: Ermm, no I don't think I can (long pause whilst he pondered).
P: Exactly, the basket is neither good nor bad. So think how can we do this with people who possess a magnitude of characteristics that are ever changing?
C: Yeah I guess you are right. We can't, however, I do it all the time (laughing).
P: We have all been guilty of it at times (smile).

This was a snippet of useful analogy used to clarify and bring meaning to the concept of USA. Notice in this example how I do not tailor this education to Brian's needs just yet, as I am trying to educate more generally about irrational beliefs.

Establishing potential ABCs

The initial interview helped highlight potential irrational beliefs, and from this I could detect that Brian possessed irrational beliefs in reference to adherence of structures or plans. This was due to his constant mention of importance of his plans, and him identifying himself as a structured person relentlessly. To my practitioner's ear it sounded more like a demand for structure rather than prefer-ence, with structure potentially being a means of achieving success. However, this notion required more substance. Prior to the sessions I decided that I would utilize the data collected from the iPBI, to ascertain greater insight to his irra-tional beliefs and overall issues. Therefore, I presented to Brian his three highest scoring beliefs, and I then asked Brian to express the one that was most prevalent in his life and the reasons why. Given the complexity and novelty of the issue, it required innovative methods to elicit information – if you are dealing with a rather delicate issue and difficult context and require a starting point without fear of rupturing therapeutic alliance I would recommend this exercise. The following conversation demonstrates this interaction:

P: So, Brian, of the three beliefs here can you say which one is most frequent in your life both general and exercise related?
     The client took the time to ponder upon his thoughts.
C: Improving my competency is the one that is most involved in my life.
     The actual statement on the iPBI is "If my competencies did not continually develop and improve, it would show what a failure I am".
P: Okay, thanks for that. Brian, can I ask you a question?
C: Yeah sure.
P: Am I right in saying that progression is important in your life?

A benefit of REBT is it allows for a directive-active practice approach, in this instance hypothesizing.

C: Yeah you are right, progression is very important to me. If I were not to go to the gym, and not keep to my structure, I would not be progressing. This works for me; I like my structure. I like where I am in life and I do not allow any negative entities in my life that prevent me from my goals. I want to hold onto beliefs like these as for now they are working for me and get me where I need to be.

Cognitive dissonance taking place here. I felt Brian became resistant to my questioning on highlighting his requirement for progression. His previous statement came across as defensive, and it was apparent that his belief regarding progression was well-rehearsed and that this was at all costs and at the core of his beliefs.

This was an extremely useful exercise for ascertaining potential ABCs. Exploring his beliefs through his results and asking about which beliefs he felt were most prevalent not only in his general life but exercise life provided me with an understanding of potential irrational beliefs that may contribute to his exercise dependence.

Establishing therapeutic goals

REBT advocates the importance of establishing therapeutic goals. This aids therapeutic alliance as practitioner and client work towards a common goal; additionally, goals allow the practitioner to clarify what is achievable and therefore clarify client expectations.

Brian's previous statement about holding onto his beliefs was delivered in a somewhat defensive and brazen manner, and due to this I was intrigued to see how compliant and collaborative he would be when setting therapeutic goals and setting homework assignments. His response was sharp and strong but unsurprising; his current belief set had served him for as long as he could remember. It seemed to me that his beliefs were well-rehearsed and unshakable. Therefore, to avoid alliance rupture, I deemed it best to express that I accepted him as he was now, and to make it clear why we were here. The following conversation demonstrates this:

P: Just to make this clear Brian, the purpose of these sessions is not to change you in any way, shape or form, however, to bring better insight to how your current beliefs are shaping your behaviors and emotions, and if you change as a by-product then it's up to you.

I could see that this statement put Brian at ease.

C: Well, I guess sometimes I'm referred to as selfish as I don't allow people in my life who will affect my goals, and sometimes I'm called arrogant at times, so I guess I'd like to work on behaving less like that.

Although this wasn't something solid, it displayed that although Brian appeared to be highly resilient in keeping his current beliefs, however, there appeared to be negative consequences for holding them.

At the end of the session we set a cognitive homework assignment. I requested that Brian fill in an ABC self-help sheet with the A (i.e., not improving upon his incompetences/not developing) we had discussed. The session came to an end, and I found myself ruminating. I recalled from my readings and teachings that one of the greatest challenges an REBT practitioner may have to circumvent is to work with a client that possesses similar irrationalities as them. Indeed, I've been practicing REBT for some time, and therefore am proficient in challenging such beliefs, however, I still recall the days when I too felt plagued by the most menacing of irrational beliefs: "I must be successful".

Thus, due to Brian's apparent resistance to change, this had the potential of triggering my most menacing irrational belief; I could sense that over the course of these sessions working with Brian would not only be insightful for him, but would also offer insight to the development and depth of my own rationality. One particular caveat for this kind of situation is the role of countertransference (i.e., reactions from the therapist in reference to the client's statements). Albeit, my cognitive patterns were no longer like Brian's, at one time they were, and therefore it was imperative that I be mindful of offering any non-verbal cues that might be comprehended as reinforcement of his irrational beliefs.

Session 2

The second session began with a review of the set homework. Brian was requested to fill in an ABC self-help sheet to the best of his ability. The ABC self-help sheets are particular useful in early sessions for many reasons, including aiding comprehension of REBT principles, increasing the client's awareness of current thinking patterns and the consequences of them, and assisting the therapist with greater insight to potential As, Bs and Cs. Brian's first ABC self-help sheet looked as follows:

A   Potential reoccurrence of failure.
B   If I fail again, I won't find the motivation for further attempts.
C   Fear of failure.

REBT and other cognitive behavioral approaches endorse the importance of homework assignments, and this information encapsulates the level of rich data that such tasks can provide. Brian's ABC sheet did not adhere to REBT principles (it contains no explicit irrational beliefs), but it allowed me to comprehend Brian's source of dysfunctionality and, furthermore, his current level of REBT comprehension.

Identifying A and C

So far, Brian had provided me with a plethora of rich data allowing me to develop a hypothesis of what I believed his activating event and emotional/behavioral consequences might be. However, at present, this was all it was, a hypothesis, so rigorous analysis was required to corroborate my practitioner's hypothesis. To do so, I called upon a trusted REBT tool, referred to as rational emotive imagery (REI; Maultsby & Ellis, 1974). REI is an elegant combination of imagery and REBT. However, distinct from traditional imagery, in REI the client is requested to consider the problem situation (A), and is then encouraged to experience the usual emotional arousal that comes with this (C). Once accomplished, the client is required to finely tune into their inner dialogue to establish their cognitive patterns (insight to B). REI is typically utilized to challenge their beliefs, and therefore change their UNEs to HNEs, or to imagine oneself behaving and feeling completely different in the problem situation (e.g., missing the gym and feeling concerned rather than anxious). However, in this instance, I only wished to use REI to meticulously scan the situation to bring greater insight to the activating event, and in addition evoke the emotions (C) that occur.

Up until this point, one trend that I had identified was Brian's commitment to his exercise schedules, and the importance of exercise to him. Therefore, the opposite of this (e.g., plans sabotaged and missing an exercise bout) provided a fitting scenario, to draw greater clarity to his activating event (A) and accompanying consequences (C). The conversation occurred as follows:

P: Brian, I want you to close your eyes, take a deep breath and imagine the following. It's Saturday and you've only been to the gym once this week, which is less than your usual; furthermore, you are unable to go today. Now take your time to get there, really put yourself in the situation; once you are there let me know.

    Brian closed his eyes and took a deep breath as he immersed himself in this image . . .

C: Okay, I'm there.

P: Great, how are you feeling at present?

C: I feel tense, irritated and very agitated.

P: I see; now, what is it that is most troubling about this situation?

C: That I haven't stuck to my plans!

P: Is this the only troubling aspect of the situation?

C: Yes, I haven't stuck to my plans and now this week has been wasted!

REI is a simple yet effective tool in bringing rich information to a client's potential ABCs. In this instance, it allowed me to identify Brian's A (not sticking to his plans, rather than not exercising). This made more sense as this rigidity of adherence filtered out into every important aspect of his life (academia, work, soccer). So with this novel insight, I proposed to Brian that perhaps his activating event was not adhering to his plans/routines, which he agreed with. Next, we delved into his emotions to bring come clarity to their conceptualization. Brian expressed feelings of irritation and tension. I requested that he identify which emotion he believed this to be, given his newfound knowledge base of emotions. He successful attributed such feelings to anxiety. At this point, my ABC appraisal was that Brian's activating event (not sticking to his plans) was subject to an irrational demand of success (one of the three common irrational beliefs) or some variation of success or accomplishment; his rigid plans would facilitate his demand to be successful; consequently thoughts of being unsuccessful and therefore not adhering to his plans would invoke a state of anxiety, which he strived to avoid.

Getting to the B

Irrational beliefs represent hot cognitions which are somewhat like schemas, thus they are at the core of our thoughts, and therefore not easily accessible. Due to their schema-like quality, they are often below conscious levels, over-rehearsed and therefore autonomous (DiGiuseppe, 1986). Hence, when I asked Brian earlier what he was thinking he expressed a conscious thought (not sticking to his plan), rather than an irrational belief. Often, asking clients what their beliefs are can yield vague answers. One tool that is highly effective in drawing unconscious automatic cognitive patterns is the "inference chain". For those new to inference chains, they merely entail asking the client to consider A (e.g., not sticking to their plans) and then asking "so what?" or "and what would that mean?" in a concise manner until a potential critical A is revealed. Brian's inference chain appeared as follows:

P: So, Brian, let's go back to considering the situation that you have not adhered to your plans.
C: Okay.
P: Now, I will ask you a series of questions that I want you to answer as soon as you can; the question I will ask you will be the same question again, and again. Does that make sense?
C: Ha ha, yes sure.
P: Brilliant, so you've failed to keep to your plans. What would this mean?
C: I haven't reached my goal.
P: And what would it mean to not reach a goal?
C: I'm not going to get where I want in my life.
P: Let's say you don't get where you want in life; what would this mean?
C: Well I pride myself on being successful!
P: Okay, so what if you were not successful; what would this mean?
C: That I'd let myself and others down!
P: Okay, thanks Brian. So what we have here is the idea that if you did not stick to your plans, you would have not reached your goal, which would mean you wouldn't get where you wanted in life, and because you pride yourself on success, you would be letting yourself and others down.

Inference chains can be powerful and insightful tools, as they often access deeper cognitions about the event. Clients are often left bewildered after inference chains, because they are astonished how one situation can lead them to think so drastically (e.g., how missing your plans equates to not being successful at all and letting yourself and others down). Furthermore, once the chains are presented to the client in a manner where they can see the steps, it provides greater insight into the critical A, and often, irrational beliefs. Therefore, it's a key point to discuss what they think about this insight. The conversation occurred as follows:

P: So, Brian, we have insight into your adversity and consequences. The activity we just did was to help us get to the depths of your beliefs, which if you recall is what is causing your emotional distress. So, correct me if I'm wrong, but I believe that your anxiety about this situation may be due to a demand that you must be successful. How does that thought sound to you?

C: Yeah, I'd say that was pretty much right . . . but when I say successful it's not what others may think of as successful, rich, etc., but I mean it in terms as successful as I can be, as in me being the best I can be.

P: Yes, I see, the word successful is rather subjective and means something different from person to person. Okay, would reaching your full potential be more fitting with your beliefs?

C: Yeah, that's more what it is like.

   I had now established an irrational demand; it was now time to proceed with analysis of any derivatives (i.e., awfulizing, low frustration tolerance, depreciation).

P: Brilliant, okay let's explore this belief more. When you think of not reaching your potential, if you went into the future, let's say 20 years in the future, and you hadn't reached your full potential in any way, shape or form, would you consider this bad?

   I used the future as Brian's C is anxiety; anxiety occurs from future-orientated cognitions so to fully comprehend his B it seemed the best course of action.

C: Absolutely! It would be terrible.

P: Okay, let's hold onto that vision, so we are aware that you think it would be terrible, but do you think you could tolerate this future where you had not reached your full potential?

C: I'll be honest, NO! I'd feel like I had wasted my whole life, if I hadn't reached my own success or full potential.

P: I appreciate your honesty; now one last question. The thought of not reaching your full potential, does this have any implications to how you feel about yourself?

C: Hmmm, well if I was not to be successful this would make me question my value to myself and to the world as I strongly believe that we should all come and give 100%!

P: Sure, so am I right in believing that you would feel less worth or value to yourself and potentially to the world if you were not successful?

C: Yeah, I'd say so.

The conversation ended at this point; Brian and I clarified and agreed on aspects of his B, and we arrived at a precise irrational belief statement.

I must reach my full potential; if I do not it is awful, I can't stand it, and it means that I am not as valuable as I must be.

B-C connection

A fundamental part of the process of change is highlighting the B-C connection. The client is unlikely to attribute their disturbance to their beliefs if they cannot see that B causes C. We discussed this matter, and Brian discovered that his current beliefs were in fact impeding his ability to do what he desired so greatly and be the best he could be. Brian expressed that on reflection he had been applying too much pressure upon himself, and at times his anxiety was debilitating, due to feeling overwhelmed, which further led to procrastination. Brian identified that his "I have to do it" cognitive pattern was the cause of his behavior and emotions, as he felt like there was no other option but to be the best he can. It was this self-discovery that fostered his desire to tackle his anxiety as he could see that his current beliefs were not serving him. What was apparent in this session was that Brain had become more open with me, and where earlier on he was defensive, he was now able to offer introspections and details about his thoughts and feelings. Client resistance in early stages of therapy is common, however, developing a strong therapeutic alliance early on, and providing a model of acceptance, fosters the client's volition and therefore inclination to change.

Ascertaining an emotional and behavioral goal

As outlined earlier, goal setting is not only important within performance, but a vital part of therapy. Setting goals relates to emotional and behavioral targets that allow the client and practitioner to work towards what is realistic, time-specific, yet challenging and motivational. It allows the client to understand what outcome we are aiming for, and what the processes will entail to get there. Brian's UNE was "anxiety", with his behavioral consequence being safety behavior manifested as rigid plans. Therefore, our agreed goal was for Brian to feel concerned, rather than anxious, and to have greater flexibility with his planning. For homework, we set a cognitive assignment for Brian to complete an ABC self-help sheet, however, distinct from the previous session I required he utilize REBT vocabulary to assess his comprehension of the content, and assist his semantic processing of his issues.

Session 3

Preparing for disputation (D)

So far, I had played the role of diagnostician; searching for and highlighting the dynamics of Brian's problem (see Figure 7.1). ABCs are all assessment-based,

---

Activating Event (A)

Situation: Missing an exercise bout
Adversity (e.g., the inference drawn about what is most difficult about the situation): Not sticking to plans

Irrational Beliefs (iB)	Rational Beliefs (rB)
Demand: I must reach my full potential	**Preference:** I want to reach my full potential
Awfulizing: If I do not it's awful	**Non-Awfulizing:** If I do not it's not the end of the world
Low Frustration Tolerance: I can't stand it	**High Frustration Tolerance:** I can cope
Depreciation (self/other/life): I'm not valuable	**Acceptance (self/other/life):** It proves that I am a fallible human being
Unhelpful Consequences (C)	**Helpful Consequences (C)**
Emotional Consequence: Anxiety	**Emotional Consequence:** Concern
Behavioral Consequence: Rigid regimes	**Behavioral Consequence:** Flexible regimes
Cognitive Consequence: Overthinking, procrastination	**Cognitive Consequence:** Greater focus

---

Figure 7.1 Completed ABCDE form

however, changing beliefs through stages D and E is where the intervention work begins. Brian's ABC can be summarized as follows:

A: Failing to stick to my plans.
B: I must reach my full potential; if I do not it is awful, I can't stand it, and it means that I am not as valuable as I must be.
C: Anxiety, rigid plan structure, avoidance behavior, procrastination.

Pragmatic style

Disputation occurs in three styles including questions of empiricism (i.e., Is there any evidence that you must?), logic (Does it seem logical that you must?) and pragmatic (Where will it get you if you believe you must?). The one that I have found most effective is pragmatic disputation. Irrational beliefs impede individuals from attaining their goals, whereas rational beliefs help individuals attain their goals. Therefore, beliefs are considered with regards to their functionality. Does the belief help them solve their problem, facilitate them in attaining a desired goal or mitigate emotional disturbance? Pragmatic disputation with Brian is demonstrated here:

P: Okay Brian, now that we have identified that this specific belief is causing problems, let's explore this belief. So, I know that reaching your full potential is important to you, however, has this demand that you must do so helped you fulfil this goal?

C: No, but at the moment it's just how I feel, that it's something I must do. *There is difference between intellectual and emotional insight. Brian intellectually understands his "must" is not helping him reach his goals, but he still feels compelled to hold his irrational beliefs.*

P: Okay, when you think that way how do you feel?

C: I'm always over thinking and can't concentrate. A lot of the times I procrastinate and feel anxious.

P: I see, so it appears that the very belief that you think helps you reach your full potential in fact is the very thing that is preventing you from doing so.

It's time to get rational

It is somewhat difficult to eliminate or suppress dysfunctional beliefs; instead the best course of action is to create alternative ideas. Therefore, one of REBT's integral components is formulating new alternative rational beliefs to help the client refute their irrational belief. In collaboration, we assembled Brian's rational alternative (see Figure 7.1). I advised Brian about the benefits of investing in this belief, as seen in the following conversation:

C: See, even looking at this sentence, I can see how it will allow me to reach my goals rather than feeling stressed about reaching them.

P: Can you see how this will lead you to a healthier emotion of concern rather than anxiety?

C: Completely. When I see both beliefs I can see how the first one [irrational belief] is leading me to more pressure, which just isn't helping me at all.

P: Exactly, the demands which you have placed on yourself make you feel that there is no other option but to reach your full potential. Can you see how this belief (rational belief) provides you with greater resilience to bounce back if you were not to reach you goals?

C: Yeah, absolutely, because I wouldn't be applying a label to myself.

As a behavioral assignment, I asked Brian to rehearse the rational belief in the face of adversity. As I mentioned earlier, Brian had gained intellectual insight towards his irrational and rational beliefs, however, for him to fully invest in his new rational belief, it was important for him to gain emotional insight through behavioral change.

Session 4

Unconditional self-acceptance (USA)

As mentioned previously, Ellis in his one formal contribution to sport and exercise psychology conceived the notion that irrational beliefs lead to compulsive exercise behavior (i.e., exercise dependence). Furthermore, Ellis proposed that the best means of resolving the matter was through investment in USA. To corroborate this notion, Hall et al. (2009) highlighted the role of USA upon exercise dependence, defining it as a mediator of exercise dependence, in that low USA is related to high exercise dependence. This interaction can be understood in terms of self-worth. Individuals who self-rate themselves, instead of unconditionally accepting themselves, may have a contingent sense of self-worth. Exercise may act as a form of validation to those driven by aesthetics or fitness. Therefore, for such individuals not exercising may cause difficulties in them accepting themselves. Given such insights, I decided to construct the second half of the therapeutic journey with great emphasis on education and investment in USA, whilst still following the traditional REBT structure (ABCDE). This began with meticulously outlining USA.

USA vs. "the self"

The self can be conceptualized in a variety of ways, however, one particularly well-rehearsed concept within western society is self-esteem, which refers to the appraisal of one's self-worth and/or value. Western society places great emphasis on self-esteem, highlighting the importance of high self-esteem; therefore, from an early age individuals begin their conquest of "attaining high self-esteem". However, regardless of how the "self" is conceptualized, a prerequisite of appraising or rating oneself must occur. If the appraisal is of low value (e.g., "I am rubbish"), this will precede low self-esteem and the individual is likely to experience a plethora of psychological problems (Chamberlain & Haaga, 2001). Even in the event of making a high-value appraisal ("I am fantastic"), and therefore preceding high self-esteem, this is too associated with a variety of psychological problems (e.g., perfectionism, narcissism, aggression; Chamberlain & Haaga, 2001). To this end, self-esteem poses a threat to psychological well-being regardless of its direction. Self-worth beliefs are complex and can be difficult to change; they are characterized by global evaluations in which the individual globally appraises their entire entity based on one behavior (e.g., "I'm a failure because I failed my exam"). REBT holds that there is no logical or scientific way of proving conclusively that one human has more worth than any other. Due to this lack of ability to scientifically appraise self-worth it leaves us with a null hypothesis that we are all equal. Therefore, REBT's solution to the problem of the self-rating is through investment of USA, implying that we take a radical stance where the individual fully and unconditionally accepts himself whether or not he behaves intelligently, correctly or competently and whether or not other people approve of, respect or love him. As you can imagine, this may be rather difficult to convince clients of when the very fabric of our linguistics is riddled with global evaluations from early childhood through to adulthood (e.g., good girl, rather than well-behaved girl, or good man, top guy, rather than a man who behaved well). Such terminology is endorsed daily. However, it is important to stress to clients that people are not their behaviors, and investment in such beliefs can be detrimental to their long-term psychological health.

In the next part of the session, we conducted an exercise designed to foster USA: "Big I, Little i". This task requires the client to draw a big "I" on piece of paper, and then using little "i"s the client fills the big "I" with behaviors both good and bad. The point here is that the client is multi-faceted, and cannot be boiled down into one rating or behavior. They are capable of good and bad behaviors, but cannot be labelled wholly "good" or "bad". For homework, I asked Brian to undertake a cognitive assignment of reading a work-sheet designed for overcoming self-esteem. This further validated the distinction between self-worth/self-esteem and USA. Additionally, Brian was requested over the course of the week to write down each time he placed a global evaluation upon himself (negative or positive), and to record what feelings followed.

Session 5

The USA credo

A credo can be defined as a statement of the beliefs or aims, which guide someone's actions. Dryden (2009) has conceived several "credos" relating to REBT theory conceptualization, including a realistic unconditional self-acceptance credo. Credos are particularly useful for giving realistic appraisals of difficulties that individuals may encounter and have to circumvent on their journey towards rationality. The USA credo acknowledges that one may still have depreciation beliefs, and therefore might rate one's whole self greatly or lowly, however, this is testimony to our human fallibility. Therefore, one should strive towards USA, although not rigidly demand that one must never succumb to global evaluations. Dryden's Credo is a lengthy text, so to aid meaning and value we tailored it. This session entailed meticulously deciphering the credo to ensure Brian fully comprehended the principles of USA and how they related to real-life application. Working in collaboration we refined it to develop Brian's own tailored USA credo (see Figure 7.2).

The last homework assignment

For Brian's final assignment, I set him a behavioral task. This was to test not only his investment in his new belief, but also his conviction. I wanted to test his rational belief to its full capacity, so a suitable situation would be for him to attend the gym and not exercise. If he was invested in his irrational belief, "I must reach my full potential; if I do not it's awful as I won't be as valued as I must be", such a situation would invoke anxiety. Prior to the sessions, the very premise of the not exercising was quite simply not an option due to his demand to reach his potential and therefore demand to exercise, with failing to exercise bringing about feelings of anxiety. Putting Brian in the face of adversity provided a perfect opportunity to test his rational belief that "I want to reach my full potential, however, this does not mean I must; it will not be the end of the world, I can cope, and it only proves I'm a fallible human being". I hoped that his rationality

In the journey towards unconditional self-acceptance I may well do many things to deal with my disturbed feelings, which may help me in the short term but not in the long term. While I recognize that I can do this, I also acknowledge that there will be times when I won't. The path towards holding unconditional self-acceptance beliefs is a rocky one.

When I do eventually think in this non-extreme, self-accepting way, I will accept that when adversities happen and I am responsible for them, I will feel badly about my behavior, but not about myself. Rather, I will see that I am unique, fallible, unrateable, complex, and ever-changing and can choose to accept myself as such even though I will continue to dislike my bad behavior.

While self-acceptance beliefs will help me to move toward greater psychological health, I recognize that even when I work hard to develop such beliefs, I will often return to thinking in a self-depreciating manner. Similarly, I acknowledge that as I work to internalize this realistic credo, I will experience many lapses along the way. The best way of dealing with these lapses is to accept them, without liking them, learn specific things from them and act on such specific learning for future situations.

When I acknowledge that holding self-acceptance beliefs is healthy this becomes another positive in my life. Sometimes I may find that I may in fact begin to depreciate myself about having irrational or self-depreciating thoughts; when this occurs I realize that in fact I am acting in an irrational way about having such thoughts and understand that it is natural at times to think irrational. I will do this by showing myself that while it is bad to depreciate myself, doing so does not define me, and that I am a fallible human being who may lapse into self-depreciation even though I know it is irrational to do so. Doing this will help me get back on the path towards greater self-acceptance.

Figure 7.2 Brian's realistic unconditional self-acceptance credo

would allow him to feel concerned about not exercising and therefore controlling his urge to exercise. For clarity, the sessions were never to discourage Brian from exercising, rather to provide rational motives for more flexible patterns of behavior. The conversation went as follows:

P: For your last assignment I really want to see how you cope in the face of your adversity, to see how it feels when you don't do what you once thought you needed to do.
C: Okay, sure.
P: So, what I want you to do is to go to the gym, however, not exercise. Just passively, stand observing others exercise, yet doing completely nothing. How does that sound to you?
C: Ha ha ha! Wow, that will be difficult, as I'm going on holiday in a few weeks also, so I want to look good for that, however, I'm open to do it. It's going to be tough but I'm happy to try.

Notice the use of his language "want" to look good rather than "need"; nuances like these embody the rational philosophy.

Session 6

The session began with a review of the final homework assignment. The sessions had been working towards testing Brian's rational belief, in his real-life settings, in the face of adversity. This was essentially to see how far he had come. The conversation went as follows:

P: So Brian how did you get on with the assignment?
C: Well, I went and I did exercise. But! When I'm at the gym now, I don't feel like I need to be there. I genuinely want to be there to exercise. My mindset in the gym is totally different to before and I just enjoy being there.

Although, Brian was unable to complete the homework, his response was positive. The aim was never to deter the client from exercise, but to bring about a healthier mindset to exercise, thus being more preferential, emotionally and behavioral functional, rather than driven by demandingness.

ABCDE recap

Here I wanted to make sure Brian was comfortable and competent in applying the ABCDE framework. Brian expressed how he would challenge his irrational belief through pragmatic, empirical and logical reasoning. He was then easily able to explain how he constructed his rational belief and most importantly explain why his rational belief was in fact rational (i.e., logical, helpful and evidence-based). Finally, he was able to bring himself to his emotional and behavioral goal through investment in this rational belief. Brian's new found rationality could be encapsulated from the following statement:

C: When I look at my previous beliefs they look foreign to me, as I'm so used now to being invested in my rational belief. Because I've been in this situation with my A-levels these sessions have been useful and a real eye-opener. I really feel like I want to do well rather than having to do well. The other week I was speaking to my Mum, just telling her how it would not be end of the world if I did not reach my full potential. I know I want to but at the end of the day if I were not to I would be able to deal with it.
    Here we can see that Brian has been able to apply the framework to other important facets of his life (e.g., academia).

Helping Leon

I believe knowledge is best expressed through application and your ability to teach or assist others, so what better way to assess Brian's rationality than to aid me with one of my own irrational beliefs. Therefore, Brian was requested to assist me through the ABCDE model. The following conversation captures elements of his attempt:

P: So, when I'm driving, I find myself getting so angry due to other drivers driving poorly on the road, I can't stand their driving! I find myself verbally outbursting!

C: Okay, so the problem here is with others' driving, which I believe is due to a belief that they must not be driving like this, which causes you to feel angry. Is that right?

P: Well yeah I guess so; they shouldn't be driving like that and I just can't stand it!

C: Okay, so first of all does it seem realistic for everyone on the road to drive the way you want? Is there any reason why they must?
       Brian utilized logical disputation at this point.

After disputing my irrational belief both pragmatically and logically, Brian successfully developed and encouraged me to invest in my rational belief, in doing so taking me fully through the ABCDE model. Although this conversation has elements of hypothetical role-play, it was useful for me to see if Brian could apply what he had learned.

The sessions had come to an end; I applauded Brian's work in helping me through my own irrationality, and his work through all the sessions. I left some time available for him to ask any final questions, and to reflect on how he found the sessions. Brian expressed feeling liberated, empowered, that the sessions had been a real eye opener for him at a suitable time, and he advised that he intends to continue to utilize what he had learnt, building upon his skill set.

Outcome analysis

After six sessions, it was apparent to both Brian and I that he had experienced significant change cognitively, behaviorally and emotionally. Brian began the sessions a highly rigid, defensive and tense individual at the mercy of his irrational beliefs. However, post-REBT, Brian now appeared a flexible, open, energetic and resilient individual ready for the good, neutral and bad that life had to offer. The data supported this notion illustrating that REBT brought about large reductions in irrational beliefs with Brian scoring pre-intervention 21.36 and post-intervention 15.60 (out of 35). Finally, REBT brought about reductions in symptoms of exercise dependence, with Brian scoring 3.28 pre-intervention and 2.71 post-intervention, suggesting that he transitioned from exercise dependent symptomatic (i.e., displaying symptoms of exercise dependence) to exercise dependent asymptomatic (i.e., displaying no such symptoms of exercise dependence). Moreover, these changes were upheld and even reduced at a 4-week follow-up, illustrating REBT's capacity to bring about long-term changes. Scores for irrational beliefs and exercise dependence have been graphed in Figures 7.3 and 7.4.

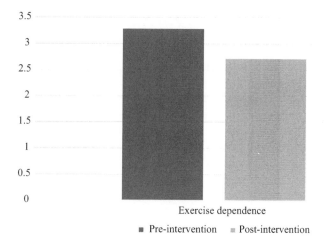

Figure 7.3 Changes in exercise dependence symptoms from pre- to post-REBT

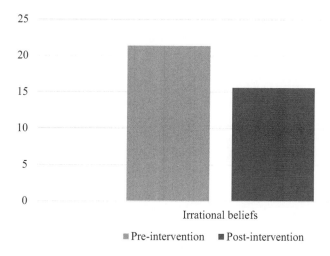

Figure 7.4 Changes in irrational beliefs from pre- to post-REBT

Practitioner reflections

This case is the first to document the use of REBT in addressing exercise dependence symptoms. Therefore, for practitioners considering its use, there are some important considerations. First, the concept of excessive, overindulgent or addictive exercise may seem unproblematic or paradoxical for exercisers, given the well-documented (e.g., Bouchard, et al., 1994) benefits of exercise participation upon physical and psychological well-being. To this end, exercisers may not be fully cognizant of just how dependent they are on exercise and the extent to which their exercise habits are dysfunctional (Johnston, et al., 2011). Thus, without recognition of their maladaptive exercise behavior they may not appraise it as worthy of attention. Therefore, practitioners need to be innovative when designing programmes (e.g., Intelligent Development) to ensure the palatability of the content, especially when considering it in exercise contexts, where establishments may not see the importance of regulating exercise dependence, or may choose to not see it, due to conflicting interests. However, it is the role of the psychologist to raise awareness of such issues and advise all concerned of the problems connected with excessive exercise. To be clear, this is not intended to deter people from exercise but to provide healthier motivations to exercise, therefore allowing for greater psychological health. The difference between wanting to exercise and needing to exercise represents a thin line between psychological health and psychological dysfunction. It is, therefore, a sport and exercise psychologist's role to educate not only the individuals at risk, but also the fitness industry, of the importance of psychological health as well as physical health.

The potential role of irrational and rational beliefs in exercise dependence is an important area for future practice to explore, due to the many deleterious effects of exercise dependence (Hausenblas & Symons-Downs, 2002) that can undermine the plethora of positive aspects of exercise participation (e.g., Bouchard, et al., 1994). This case has highlighted the role of irrational beliefs. Brian's irrational belief, "I must reach my full potential", played a role in many facets of his life (academia, sport and social life). REBT enabled us to get to the core of his irrationality and produce more flexible, functional beliefs, which had a knock-on effect on all these domains. Therefore, I encourage fellow practitioners to use REBT within such settings more. An unhealthy mind in a healthy body still yields an unhealthy individual.

References

Bouchard, C., Shephard, R. J., & Stephens, T. (1994). *Physical activity, fitness and health: International proceedings and consensus statement.* Champaign, IL: Human Kinetics.

Çardak, M., Koc, M., & Çolak, T. S. (2009). The effect of a Rational Emotional Behavior Therapy (REBT) group counseling program on the internet addiction among university students. *International Conference on Foreign Language Teaching and Applied Linguistics, 11,* 5–7.

Chamberlain, J. M. & Haaga, D. A. F. (2001). Unconditional self-acceptance and psychological health. *Journal of Rational-Emotive & Cognitive-Behavior Therapy, 19,* 163–176.

DiGiuseppe, R. (1986). The implication of the philosophy of science for Rational-Emotive Theory and Therapy. *Psychotherapy, 23,* 634–639.

Dryden, W. (2009). *How to think and intervene like an REBT therapist.* London: Routledge.

Ellis, A. (1994). The sport of avoiding sports and exercise: The Rational Emotive Behavioural Therapy perspective. *The Sports Psychologist, 8,* 248–261.

Glasser, W. (1976). *Positive addiction.* New York: Harper and Row.

Hall, H., Hill, A., & Kozub, S. (2009). The mediating influence of unconditional self-acceptance and labile self-esteem on the relationship between multidimensional perfectionism and exercise dependence. *Psychology of Sports and Exercise, 10*(1), 35–44.

Hausenblas, H. A., & Symons-Downs, D. (2002). Exercise dependence: A systematic review. *Psychology of Sport and Exercise, 3*, 89–123.

Johnston, O., Reilly, J., & Kremer, J. (2011). Excessive exercise: From quantitative categorisation to a qualitative continuum approach. *European Eating Disorders Review, 19*, 237–248.

Maultsby, M. C., Jr., & Ellis, A. (1974). *Technique for using rational emotive imagery.* New York, NY: Institute for Rational Living.

Turner, M. J. (2016). Rational Emotive Behavior Therapy (REBT), irrational and rational beliefs, and the mental health of athletes, *Frontiers: Movement Science and Sport Psychology,* doi: 10.3389/fpsyg.2016.01423.

Turner, M. J., Allen, M. S., Slater, M. J., Barker, J. B., Woodcock, C., Harwood, C. G., & McFayden, K. (2016). The development and initial validation of the irrational performance beliefs inventory (iPBI). *European Journal of Psychological Assessment.*

Editors' commentary on Chapter 7: "The use of Rational Emotive Behavior Therapy (REBT) to address symptoms of exercise dependence"

One of the most important aspects of this chapter is the contribution to REBT in exercise psychology literature. There are precious few studies applying REBT with exercisers, and Leon's focus on exercise dependence opens up a useful debate concerning how irrational beliefs may contribute to our understanding of overindulgence in exercise. The clear goal of Leon's work here was to help the client to gain more control over his exercise behavior, not to exercise less. In other words, Leon did not set about challenging the merits of exercise per se, but rather, Leon challenged the irrational beliefs associated with exercise in order to lift demandingness and promote preferences.

As part of the intervention, Leon encouraged the client to endorse and hold rational USA beliefs. This is important for at least two reasons. First, irrational and rational beliefs are considered to be relatively orthogonal, in that low irrational beliefs do not necessarily mean high rational beliefs (e.g., Ellis, et al., 2010). So whilst reducing irrational beliefs in the client is an important part of REBT, promoting rational beliefs is also necessary. An equitable research base does not exist for the use of REBT to increase rational beliefs compared to decreasing irrational beliefs. This obviously needs to be, and is being, addressed by researchers (e.g., Cunningham & Turner, 2016), and Leon's focus on USA here is good practice for sure. Second, self-esteem is considered an important risk factor for exercise dependence (Chen, 2016), but REBT considers the notion of valuing the self rather problematic. REBT suggests that, rather than trying to help the client enhance their self-esteem, a practitioner should encourage the client to unconditionally accept oneself, whilst valuing actions and behaviors, rather than the self. This approach works with Leon's client, but further work is needed to help understand this issue in more detail in exercisers.

References

Chen, W. (2016). Frequent exercise: A healthy habit or a behavioral addiction? *Chronic Diseases and Translational Medicine, 2*(4), 235–240.

Cunningham, R., & Turner, M. J. (2016). Using Rational Emotive Behavior Therapy (REBT) with Mixed Martial Arts (MMA) athletes to reduce irrational beliefs and increase unconditional self-acceptance. *Journal of Rational-Emotive & Cognitive-Behavior Therapy, 34*(4), 289–309.

Ellis, A., David, D., & Lynn, S. J. (2010). Rational and irrational beliefs: A historical and conceptual perspective. In David, D., Lynn, S. J., & A. Ellis (Ed.), *Rational and irrational beliefs: Research, theory, and clinical practice* (pp 3–22). New York, NY: Oxford University Press.

8 Mixed Martial Arts and the paradox between self-improvement and self-acceptance

A Rational Emotive Behavior Therapy (REBT) intervention

Rachel Cunningham

Introduction and practitioner philosophy

At the heart of both REBT and Person-Centered Therapy (PCT) is the appreciation of what makes us human, and the end goal for clients of being a fully functioning person. It was Ellis who initially referred to his approach as "Rational Psychotherapy" (Ellis, 1957). There is something inherently practical about the REBT model as an action-oriented therapeutic approach, and this is what really grabbed my attention at first. I have always been an advocate for a person-centered approach in practice, and my own work is influenced by Rogerian philosophy. In addition, what I have found is that REBT is both capable of being mindful of the individual's place in their own development and promoting collaborative cognitive restructuring.

Context

I had been interested in the culture of Mixed Martial Arts (MMA) for some time and so through a connection at a local club, I started going to watch fights and approached the coach to have an initial discussion about the sport. From our initial discussions, it appeared that his MMA athletes were prone to perfectionistic tendencies. He explained how the athletes consistently put themselves down for the slightest mistake, always wishing to be better, faster, or stronger. I informed him that I was interested in working with his club members. He was very open to the idea and explained that he was always keen to develop the profile of MMA in this domain. I gained permission to observe the athletes in training and was introduced to them.

In my first talk with the coach he had mentioned that he had a few athletes in mind that he thought would really benefit from some 'mental' training. Without naming anyone, he asked that I come back to him after my observations and see if we could come to a consensus on who might be good candidates for my study. What I witnessed in training sessions was a variety of non-verbal examples of what appeared to be perfectionism. For instance, the athletes would refuse to stop until they got what they were practicing right (e.g., a move such as grappling, or a kicking technique). I agreed to work with four of the athletes, and the coach communicated to the athletes that if they were interested in working with me, they should get in touch. After making initial contact, I arranged to meet each of the four athletes on a one-to-one basis to discuss the work.

In talking with them I started to hear common phrases about how the individuals felt they *had* to train, and the limits to which they *had* to push themselves. Winning was the only thing they saw as a measure of a good fighter. Many of them also found it difficult to bounce back after a loss, no matter how well they performed. Often, there were also external pressures to deal with. For instance, most of these athletes held full-time jobs whilst also training for an equal amount of time. Many of them had family responsibilities or were in education. In addition, they had to meet a specific weight category to compete at a desired level. What I observed because of this were very restrictive eating behaviors, often putting individuals in both nutritional and calorie deficits. Psychophysiologically they were under a lot of stress.

In the time that I spent observing MMA, I witnessed what has been referred to as a "culture of fear" (Harpold, 2008; Vaccaro, et al., 2011). Research has indicated that accepting pain and psychological distress is perceived as part of the development process for an MMA athlete (Massey, et al., 2013). Two of the main concerns that were identified for these individuals were fear of failure and trying to make other fighters fear them (Harpold, 2008; Vaccaro et.al, 2011).

I continued to work with all four athletes, but for the present case study I have selected one of the four athletes to detail my work, an amateur MMA athlete named Mark (pseudonym). In this way, I can provide specific details of the work done, and the idiosyncratic nature of the work that unfolded. Mark had been training for approximately five years, was a full-time student completing his undergraduate degree, and he expressed a real love for his sport, prioritizing training above all other aspects of his life.

Presenting issue

In the initial consultation, Mark discussed how much time he spent working on his goal of becoming an elite MMA fighter. He was engaging in hours of extensive training both in the MMA gym and in his own time. In addition to this he was on a very restrictive eating plan. He expressed how this training was going well but just wasn't enough to progress. He was also coming back from a series of injuries, which he believed were to blame for the stall in his progress. His initial thoughts were that training as hard as he was, and being so disciplined with his diet, was all worth nothing unless he could win in competition. He commented that he "had" to be at his best before signing up for a competition. This meant that he had to get his training and nutrition "right" otherwise he "would not reach his full potential". He was feeling frustrated and angry at his lack of perceived progress towards his present goal of being an elite athlete. He felt he should not lose to amateur or semi-professional athletes, since he "should be better than them".

Needs analysis

From this first interview, what the athlete seemed to display were conditional self-depreciation (SD) beliefs (e.g., I am useless/worthless/a failure if. . .) and he was also placing a lot of demands on himself. He feared that not being able to meet these expectations of his performance goals would negate any chance he had of reaching an optimal level of performance. This is akin to the concept of 'fear of failure' and is also considered an irrational cognitive appraisal (Ellis, 1985). To assess the presence of SD beliefs, he was asked to complete the Shortened General Attitudes and Beliefs Scale (SGABS; Lindner, et al., 1999) and Unconditional Self-Acceptance Questionnaire (USAQ; Chamberlain & Haaga, 2001) over a four-week period, prior to any formal REBT intervention work. USA was measured to indicate rational beliefs opposing SD. USA was developed by Ellis to contrast irrational beliefs as an alternative, healthy psychological perspective on self-esteem. USA means that "the individual fully and unconditionally accepts himself whether or not he behaves intelligently, correctly, or competently and whether or not other people approve, respect, or love him" (Ellis, 1977, p. 101). During these initial four weeks Mark was also encouraged to keep a diary of his thoughts and experiences related to training and performance. This baseline data could then be used to determine if changes in scores were attributable to the introduction of the intervention. Following this baseline data collection, Mark's scores did indicate the presence of SD beliefs above the population mean ($M = 4.00$, $SD = .00$) and USAQ scores marginally higher than the population mean (84). That is, according to Lindner et al. (1999), SD beliefs scores above 1.47 indicate that self-depreciation is above the population mean and normative data suggests that USA scores below 82.78 represent low USA (Chamberlain & Haaga, 2001).

More specifically, Mark did not perceive any forms of progress in training to be an achievement. He believed he was only good enough when winning in competition. As a result, Mark consistently doubted his ability to compete at elite level and this was leading to low mood. He also indicated that despite the support from his coach and being reminded that recovery from injury takes time, he never felt 'good enough' and that he could always be better. As a result, Mark was consistently pushing himself without adequate rest and therefore his energy in subsequent training sessions was diminished. As a result of the needs analysis, Mark was invited to receive the REBT intervention, and we discussed what this would entail, and the time commitment required.

The intervention

Unlike much of the research portraying the use of REBT with athletes, the present REBT intervention was delivered using Skype. Skype is a form of online communication software that facilitates video calling at no cost to the practitioner or the individual and has received recent consideration for use in applied sport psychology contexts (Cotterill & Symes, 2014). The advantage of Skype over other forms of electronic communication (e.g., e-mail consultations) in this case was that it provided face-to-face interaction (Bergman, Magnusson, & El Khouri, 2003). The REBT sessions were structured based on guidelines from REBT practitioner handbooks (e.g., David, et al., 2010; Dryden & Branch, 2008), and under the supervision of a certified REBT practitioner. In addition, the reader should note that in my work with Mark I often chose to challenge his As, as well as dispute his Bs. Although the chief aim of REBT is to work with Bs, I found that with Mark it was sometimes very effective to challenge As that were clearly hindering his progress.

Identifying the issue(s) – the 'A'

We began with a training (or psycho-educational) phase in which the athlete received detailed information on the ABCDE process. It appeared he had grasped the concepts and so we moved on to identifying his A in the second session. Mark was encouraged to review his diary in advance of this session and to bring any examples he had recorded during baseline. He appeared to find the exercise challenging, saying he found it, "quite hard to fill in . . . just trying to work out exactly what event led me to thinking, well worrying about failing. . . . It happens literally when anyone brings up a competition or something." Whenever competition was brought up in conversation, Mark said that he would immediately start thinking about what it would be like to lose, what could go wrong, and if he lost, why this might happen. He added, "As soon as I thought about it, you know what if I'm not in the right shape, if I'm not in the right mind-set . . . in the right everything . . . and it's not necessarily just in the gym, it happens at home as well, that I'd be thinking about it [competition]."

Exploring beliefs

We began by looking more specifically at what was causing his self-depreciation belief of being 'not good enough as an athlete'. His comments referred to how hard he was training, his rigorous dietary regime, and his dissatisfaction with the effects of both behaviors on his overall performance. I encouraged him to identify a specific time where he experienced this dissatisfaction. He explained that recently in training, he and some fellow athletes were talking about their plans to compete or not. When he informed them that he would not be registering for a forthcoming competition, they questioned this. He said that he got really frustrated and angry at the fact he didn't feel up to standard, and tried to shift the conversation onto something else. We explored how debilitating this anger was and the impact on his ability to perform. In this specific example he also avoided responding to the question. It appeared that his anger at himself was linked to the subject of competing or not. He also felt ashamed that he got angry in this way in front of the athletes he trained with. I felt that the first step in helping him was for him to better understand this shame.

When feeling shame about getting angry with himself, he was thinking things such as, "The others won't believe me" (inference) and they would also think that he was being ridiculous for thinking that he wasn't fit enough. This, he believed, would also make him feel worse about his lack of ability to compete at elite level. He thought that he should not feel ashamed in front of these people since he has known them for a long time and never felt unable to talk to them in the past. This emotional response to existing negative emotions is an example of a meta-emotional response (e.g., feeling one emotion in response to another; Ellis, 1980). This can be problematic when working with clients. If the meta-emotion is preventing the client from dealing with their primary emotion then it is normally best to deal with the meta-emotion first. We identified that he was angry (primary emotion) at his inability to compete at elite level and that he felt ashamed (secondary emotion) about this anger towards himself, especially in the company of his training peers.

Working with the secondary emotion

The process began by encouraging the athlete to assess his inferences (A) relating to his feelings of shame. We targeted this secondary emotion through empirical investigation of the A with questions such as, "Where are these ideas about the others thinking you're ridiculous coming from?" He was adamant that others would think this way and that he just knew this to be the case, despite a lack of empirical examples. It seemed he was unable to accept that his perceived 'inability to perform at elite level' was actually a part of a process: in order to fight at elite level the athlete may need to experience both success and failure in training and competition. By consistently setting unrealistic expectations of his own performance he was struggling to accept that others might perceive his current standard of performance as 'good enough'. Ellis suggests that self-acceptance is a more functional belief that should be fostered in the therapeutic process. This contrasts with working towards high self-esteem, which he proposed is often conditional upon some form of achievement or positive behavior.

The athlete was also placing rigid demands upon himself (B). We put this experience in context and Mark was asked to list the number of times others had expressed that he was not good enough. He could only recall two instances, one of which was when he didn't know the other people as well as he does now. So, we discounted this as a different situation. Using the second example, we targeted his feeling ashamed of being angry. I asked Mark for the evidence in his example that the others were thinking he was ridiculous (I was challenging the A here). At first his responses were centered on the fact that "he just knew" so I asked again what evidence there was for this and provided examples such as things people had said, how they had reacted to him, etc. He still tried to justify his response but in the end was unable to provide actual instances whereby others had expressed that he was ridiculous. This also helped him to see that his feeling ashamed was only making his anger worse. We explored this a little further. I asked Mark to consider how feeling ashamed was helping him deal with his anger and this appeared difficult for him to understand. Sometimes it is useful to present the relationship between the emotions in a diagram to avoid confusing the primary and the secondary beliefs. This also helps ensure the client is focusing on the same belief as the practitioner. He agreed that it was not helping and I asked what would be a more helpful response to his anger. Again, this was difficult for him so I gave an example. I asked him what would help him be able to start to deal with his anger and he responded with "by not being ashamed". I asked him if other people he knows get angry and if he thinks this is a shameful emotion to have. He did not think so and said that it was okay for them to be angry. He agreed that it was also okay for him to be angry. In essence here, I helped Mark to address A, and challenged it in a way that is more consistent with Cognitive Therapy (CT) than REBT. Mark arrives at some acceptance of his anger, and I did not deem it necessary to dispute his irrational beliefs at this stage.

In preparation for the next session, we agreed to look at his anger towards his inability to compete at elite level. We came up with a scenario involving another athlete who was in his position. He had to pretend to be the one asking why they were angry about not feeling good enough to compete. He was asked to write down what this led him to think about the person. We came up with some initial statements to ensure he understood the task. Before our next meeting, I asked him to continue working on this and to add to these statements. If he was asked about his intentions to compete before our next meeting, I also asked him to think about this scenario to see if he could respond differently and to record any thoughts, feelings, and behaviors that occurred in his diary.

Working with the primary emotion

We began by re-capping on the homework exercise, and it appeared that he was starting to think that he would not think badly of someone for not wanting to compete, nor would he think they were ridiculous for being angry. We moved on to explore what he had previously referred to as the "right everything" that he was expecting of himself to compete at elite level, which was leading to him feeling angry. He was thinking that he ought to be doing better than he was, given how much time he spent training and his ability to stick to his diet. He also thought showing weakness or losing in training would determine whether his coaches thought he was worthy of fighting at elite level in MMA. This was causing him to often over train, therefore leading to fatigue, aches, and pains, and indications that his injuries had not healed completely. He believed he should meet the expectations he had set for himself to be considered an elite athlete and that he should not be losing fights to semi-professional/amateur athletes. To get a better sense of his personal expectations, I asked him to outline the key components that he thought were required of an elite MMA fighter. These were: strong mind-set, good nutrition, and progression in training and competition. In addition, despite the athlete's description previously of not being good enough, when asked about how his training was going, he did show enthusiasm and enjoy-ment. However, due to his recent minor injuries, he also doubted whether he was as good as he was before, stating, "I feel a little bit slower, a little bit weaker almost." So it appeared that he had lost some of his self-belief as a result of these setbacks. He expressed his need to attend every training session on offer to get back to 'peak' level performance.

What we discovered is that aside from the attributes he listed, he had no clear picture of what he was striving for, just that he was not as good as he needed to be to win. When asked what he believed he was capable of, he did believe he could fight professionally and therefore should not lose any fights at semi-professional level. He agreed that this was leading to his worries about losing. He was only able to focus on the fact that he was not yet at professional level and that unless this was the case, he was no good as an MMA athlete. We discussed this belief. He thought he was a long way behind where he needed to be in terms of training despite completing two workout sessions each day of the week. Therefore, his beliefs about his performance appeared unrealistic, and due to his constant self-evaluation, he was only perpetuating this unhealthy belief system. This was lead-ing to fatigue and what appeared to be depressive mood states. Mark expressed that he was lacking enjoyment in the things he previously loved. It seemed that this mind-set was becoming detrimental to his wellbeing. Indeed, past research suggests that over time, high irrational beliefs can lead to physical and emotional exhaustion and burnout (Turner & Moore, 2016).

The fatigue was also affecting his capacity for training. For instance, he was lacking coordination when sparring, missing the pads more than he 'should' be. Despite receiving positive feedback from the coaches, he felt this was not condu-cive to progressing. He felt he needed his coaches to tell him where he was going wrong more often. This appeared to be a second A. I thought at this stage it would be best to focus on the athlete's SD beliefs given the brevity of the intervention.

Disputation

With reference to Figure 8.1, we used inference chaining to explore what would be the worst thing about not doing as well as he thought he ought to do. He responded with, "I would lose in front of everyone." Taking this a step further we assessed what was so awful about this and what it meant about him as a person. His global evaluation was that he would be a failure as a person. It was clear that his identity as an MMA athlete was contributing to a large proportion of his sense of self-worth as a person. I asked him to think of a very similar MMA athlete to himself, who was training hard and following all his dietary guidelines strictly, and whether he thought that he/she should ever lose at elite level. He commented that he knew lots of others in his gym like this who did lose fights. I asked what he thought of them and he described them as committed, talented, and sometimes just unlucky or as having a dip in performance. With this ques-tioning I was trying to dispute the SD belief using a logical argument. Mark was applying one rule to himself, and another rule to others. Finally, as a homework

---

Activating Event (A)

Situation (A^1): Losing a fight
Adversity (A^2): "I would lose in front of everyone"

Irrational Beliefs (iB)	Rational Beliefs (rB)
Demand: "I really want to win and people must not see me lose"	**Preference:** "I really want to win but I don't absolutely have to"
Awfulizing: "It would be awful if this were to happen"	**Anti-Awfulizing:** "It would be bad but it would not be awful"
Self-Depreciation: "I would be a failure as a person"	**Unconditional Self-Acceptance:** "It is never nice to lose but failing at an event does not equal failure as a person. My worth does not diminish if I lose one fight"
Unhelpful Consequences (C)	**Helpful Consequences (C)**
Emotional Consequences: Anxiety (about anticipated shame)	**Emotional Consequences:** Healthy concern
Behavioral Consequences: Reduced performance in training	**Behavioral Consequences:** Better performance in training
Cognitive Consequences: Repeatedly worrying about failure, comparisons with others, and his progress as an athlete	**Cognitive Consequences:** Thinking constructively about failure, comparisons with others, and his progress as an athlete

---

Figure 8.1 ABC form relating to the primary emotion

task, I asked him to write down an example of when he has to confront the idea of competing in his mind (preferably if he could identify one in the period before the next session) and to think about his 'shoulds' in this experience.

Reinforcing new beliefs

At our next meeting, Mark seemed to have been able to identify how his beliefs were impacting his feelings and behaviors. One of the other MMA fighters had asked him whether he was going to compete. He said his response was, "No, because of my fitness and mental frustration. As well, six weeks isn't enough. I . . . I didn't have much confidence." The other athlete responded by saying that six weeks is plenty of time to get in shape. At this point the client's immediate reaction was that this other athlete was just stating what he thought was "an acceptable level of fitness but not one that was good enough for me". However, then he moved on to say that he could see that every situation could be completely unique. He explained:

> The level he's at, well, is different to the one I'm at. I started to then think
> about my beliefs, where my beliefs were coming from, and I think I get these

from the media. From watching the best in the world compete . . . and well, obviously, I'm not at that level . . . I'm not at the level of UFC, which is the equivalent of say the "Premiership", say in football. . . . I was putting myself up against them, and what shape I should be in for my next fight, that sort of thing. Most of the athletes in MMA are, well they're in really top condition. But I was thinking were they doing that at this level, or were they just getting the competitions in? Because, there's a massive difference between the two levels, and of course with the top level they've got access to the best equipment money can buy, they've got . . . it's completely different. I don't know, it's a completely different game . . . I was thinking maybe I shouldn't worry too much, or at least not as much as I am because . . . for my level of competition, I'm in very good shape. But for the absolute elite maybe I wouldn't be. But maybe I don't need to worry about that until . . . I've progressed up.

Two things are happening here. First, Mark's A is shifting from not being good enough, to taking a more balanced view of what level he is at compared to others. Second, Mark's beliefs are shifting in the direction of preferences rather than demands, and it appears that his new ways of dealing with irrational thought patterns are allowing him to have more functional responses to activating events. He realized that his 'should' was based on an unfair comparison with highly elite fighters.

We discussed how the ABC model had allowed him to have a structure to think about his unhealthy emotions. He commented that he could see that he was progressing and "eventually I'm going to get there". He seemed much less 'stuck' and more able to focus on his long-term aspiration of being as good as a UFC fighter "one day" by understanding that this might mean that he also has to lose some fights along the way, but that losing does not mean he is a failure as a person. Instead, competing against a variety of opponents would provide him with the adaptability to fight "better in the long run". We discussed how he felt he was now able to 'unpack' his thought processes and no longer felt he was stuck worrying about his performance in training, but rather he was focusing on just getting better and not thinking, "Why am I not doing this yet, and this yet, and this yet . . .?" He felt that he was still 'moving forward'. Prior to this, he had been asking too much of himself. He agreed that he had set unrealistic, demanding, and rigid expectations of his performance standards.

The second ABC

We had time to revisit the issue around his coaches telling him (or not) where he was going wrong. He commented that it still mattered what they said because they had "seen so much in the sport" and would rather that they provided him with what he was looking for but that he could still progress even if they didn't offer him the support he was anticipating. This was a strategy the athlete came up with on his own and he commented that the ABC process had been useful for him here in understanding why he was allowing his beliefs about their behaviors to have a negative impact on his training. He also felt more capable of changing his own behavior by just asking them instead of waiting for them to provide him with feedback. He felt that he could do this in a way that still maintained respect for the coaches. I felt that this was no longer a distressing issue for him. However, he did comment that he still had worries about losing in certain situations, for example, if the referee stopped the match due to a technicality and therefore having no control over the outcome of the match. To conclude this session, I asked the athlete to find examples of when the referee has stopped matches in the UFC context and to consider his view of these athletes and their overall performance record, as a means of further assessing his beliefs about such situations and establishing a B-C connection, given his stated anxiety. Again, here I was working with and questioning the A, rather than B, because I felt that this challenge might be sufficient to deal with Mark's perspective on referee decisions.

Disputing the second ABC

In the next meeting the athlete brought his examples of referee stoppage. We explored to what degree these impacted the athlete's overall ranking. He agreed that it had had minimal impact. We then established that the referee is also a human being, and he commented that "fighting is like a game of chess, you know . . . it goes wrong sometimes and there's not much you can do about it". He agreed that referee stoppage was one such event. So, I questioned the athlete about what he would do when faced with this worrying scenario. He said he that he wouldn't be able to do anything. When asked what he could do (C) in response to this situation (A), he said that he could move on and start looking towards his next fight, as it wouldn't be helpful for him to dwell on something that he had no control over. He could recognize that in the long run, it's not something that happens very often and would not have a noticeable impact on his ranking, and that even if it did, adopting a preferential and accepting philosophy at B would help produce more functional behavior at C. Thus, Mark found a solution to this issue by adopting more flexible and logical Bs.

Summarizing and reinforcing rational beliefs

It was felt that at this point the athlete had changed his perspective enough that he would be able to approach the subject of competition and competing without getting himself angry or embarrassed. He still appeared to have challenges but was also more capable of dealing with these. He demonstrated an increased capacity to come up with more functional ways of dealing with these. We had one final session where we re-capped on what had been covered, and reinforced his new methods of dealing with events in which he made himself angry or frustrated. We met for a final time to carry out a social validation interview to assess the perceived impact of the intervention on his beliefs about performance. The questionnaires were administered once more to assess the athlete's scores at a post-intervention phase.

Outcome analysis

The data that was collected through the SGABS and USA questionnaires did appear to reflect positive changes from baseline to post-intervention in general irrational beliefs, SD, and USA (see Figures 8.2, 8.3, and 8.4).

Visual analysis

To determine whether REBT had an effect on irrational beliefs, SD, and USA, data was visually analyzed (Ottenbacher, 1986), based on the recommendations (Barker et al., 2013).

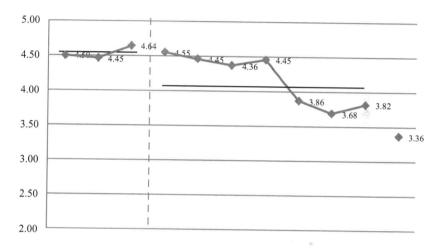

Figure 8.2 Total Irrational Beliefs scores from pre- to post-intervention

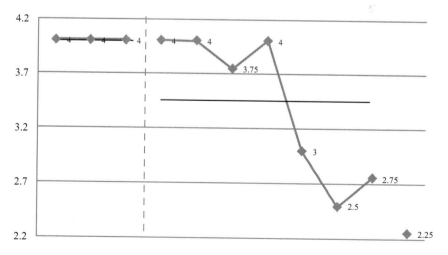

Figure 8.3 Self-Depreciation Beliefs scores from pre- to post-intervention

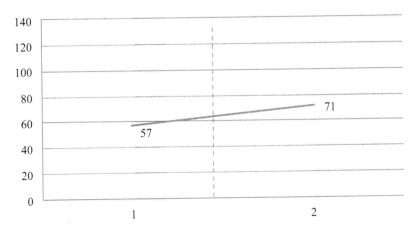

Figure 8.4 Unconditional Self-Acceptance scores from pre- to post-intervention

Statistical analysis

Since visual analysis is susceptible to subjective interpretation the data was assessed statistically. Effect Size (ES) was calculated using Cohen's *d* where $M_1 - M_2$ provides the difference between the mean pre- and post-test scores. SD_1 refers to the mean standard deviation of pre-intervention scores and SD_2 is the mean standard deviation of post-intervention scores:

Cohen's $d = M_1 - M_2 / SD_{pooled}$
(where $SD_{pooled} = \sqrt{(SD_1^2 + SD_2^2) / 2}$)

In an assessment of single-case AB designs, Parker and Vannest (2009) determined that <.87 indicates a small effect whilst .87–2.67 suggests a medium effect with a large effect being anything >2.67.

The athlete showed a medium decrease in total irrational beliefs from pre- (M = 4.53, SD = 0) to post-REBT (M = 4.18, SD = .66; *d* = 1.32). There was also a medium decrease in SD beliefs from pre- (M = 4, SD = 0) to post-REBT (M = 3.43, SD = .66; *d* = 1.22), and a 34% decrease from post- to follow-up phases. The athlete also demonstrated an increase in USA scores (pre = 84, post = 118). At the six-month follow-up phase, his USA scores increased slightly (122).

Practitioner reflections

Although it was felt that the intervention had an overall positive effect on the athlete, I would like to outline some key considerations for the future application of REBT. First, I chose to use Skype to deliver therapy as it allows for a degree of geographical distance between yourself and the athlete (Cotterill &

Symes, 2014). However, the efficiency of these sessions was subject to having a good Internet connection at both sides of the communications. Some sessions were interrupted to fix video and sound problems, thus breaking the flow in the session. One session had to be cut short, as we were unable to resolve the audio quality. However, due to Skype, the sessions could be arranged to take place at a convenient time for the athlete who had a lot of external responsibilities and sessions could be changed at short notice.

Engaging with the athlete in his process of evaluating activating events did add valuable detail to the questionnaire results. The interactive component provided greater depth of understanding of the athlete's experience. It also encouraged me to look at the whole picture and to not be overly concerned with the significance or reliability of change in irrational beliefs and SD. Indeed, it was often effective to help Mark dispute his As. It helped to reinforce that the aim of implementing the REBT approach with this athlete was to help him to be able to approach challenges that were once leading to ineffective behaviors and emotions, and to deal with these in a way that was conducive to better performance outcomes rather than dogmatically stick to REBT no matter what. Therefore, reflecting on reflections has been useful in my self-development as a scientist-practitioner (Shapiro, 2002) in which theory has guided practice. By recording my thoughts immediately following each session I was then able to re-visit these at the end of the whole process. I believe this helped to enhance and consolidate my learning as an REBT practitioner and helped to better understand the root of this athlete's issue. Within applied sport psychology, intervention effectiveness is believed to rely on providing individualized treatment in a systematic way (Barker, et al., 2011). It was felt that this was achieved in the present case through continual evaluation of practice.

Nonetheless, I am aware that credible results in applied sport psychology are important but that it is important not to lose sight of client expectations whilst still aiming for 'significant' results. I believe that in relation to REBT specifically, this could be aided using more sport-specific measures (irrational Performance Beliefs Inventory; Turner et al., 2016). In the present study, being transparent about the findings was a conscious decision. It not only allowed for practitioner development but also for an accurate reflection of how future research might learn from this case study. Sharing honest experiences in applied practice may prove beneficial to enhancing practice, therefore not only advancing theory, but also creating a more established network of REBT practitioners in sport psychology.

Applying REBT to my own thoughts, cognitions, and behaviors

The more I use REBT with others the more I feel I adopt the same disputation of unhealthy beliefs myself. What I have experienced is an almost subconscious internalization of statements such as, "It's not the end of the world". I have consciously heard myself say these things and realized that, "that's that REBT stuff". Admittedly this can sometimes be a painstaking experience, as it seems to heighten personal awareness of my responses to events. For example, when in session with a client, I have experienced an over-evaluation of my responses to them. This can result in less time spent focusing on just dealing with the client's issue. In these cases, I do not always know the depth of the client's issue until I listen to the recording. Nonetheless, these experiences are infrequent, and generally with experience, they are becoming less of a problem.

REBT has at the same time encouraged me to not try so hard to do what is 'right', both in practice and in my other role as a researcher. I feel less compelled to appease the needs of others and certainly engage in a lot more self-care than I ever have. It does feel like the REBT process has helped me be more accepting of the days when things don't quite work out, or when I just cannot be bothered for whatever reason. What the REBT process has also taught me is to take more responsibility in these situations: to accept that if I behave in a certain way then it will have certain consequences that won't always necessarily be positive, but that that is okay. I like to consider these experiences by asking myself, "Would your 80 year old self care about 'x'?" and generally I find the answer to be no. In some ways I feel like I have really been able to engage in my roots in existentialism and phenomenology: by living more authentically through REBT.

References

Barker, J., McCarthy, P., Jones, M., & Moran, A. (2011). *Single case research methods in sport and exercise.* Oxford: Routledge.

Barker, J. B., Mellalieu, S. D., McCarthy, P. J., Jones, M. V., & Moran, A. (2013). A review of single-case research in sport psychology 1997–2012: Research trends and future directions. *Journal of Applied Sport Psychology, 25*(1), 4–32. doi:10.1080/10413200.20 12.709579.

Bergman, L. R., Magnusson, D., & El Khouri, B. M. (2003). *Studying individual development in an interindividual context: A person-oriented approach.* Mahwah, NJ: Lawrence Erlbaum.

Chamberlain, J. M., & Haaga, D. A. (2001). Unconditional self-acceptance and psychological health. *Journal of Rational-Emotive and Cognitive-Behavior Therapy, 19*(3), 163–176.

Cotterill, S. T., & Symes, R. (2014). Integrating social media and new technologies into your practice as a sport psychology consultant. *Sport & Exercise Psychology Review, 10*(1), 55–64.

David, D., Lynn, S. J., & Ellis, A. (Eds.) (2010). *Rational and irrational beliefs: Research, theory, and clinical practice.* Oxford: Oxford University Press.

Dryden, W. (2009). *How to think and intervene like an REBT therapist.* London: Routledge.

Dryden, W., & Branch, R. (2008). *Fundamentals of rational emotive behaviour therapy: A training handbook.* Chichester: John Wiley & Sons.

Ellis, A. (1957). Rational psychotherapy and individual psychology. *Journal of Individual Psychology, 13,* 38–44.

Ellis, A. (1977). Psychotherapy and the value of a human being. In A. Ellis, & R. Greiger (Eds.), *Handbook of rational emotive therapy.* New York, NY: Springer.

Ellis, A. (1980). Rational-Emotive Therapy and cognitive behavior therapy: Similarities and differences. *Cognitive Therapy and Research, 4*(4), 325–340.

Ellis, A. (1985). Intellectual fascism. *Journal of Rational Emotive Therapy, 3*(1), 3–12.

Ellis, A., David, D., & Lynn, S. J. (2010). Rational and irrational beliefs: A historical and conceptual perspective. *Rational and irrational beliefs: Research, theory, and clinical practice*, 3–22.

Ellis, A., & Dryden, W. (1997). *The practice of rational-emotive behavior therapy*. New York, NY: Springer Publishing Company.

Harpold, M. E. (2008). *The mental cage: A qualitative analysis of the mental game in the sport of mixed martial arts* (Unpublished master's thesis). Georgia Southern University, Statesboro, Georgia.

Lindner, H., Kirkby, R., Wertheim, E., & Birch, P. (1999). A brief assessment of irrational thinking: The shortened general attitude and belief scale. *Cognitive Therapy and Research, 23*, 651–663. doi: 10.1023/A:1018741009293.

Little, John (1996). *The Warrior Within – The philosophies of Bruce Lee to better understand the world around you and achieve a rewarding life* (illustrated ed.). New York, NY: McGraw-Hill.

Massey, W. V., Meyer, B. B., & Naylor, A. H. (2013). Toward a grounded theory of self-regulation in mixed martial arts. *Psychology of Sport and Exercise, 14*(1), 12–20.

Ottenbacher, K. J. (1986). Reliability and accuracy of visually analyzing graphed data from single-subject designs. *American Journal of Occupational Therapy, 40*(7), 464–469.

Parker, R. I., & Vannest, K. (2009). An improved effect size for single-case research: Non-overlap of all pairs. *Behavior Therapy, 40*(4), 357–367.

Russell, M. (2000). Summarizing change in test scores: shortcomings of three common methods. *Practical Assessment, Research & Evaluation, 7*(5), 1–4.

Shapiro S, D. (2002). Renewing the scientist-practitioner model. *The Psychologist, 15*(5), 232–235.

Turner, M. J., Allen, M., Slater, M. J., Barker, J. B., Woodcock, C., Harwood, C. G., & McFadyen, K. (2016). The development and initial validation of the irrational performance beliefs inventory (iPBI). *European Journal of Psychological Assessment*, ahead of print issue.

Turner, M. J., & Moore, M. (2016). Irrational beliefs predict increased emotional and physical exhaustion in Gaelic football athletes. *International Journal of Sport Psychology, 47*(2), 187–199.

Vaccaro, C. A., Schrock, D. P., & McCabe, J. M. (2011). Managing emotional manhood fighting and fostering fear in mixed martial arts. *Social Psychology Quarterly, 74*(4), 414–437.

Editors' commentary on Chapter 8: "Mixed Martial Arts and the paradox between self-improvement and self-acceptance: a Rational Emotive Behavior Therapy (REBT) intervention"

Rachel's chapter successfully highlights the impact that negative global self-evaluations can have on the pursuit of an individual's values and goals, and how difficult such issues can be to talk openly about. In clinical practice, it is striking how often emotional disturbance, whatever the diagnostic label that has been attached, can be traced back to difficulties with self-acceptance and a demand that the individual be better, or closer to perfect, than he or she perceives themselves to be (Bennett, 2017). It is no surprise to see this issue arising in a sport and exercise context, since athletes are human too. What Rachel expertly notes in this chapter is the centrality of these beliefs in coming to an understanding of Mark's perceived lack of progress. Whilst the coach identified Mark as one of those who might benefit from "mental training", it is unlikely that the coach or even Mark himself anticipated that the subsequent intervention would end up addressing fundamental existential questions such as, "Am I good enough?" Yet, this is exactly where the intervention ended up, identifying a demand for perfection and the depreciating belief that to fail in an MMA event would indicate that Mark was *a failure as a person*.

Human evolution, and our history of living together in social groups for hundreds of thousands of years, has led us to develop a very keen awareness of whether we are 'good enough', when compared to our peer groups. We are incredibly skilled at noticing even the slightest indication of disapproval or rejection, and the cost of this talent is that our minds can suggest rejection to us when it is not even present. Practitioners using REBT are well advised that this approach has the potential to get very deep very quickly. The ABC model, with its focus on self-acceptance, is an excellent technique for uncovering long-standing negative beliefs about the self. Whilst clients presenting for therapy in clinical contexts might be prepared for this type of soul-searching, it seems reasonable to assume that many athletes might not be, and they can quickly find themselves in a position of revealing more than they had bargained for. This is not necessarily a problem, and as in Mark's case, may ultimately be beneficial, but practitioners will benefit from keeping this in mind, and ensuring that they handle such issues with skill and sensitivity, particularly in certain sporting contexts where self-disclosure and expression of painful thoughts and emotions may be actively discouraged.

Reference

Bennett, R. (2017). From esteem to acceptance: Contemporary perspectives on the self. *BPS Psychotherapy Section Review, 59*, 8–15.

9 The use of Rational Emotive Behavior Therapy (REBT) with an anxious sub-elite fencer

Evangelos Vertopoulos

Introduction

Fencing is an individual sport with a variety of complex characteristics. Apart from the fitness, strength, and endurance it requires, fencing also requires very fine motor skills. It requires the ability to sustain the focus of attention, an ability to perceive, to elaborate and react very fast to rapidly occurring and changing visual cues, an ability for instant decisions, tactical thinking, as well as high inhibition of action and purposeful change of decision while already executing an action (Czajkowski, 2005). In addition, fencing is an individual sport in which the athlete does not share victory or defeat with his or her co-athletes. Moreover, fencing brings the athlete opposite to an opponent and this gives a character of personal confrontation to many athletes (Czajkowski, 2005). As far as this interests the REBT sport psychologist, the element of personal confrontation may raise issues of conditional self-acceptance or self-depreciation. In case of a defeat or a failure to meet one's objectives, this may result in self-defeating emotions, thoughts, and behaviors. In case of winning, conditional self-acceptance may result in arrogance, a trait that does not seem to help the athlete in the long-term (Turner & Barker, 2014).

Introductory information

For the purposes of this chapter the client's name will be Chris (pseudonym). Chris was a female fencing athlete who contacted me to help her overcome the psychological obstacles she was experiencing. The reason for her decision to contact me was her knowledge of my previous experience as a fencing athlete and coach, apart from being a sport psychology professional. Her fencing goal was to establish herself within the top eight athletes in her country. My work with Chris took place mainly at my office, as she had approached me independently of her team. However, in some instances I observed her compete. After a point during this collaboration with her I observed some of her training sessions as well, and I had the opportunity to speak with her coach. When meeting at my office, our sessions lasted approximately fifty minutes, but when our meetings took place at the gym before or after her training, we often had only a few minutes. However, these sessions were tightly related to her training and focused on briefing or debriefing her on psychological skills that she would work on during training. We preferred to work within the office context on issues that involved emotions and disturbance, apart from specific instances when she experienced disturbed emotions at the gym.

Presenting issue

After an icebreaker conversation, a semi-structured interview was conducted so that I could gather information on her history in sport and fencing, the importance of fencing in her life, her goals and perceived obstacles, and her request for the present consultation. As is often the case with athletes who practice their sport at a competitive level, fencing had a central role in Chris's life and fencing seemed to be a major determinant of her identity, self-esteem, and mood.

Chris came to the first session with a specific agenda. She reported losing her concentration when she competed, not being able to maintain her perception of distance (which is a crucial prerequisite for fencing), and emotional outbursts when things did not go well. During the initial assessment, it seemed that the amount of training and the fencing experience of the athlete were sufficient so that the reported issues could at least partly be attributed to psychological causes as opposed to shortcomings in training quantity or quality. An interesting point was that she identified two specific situations in which her concentration and focus were disrupted. One was when she faced an opponent that she perceived to be a novice and the other was when she faced an opponent she did not like on a personal level. Lastly, she reported finding it very difficult to handle failure, although failure seemed to be an abstract concept, which was relative to each different context. For example, losing to a superior adversary was not considered a failure while losing to a novice made her "a complete failure".

Needs analysis

Observing the cues that Chris gave me from the first session allowed me to identify possible causes of the emotional and behavioral/performance disruptions she reported. Her discourse was ego-related and she seemed to attach an intense self-depreciation meaning to the examples she gave. She would become emotional when she talked about what success and failure would indicate for her as a person.

Performance profile

A performance profile was conducted within the session to assess her perceptions of her current training status and help her identify specific areas for improvement. She identified nine descriptive characteristics of a 'good fencer' and rated her status with reference to these. The areas she identified were: perception of distance, speed, reaction times, accurate point, footwork, technique, strength, concentration, and staying calm in competition. Her lowest scores were in the areas of concentration and ability to stay calm in competition. She also noted a need for improvement in distance perception and technique. Chris took a copy of her performance profile to show it to her coach and ask him to create a similar profile for her. Her coach added some characteristics, namely, control of the distance, length of attack, speed of hand, speed of feet, hand-foot coordination, hand-technique, foot-technique, and self-confidence. His scores were similar to Chris's although he gave a lower score in technique and gave a low score in the hand-foot coordination characteristic.

Chris accepted her coach's version of her performance profile without any objections. Before the profile reached me, she had discussed it with her coach and she had identified both the need for a more elaborated version which would include the additional attributes as well as the lower scores her coach gave her in technique and hand-foot coordination. She stated that receiving her coach's feedback helped her.

Cognitive ability

One thing that remained to be assessed was the client's cognitive ability, which is a prerequisite for all cognitive approaches in therapy. Early on during our sessions and meetings I identified a difficulty in thinking with analogies and metaphors. Initially I assessed this observation further, and I chose to reduce the use of abstract examples, analogies, and metaphors, as they would create confusion. Examples were used only if they were concrete and simple.

Another identified pattern of thinking emerged from the fact that her discourse did not stay focused but spread across different subjects that she perceived to be interlinked. She often recalled and linked childhood experiences to each topic. It seemed that her present performance and concentration issues were attributed to older experiences. This need to present me all the information, and to link her existing performance issues to her past experiences, was something to be further assessed.

Suitability of REBT

The needs analysis identified the need to simplify her thinking to be able to focus more on the present, on her ability to achieve her goals (internal locus of control), and to hierarchize perceived stimuli. The information that Chris shared with me either explicitly or implicitly strengthened my belief that REBT would be the preferred approach to help her build a more functional attitude towards her fencing goals and perform without experiencing dysfunctional emotions. REBT can be short-term, focuses on results, and works both with cognitions and behaviors. In addition, REBT often prefers to work with the 'worst case scenario' and this approach sets a more realistic context for the athlete who often demands, awfulizes, depreciates oneself, and expresses frustration intolerance.

Even though Chris's lack of high analogical thinking set a challenge, REBT theory suggests that flexibility in therapy is legitimate in order to customize therapy to the client's individual characteristics (Ellis, 1962; DiGiuseppe, et al., 2013). Flexibility does not mean adopting a different approach, but choosing effective techniques and using them within the REBT theory framework (Ellis, 1962). Above all, REBT is the approach that suits me and is the one I have chosen to be trained in and apply, and one of the reasons for my choice was my belief that it is a well-founded scientific approach which would be effective especially for people who are results driven, like athletes.

The intervention

REBT is an approach that comprises the cognitive as well as the behavioral component to help the person overcome emotional and behavioral dysfunction. In sport psychology literature, the cognitive and the behavioral components are often viewed independently. Relaxation techniques, imagery, self-talk, and other confidence-enhancing techniques, as well as other behavioral tools, are sometimes used in a superficial way, without consideration of the emotional factors or the irrational beliefs that cause dysfunctional emotions. So, the athlete may learn how to momentarily relax herself, but does not learn how not to be unhealthily angry or anxious. REBT focuses on irrational beliefs to change dysfunctional emotions to their functional alternatives, and, to enhance its effectiveness, it also teaches the athlete all the necessary psychological skills since they can now be founded on a healthy emotional state.

Moreover, REBT is not dogmatic. In its extensive literature, it is widely agreed that many therapeutic techniques and tools can be applied, even if these have their roots in other approaches (Ellis, 1962; DiGiuseppe et al., 2013; Dryden & Neenan, 2003). However, these tools are deployed within a framework of REBT theory. REBT may be flexible, however, its theory affects all the employed techniques in important ways. So, even if a 'person centered' approach is employed for certain reasons and for a given period, this is always channelled via an REBT point of view, resulting in a more 'rational' and empathic style, but still REBT. So, REBT is by definition a flexible, integrative, and non-dogmatic approach that directs itself according to the client's interest and individual characteristics.

From the initial sessions, it became apparent that Chris experienced unhealthy emotions both during training and competition, which had a negative effect on her performance. The identified emotions were anxiety, depression (non-clinical), and hurt, and the beliefs assessment revealed that her irrational beliefs were ego-related. See Figure 9.1 for a typical ABC form for Chris. I explained to Chris the causal relation between her beliefs and the emotions she experienced (the 'B-C connection' in REBT terminology) and then, following a Socratic approach, she understood how her performance was linked to her emotions and beliefs. It was also discussed that training in relaxation techniques and concentration skills was not very effective for her, as her emotional disturbance was cancelling out or disrupting these efforts. Chris understood the logic behind the B-C connection and

A	B	C
Perceiving that winning is not certain, e.g., "I might lose"	**Demand:** "I do not want to lose, therefore I must not lose"	**Cognitive C:** Enhancing catastrophizing
	Derivative 1 (Self-Depreciation): "And if I lose, I will be worthless"	**Behavioral C:** Focuses on the feared outcome and does not focus on the present moment and the necessary action in order to perform better
	Derivative 2 (Catastrophizing): "This will be the worst thing that could happen"	Loss of focus Quitting Maximized possibility of losing
	Derivative 3 (Frustration Intolerance): "And I can't stand losing"	**Emotional C:** Anxiety, anger, depression

Figure 9.1 ABC formulation

agreed that her irrational beliefs should be addressed first. A number of irrational beliefs were identified during the work with Chris. These included:

- *Demandingness* (e.g., "I very much want to win, therefore I must win"; "I am better than my opponent, therefore I must win this"; "I desire success and therefore I must always succeed"; "I have put in so much effort, so I have to succeed"; "I want to enjoy training and competition in order to be able to focus and put in the necessary effort, and therefore I must")
- *Frustration intolerance* (e.g., "It will be difficult for me if I lose, so I could not bear losing; "I cannot stand the pressure of the competition")
- *Self-depreciation* (e.g., "I am what I do, therefore if I fail I am a failure"; "I am worth my successes, so if I do not succeed I am unworthy"; "if important others do not approve of me then I am unworthy"; "if I lose to an inferior opponent then I am a total loser")

Early in the initial needs analysis Chris seemed to lack awareness of her emotions and thoughts, especially when in stressful conditions. A guided discovery approach was adopted to help her distinguish the existence of functional versus non-functional emotions and their relationship with a person's beliefs. This relationship had to be re-taught several times in order for her to understand it. The REBT notion of the B-C connection was explained with the use of different examples so that she understood that her beliefs are the decisive factor for her non-functional emotions. In addition, relevant between-session practice was assigned to her to increase her emotional and cognitive awareness. This between-session practice comprised keeping a log with sets of Incident/Experienced Emotion/Thoughts/Behavior or Tendency for Behavior. This homework was discussed every time in the next session and it was used to choose a specific example of her disrupted focus and emotions and to implement the REBT model.

Scope of agenda

As is often the case with athletes, the session agenda did include issues outside of her sport. This occurs for two main reasons. First, the athlete is a person, not just an athlete, whose life contains many different roles and interests and naturally he/she can ask for issues to be included in the session agenda. Moreover, athletes are affected by events surrounding their personal, family, or school/occupational lives. Second, the belief system according to which the athlete functions within his/her sports role often presents itself in other domains, and working on issues seemingly irrelevant to the sports role may be in fact quite relevant to it. However, since the client's request for our collaboration concerned her fencing career, we always linked our work on the session agenda to her fencing effort and goals.

Cognitive techniques

REBT suggests that in order to experience functional emotions – and therefore be able to perform better – one has to adopt a more functional belief system. For a more functional way of thinking to emerge one can *dispute* existing dysfunctional beliefs and create and strengthen their functional alternatives. This disputing process aims to help the person perceive and experience the flaws of his/her current thinking and adopt a new, more functional philosophy. The three main disputation styles of REBT were used with Chris. Logical disputing aims to help the person understand the illogicality of present beliefs ("I want to win, but I don't absolutely have to"). Empirical disputing brings the person to identify and accept reality, and examine demands and whether reality supports what he or she demands ("I must always win, but the truth is that there is a possibility of me losing"). Pragmatic disputation examines how helpful it is for the person to adopt a certain way of thinking ("I must always win, but if I think like this I get anxious and this does not help me at the end"). All three disputation styles were employed with Chris, however, not all were equally effective at all times.

A typical ABCDEF process for Chris which shows the perceived adversity (A), irrational belief and its three derivative beliefs (B), the belief's cognitive, emotional, and performance consequences (C), the disputation of each of the beliefs (D), the new, more effective and functional belief (E), and the emotional, cognitive, and performance consequences of the new belief (F) can be seen in Figure 9.2.

Chris found it difficult to understand logical disputing. The reason for this was partly her linguistic confusion as she was confusing the meaning of 'want to'

Activating Event (A): Facing a less experienced opponent

Adversity (the most difficult inference drawn from this event/situation): "I may lose to a less good fencer than me"

Irrational Beliefs (B)	Rational Beliefs (E)
Demand: "Since I am better than my opponent, I want to win, therefore I must win"	**Preference:** "Of course I want to beat this opponent, but I do not absolutely have to. I might as well focus on my game and do the work"
Awfulizing: "It would be the worst thing if I lost to this opponent"	**Anti-Awfulizing:** "If I lose, this is going to be a bad experience, and I will have to work harder to correct my mistakes, nevertheless it will by no means be the worst thing that could happen. I will still have the capability to work and get better, so it will be a setback but it will not be a catastrophe"
Frustration Intolerance: I could not stand losing from such an opponent	**High Frustration Tolerance:** "It will be difficult to tolerate the frustration if I lose, but it is certain that I will stand it. It will be worth standing, in the service of improving my game"
Depreciation (Self/Other/Life): "I am worthless and a failure. I am ridiculous"	**Acceptance (Self/Other/Life):** "It will be a failure, yes, but this will not make me a worthless person or a failure or ridiculous. It will make a fallible human being who has failures and successes in life, and this was one defeat. Even if I lose I will still have the ability to work on the game's feedback, and get better"
Unhelpful Consequences (C)	**Helpful Consequences (F)**
Emotional Consequence: Anxiety	**Emotional Consequence:** Concern
Behavioral Consequence: Lack of concentration, passivity when competing	**Behavioral Consequence:** Good control of movements, taking initiative during the game, accuracy
Cognitive Consequence: Negative thinking, focus on uncontrollable parameters	**Cognitive Consequence:** View game and opponent as challenge
Physiological Consequence: Threat state (trembling, increased heartbeat)	**Physiological Consequence:** Vigilant but in control

Figure 9.2 Expanded ABC formulation

and 'must'. In order to deal with this confusion, at first we clarified the meaning of each phrase, however, this proved to be more difficult than expected, so we agreed to keep her understanding that 'want' is more absolute than 'must'. As sessions moved on, Chris gradually started to understand the correct meaning and identified her initial difficulty in the rigid demandingness she had. Empirical disputation was also not producing the desired results as Chris kept resisting accepting reality and used passionately her desires as arguments that provided support for her demands.

The most effective disputing approach was pragmatic. When asked whether her irrational beliefs served her goals, Chris understood that her beliefs kept her from working for her goals in better terms. As a personal reflection on this, it seems to me that she was in a pre-contemplation stage when she first came for counselling and it would be wiser to first work towards helping her be motivated to change before getting into the ABCDE process. However, after a number of sessions, it was possible to dispute her beliefs empirically and logically but only after pragmatic disputation. If another style was attempted first, she became resistant and emotional.

As the layers of the onion gradually peeled off there was always a self-depreciation belief at the core and this became the priority and main point of focus. Chris accepted herself under certain conditions and these conditions included success and achievement. If she did not succeed then she did not consider herself worthy, which boosted her demandingness for success. Chris responded well to demandingness disputation, and gradually to frustration intolerance and catastrophizing, even though this seemed to be a superficial improvement, a so called intellectual insight, which still was a long way from reaching emotional insight (Ellis, 2002). However, when it came to self-depreciation, Chris resisted hard and even intellectual insight was difficult for her.

A number of approaches were used in order to enhance unconditional self-acceptance. The ones that seemed more effective and had a breakthrough to Chris's harsh judgment of herself were the ones that led her to distance herself from her own perspective and consider specific examples of other people. Following this tactic, she started to understand that failing does not make one a failure and worthless being, however, when she was asked to transfer this perspective to examples that concerned her, she resisted. It took quite some effort and repeated shifts to pragmatic disputation for her to start exhibiting signs of unconditional self-acceptance. Chris was often assigned with between-sessions practice that was related to unconditional self-acceptance, as her self-depreciation emerged in every problematic performance she talked about. Examples of such practices were reading related books, and considering whether other people around her were worthless or failures due to their mistakes and failure to achieve goals.

A source of difficulty resulted from her low emotional and cognitive awareness. To overcome this deficit, I chose to be as concrete as possible during sessions. Another choice was to use either only pragmatic disputing or, even if other disputation styles were employed, to always start from this functional position. This helped her identify that her best interest was to quit her usual way of thinking and motivate herself to embrace the rational alternative, even if she resisted it initially. One source of resistance was stemming from her 'psychoanalytic' thinking. Chris had a strong belief that, "My past and my experiences define my present and my future". This deterministic way of thinking had to be brought to awareness, and assessed to see if it served her goals and disputed if it did not. However, she seemed to hold on quite strongly to this 'knowledge' that she cannot escape her past experiences, and logical, as well as empirical disputing, was not effective. What was more effective was again pragmatic disputing, since it helped her to perceive that believing her past negative experiences condemned her for life does not help her achieve her goals.

Chris had undergone psychoanalysis in the past and she had adopted a psychoanalytic point of view. More specifically, she had two patterns. Either she wondered what the causes for her disturbance were, and/or she expressed the belief that her past experiences were the causes of her disturbance in the present. However, she used this knowledge in a deterministic way. She would consider her present disturbance as unavoidable, because as she believed, she was sentenced and could not do anything to deal with past traumas. Dealing with this challenge helps me value the usefulness of REBT, especially when working with clients who are goal driven in life, like athletes. It seems that REBT has specific advantages compared to a psychoanalytic approach. As Albert Ellis first noted, it is more short-term and does not focus on identifying the historical causes of the disturbance, but focuses on the present and on helping the individual achieve a positive emotional change that will help him/her function and perform better. Even if past experiences have had an impact on the person, REBT focuses on how these past experiences are elaborated in the present and deals with them rather than accepting them as deterministic misfortunes. So, REBT helps the person enhance internal locus of control and this change promotes action versus frustration and resignation.

Emotive techniques

As soon as Chris had been accustomed to the ABCDE model, and had learned how to dispute her irrational beliefs, she was taught rational emotive imagery (REI), for her to experience the discomfort and the disturbed emotion she experienced during competitions. In a specific instance, Chris was asked to imagine that she started very badly in a certain match and was behind 7–1 in score. She was asked to remember and imagine/experience all the details of this event, until she experienced the maximum anxiety possible. When she signalled that she had reached this point, she was asked to try and change her anxiety into its more functional alternative which we had named 'concerned to win, but not stressed-out to win'. Gradually Chris learned to use REI more effectively and practiced it between sessions, as a tool that would also help her be more prepared and accustomed to negative instances like being behind in score, listening to others criticizing her, and being eliminated early in a competition.

Therapist style is important in REBT. The therapist often expresses oneself in a vivid way, as in role-plays or during disputation process. This emotive style was employed with Chris, especially during disputation of her irrational beliefs, as well as when we disputed her rational beliefs. The 'zig-zag' and the 'court-room' technique were used. In both these emotive techniques the client has to defend her belief and its derivative beliefs while the therapist attacks them and tries to dispute them. Chris initially had difficulty in defending her newly formed rational beliefs and she fell back to re-adopt her irrational beliefs. When this happened, I chose to dispute again her irrational beliefs, following the three basic disputing styles (empirical, logical, pragmatic). Chris gradually started to be able to defend effectively her rational beliefs and started to exhibit a shift from intellectual insight to emotional insight, at least concerning some of her superficial beliefs and some of her core ones.

Behavioral techniques

Along with the ABCDE part of my work with Chris, several behavioral techniques were used to facilitate her concentration and reduce the tension caused by her unhealthy emotions. One such tool was learning how to breathe and use diaphragmatic breathing as a relaxation technique. Of course, relaxation did not aim to change Chris's beliefs or emotions. Instead its role was to offer her a tool to reduce the physiological tension, which was a consequence of the dysfunctional emotional arousal. Chris could learn to change her emotion from dysfunctional to its functional alternative (concern instead of anxiety), however, and especially in competition context, athletes do not always have the luxury of time in order for the effects of emotional regulation to affect positively their over-arousal. Emotional disturbance may occur and then a more adequate portfolio of techniques – cognitive, emotive, and behavioral – can be necessary to help athletes deal with the situation. Chris learned and practiced breathing, although she mentioned that she found it difficult to 'let go' of her tension. When this statement was assessed further, she replied that even when alone she 'could not' let herself relax. Further assessment revealed a fear to let go, which stemmed from the belief, "I should not rest if there are things to be done". This belief took the form of resistance when we tried to use breathing as a part of relaxation in which she would also close her eyes. She resisted that and claimed that she could not allow herself to relax. This brought new irrational beliefs to the session, which were assessed and disputed at a later point, for the session to keep focused. Such beliefs included, "I want to have control of things in my life, therefore I must be in control at any moment for everything", "I cannot bear lack of control", and "It is awful not to be in control, and I am a failure if I am not always in control". Consequences included constant tension, lethargy, and not allowing herself to rest enough.

Between-session practice

Chris was advised to practice some cognitive, emotive, and behavioral exercises between sessions. At our first sessions when it was evident that Chris lacked awareness of her emotions and thoughts, she was advised to keep a log, where she would note instances in which she became disturbed, along with her thoughts at that moment, her emotions, and her behavior. This exercise helped her to understand better the link between her thoughts and her emotions. It also helped me to have specific examples of her disturbed emotions and performance to use in the ABCDEF process. As noted earlier, Chris learned how to use REI and practiced it between sessions, as well as when mentally preparing for a competition. Reading was also suggested to her. She found the books of Windy Dryden on anxiety, self-acceptance, and hurt especially useful. Chris also practiced relaxation breathing, and muscular relaxation.

Chris also did essay writing. At the beginning these writing assignments were about helping her remember her life accomplishments in order to enhance her confidence and self-appreciation. As soon as we had worked on the ABCDEF process and we had formed a new rational belief, she was advised to write the new functional belief down, and elaborate on it critically many times per day. As Chris became more capable at disputing her irrational beliefs and defending her rational ones, she undertook zig-zag exercises, but she found it difficult to support her rational beliefs. This was indicative of the robustness of her rigid beliefs.

Effectiveness of work with Chris

Inferences on the effectiveness of the approach that was adopted in this case could be drawn from Chris's feedback, from her coach's feedback, from her competition results, from the data gathered by me via questionnaires, and from her behavior within therapy. Chris stated that her most important benefit from our work together was that she understood and accepted that, "As much as I would like it to happen, no one is going to grant me victory. Unfortunately, I have to work hard and exhaust myself in order to claim victory. So, I had better shut up and do the work. Life may be unfair, but there is no reason why it should not be".

Chris attributed her enhanced quality of training as well as her good competition results to her improved attitude. She stated that she perceived "clearer thinking" and an "ability to stay focused on the specifics of her performance" and these allowed her to be more concentrated, overcome adversities, and focus on the things that were within her control rather than to worry about uncontrollable issues. Chris's coach also gave positive feedback. According to his observations, she gradually became more cooperative, with less emotional outbursts, enhanced concentration, and "remarkably more focused during competitions". She also had a more "professional" approach in competitions, following discipline-specific pre-performance routines. Her results were also positive as she achieved and overcame her goals, establishing herself at the first four of her country's ranking for the last year.

Her irrational beliefs scores (measured using the Shortened General Attitudes and Beliefs Scale [SGABS]; Lindner, et al., 1999) also indicate a more rational way of thinking, as Chris's scores on rational beliefs improved (see Figure 9.3). Her irrational beliefs were reduced, especially self-depreciation, need for achievement, and need for approval scales. Her results were surprising to an extent as she continued to be quite resistant within sessions, especially when we had a longer period without sessions. Her feedback, when I expressed my thoughts, was that

	Start of Intervention	*After Eight Months of Intervention*
Rational Beliefs	2.00	3.50
Self-Depreciation	3.75	2.25
Other-Depreciation	1.33	1.67
Need for Achievement	4.50	3.25
Need for Approval	3.33	2.33
Need for Comfort	2.50	2.75
Demand for Fairness	2.50	2.25

Figure 9.3 Pre- and post-intervention SGABS scores

she could understand the logic behind the statements, however, when sometimes events overwhelmed her she found it more difficult to control her emotions. I considered this feedback a manifestation of intellectual awareness but still not achievement of emotional awareness, and discussed with her my suggestion that our work should be more consistent without large intervals.

Reflections on working with Chris

What made my work with Chris especially interesting was the fact that she had a complete understanding that her performance disruptions did not have simple, one-dimensional causes, but instead, they were the result of a rigid belief system that formed self-depreciation cognitions. So, we had the opportunity to work from the beginning on her beliefs and not to lose time trying to help her by teaching psychological skills. Most athletes come to my office with specific requests and some of them bring along the belief, "I want the psychologist to solve my difficulties immediately and in a practical way, therefore he must accomplish this expectation of mine". But, working on psychological parameters is exactly like training. It requires consistency, frequency, and hard work. Chris understood this from the very beginning and this helped her, even though she often became very resistant when her core irrational beliefs were tackled.

Finally, athletes' lives have many more aspects and these either affect their reported issue or are brought in the agenda autonomously. So, in working with athletes it is not enough to work only with their sport-related issues, but also to help them with their life in general. Working with Chris covered both aspects well.

References

Czajkowski, Z. (2005) Understanding fencing. *The unity of theory and practice.* New York, NY: SwordPlay Books.

DiGiuseppe, R., Doyle, K., Dryden, W., & Backx, W. (2013). *A practitioner's guide to rational-emotive therapy* (3rd Ed). New York, NY: Oxford University Press.

Dryden, W., & Neenan, M. (2003) *The rational emotive behavior therapist's pocket companion*. New York, NY: The Albert Ellis Institute.

Ellis, A. (1962). *Reason and emotion in psychotherapy*. Secaucus, NJ: Lyle Stewart.

Ellis, A. (2002) *Overcoming resistance* (2nd Ed.). New York, NY: Springer.

Lindner, H., Kirkby, R., Wertheim, E., & Birch, P. (1999). A brief assessment of irrational thinking: The shortened general attitude and belief scale. *Cognitive Therapy and Research*, *23*, 651–663.

Turner. M. J., & Barker, J. B. (2014) *What business can learn from sport psychology: Ten lessons for peak professional performance*. Oakamoor, UK: Bennion Kearny Limited.

Editors' commentary on Chapter 9: "The use of Rational Emotive Behavior Therapy (REBT) with an anxious sub-elite fencer"

When we learn about REBT and become trained in its application, it is all too easy to forget to apply the REBT philosophy to our own functioning as practitioners. In this chapter, Evangelos importantly reminds us that REBT is by definition flexible, integrative, and non-dogmatic, meaning that REBT can fit alongside and can include many other approaches to working with athletes. The use and integration of REBT with other approaches are really dependent on the client's needs, highlighting the importance of a detailed and thorough needs analysis in the early stages of our work with athletes.

As early practitioners, having learned a host of REBT skills that we were eager to use, we were probably quite 'dogmatic' about REBT too, and probably used REBT rigidly. This is common in neophyte practitioners, and is part of the learning process. But with experience, we arrive at Evangelos's idea of integration, driven by client needs, rather than our desire to implement REBT too rigidly. As REBT practitioners working in sport and exercise, we find that it is often effective to consider REBT as one's underlying theory of emotion and behavior, and in the needs analysis, try to conduct as thorough an assessment as one can. In the data collection and initial conversations and exploration with clients, if irrational beliefs emerge, then it makes sense to pursue REBT as a course of action. However, it is possible at the same time to help the client to develop other psychological skills for performance enhancement. An athlete can learn to dispute irrational beliefs, while also developing their ability to apply relaxation, for example. Being an evidence-based practitioner is really important, but it is also important to be non-dogmatic about approaches. The goal is to help the athlete, not prove or disprove theory.

10 Rebounding from injury and increasing performance using Rational Emotive Behavior Therapy (REBT)

Murat Artiran

Introduction

The main focus of this case study is work with Deniz, a 19-year-old professional Turkish basketball player. The work was completed within 4 months over ten sessions. This chapter details the use of Rational Emotive Behavior Therapy (REBT) with the client, including case formulation, and the methods and techniques used throughout the treatment process. Deniz was referred to me by the former captain of the team at her sports club. The reason she came to therapy is because she was emotionally disturbed by her injury and not able to concentrate on games. At the first session, she also brought some issues about her family and her team members, which caused her to have depressive symptoms. After the first session, I observed that she was catastrophizing her injury and that she had self-depreciation beliefs. She also had some relationship problems with her family and teammates. She was thinking about quitting basketball; however, she gave herself a chance to continue following therapy. I thought REBT could help her to overcome emotional disturbances and to help her to find the right decision regarding the continuation of her sport. After sharing the ABC model of REBT and the notion of dysfunctional emotions she had, we discussed whether it was her beliefs or events that led to her anxiety. She seemed to mostly subscribe to an A-C model. That is, Deniz believed that what had happened to her (injury, difficulties with significant people in her life, etc.) was causing her emotional and behavioral issues. In overcoming practical and emotional difficulties it is important to first understand that, "People are disturbed, not by things, but by the principles and notions which they form concerning things" (Epictetus, c. 55 – c. 135 AD). Therefore, I thought it might be helpful to use REBT, and I explained to Deniz that, in fact, events or situations may affect us but our thoughts and beliefs about those events make us disturbed (the B-C connection). She found the idea interesting and she wanted to work on this. Before initiating the session, psychometric measures were taken. These included the Attitudes and Beliefs Scale – II (DiGiuseppe, et al., 1988) for irrational beliefs but for anxiety, the Competitive State Anxiety test (CSAI – 2; Martens, et al., 1990) was used; and for self-confidence, the State Sport-Confidence Inventory (Vealey, 1986) at pre- and post-REBT.

Session 1

"Critical A"

A brief case history of the client was elicited, alongside information regarding Deniz's family, her educational background, her general activities and interests, and lastly her future plans. I then established the reasons why Deniz thought the therapy was necessary and the issues Deniz wanted to resolve. Recently, Deniz had experienced some major adversity. She had ruptured the tendons in her knee and had had surgery, which was affecting her performance in rehabilitation. She also stated that another reason for the decrease in her performance was her fear of injury and lack of self-confidence, stemming from her belief that she could never play as well as she did before. She also indicated that her family criticized her all the time after her injury, hinting at the idea that she should quit playing basketball. In addition, her club did not appear to care about her recovery and left her alone through her rehabilitation, which led Deniz to feel let down. The new team she was transferred to played in a less prestigious league, further decreasing Deniz's feelings of esteem as a competitive athlete.

Deniz dreamed of playing in Turkey's premier league, and felt she was competent enough to do so provided she "reined in" her psychological issues. Her fear of injury, however, prevented her from training as hard as she thought necessary. In addition, Deniz struggled with anger, which resulted from the overtraining that led to the injury. This issue also affected her relationships with her teammates. Her team had mocked her during practice and via Facebook by posting her photo when she was crying after a game in the locker room. According to Deniz, the other team players' attitude towards her was almost as difficult to handle as her injury, and was one of the major factors affecting her performance.

I gave Deniz some brief psycho-education about REBT, the ABC model, the four core types of irrational belief, and unhealthy negative emotions. Corresponding to the ABC model in REBT, I asked her to give me some information about the activating event (A) which was most bothering her. I then probed for a "critical A" besides an activating event in order to understand the most significant side of the event for Deniz. According to REBT theory, "A critical A is that part of the 'A' which triggers your client's irrational belief which is at the core of unhealthy negative emotion" (Dryden and Branch, 2008, p. 87). After she gave me some typical examples regarding the three problems described earlier, I started to explain the ABC model to her using a white board. As we approached the end of our first session I told her I would continue to introduce REBT to her in the following week.

Session 2

ABC model and irrational beliefs

In session 2, I continued to describe the ABC model and irrational beliefs. We tried to illustrate the model by following the activating events and emotions she recounted in the last session. I told her about the B-C link and we discussed the meaning of the aforementioned Epictetus quote. I gave her the example of "100 people and 100 different ideas", where 100 people with a very similar problem (like an injury or losing a game) evaluate the situation in 100 different ways. When she said she understood the B-C connection, we started to do in-session role-play. I explained the role-play process to Deniz and asked her to take my place and become a therapist. During the role-play she asked me to give an activating event that had triggered her unhealthy negative emotions last week. I told her my car had broken down on the way to work and I was late, which caused me to have feelings of anger and frustration.

Deniz's irrational beliefs

According to DiGiuseppe, et al. (2014), the four irrational beliefs are defined thus: *Demandingness* is an unrealistic and absolute expectation of events or individuals being the way a person desires them to be. *Awfulizing* is an exaggeration of the negative consequences of a situation to an extreme degree, so that an unfortunate occurrence becomes "terrible". Low frustration tolerance (LFT) stems from demands for ease and comfort, and reflects an intolerance of discomfort. Finally, *Global Depreciation* of human worth, of life, the self, or others, implies that human beings can be globally rated, and that some people are worthless or, at least, less valuable than others. I formulated the case in these terms. We talked about this in the session, and I tried to uncover the irrational beliefs using the inference chaining technique:

C (Deniz):   I felt a pain in my knee the other day while I was doing circuit training (A).

T (M.A.):   What is the most significant thing about this particular "A" that is bothering you?

C: I felt as if my injury would relapse and some thoughts came to my mind such as, "I won't be able to get in the team and I won't play basketball anymore".

T: Let's just assume for a moment that your injury will really re-occur and you really won't be able to play in the first five and maybe you will never be able to play basketball in the professional league. What would this mean to you? (inference chaining)

C: My career would collapse and I would have no goal in my life.

Deniz's initial ABC is detailed in Figure 10.1. As we continued inference chaining, we determined that Deniz's irrational beliefs reflected demandingness, awfulizing, and self-depreciation ("I must be able to continue to play as a professional basketball player otherwise it will be catastrophic, and I will be a failure"). The fact that her leg was not the same as before seemed to be the end of the world for her. Her demand was that her leg and her ability to train with her full force should go back to the way they were before the injury. I identified this as

Situation: Felt pain in the context of a prior injury
Adversity: "I'm going to relapse and I won't get into the team. My career will collapse"

Rational Beliefs	Irrational Beliefs
Demand: "I want my career to continue and therefore it absolutely has to"	**Preference:** "I want my career to continue but it does not absolutely have to"
Awfulizing: "If it does not continue, it will be a catastrophe"	**Anti-Awfulizing:** "If it does not continue, it will be bad but it will not be catastrophic"
Self-Depreciation: "If it does not continue, I will be a failure"	**Self-Acceptance:** "If it does not continue, that would not make me a failure as a person"

Unhelpful Consequences	Helpful Consequences
Emotional:	**Emotional:**
Depression/anxiety	Sadness/concern
Behavioral:	**Behavioral:**
Difficulty concentrating	Improved concentration
Urge to quit basketball	Motivation to continue playing
Avoiding certain positions when playing	Playing with greater freedom

Figure 10.1 ABC formulation of presenting problem

the primary irrational belief we would work to change. I hypothesized she was demanding fairness and comfort (DiGiuseppe et al. 2014), and I understood from her statement, "I shouldn't be injured and I must be recovered fully to play as well as in the past".

In the session, two further major issues appeared when we talked about her emotional state. One of the problems besides injury was the hostile attitude of her friends, and her family's attitude towards her basketball career. Also, her parents' statements that she should quit playing basketball really bothered her. This was another example of demandingness. Deniz had a firm idea about what other people should think about her ("My parents should agree with me about my basketball career, and I must have their support"), greatly adding to the emotional disturbance that she had already experienced due to her injury. She suggested that she had feelings of disappointment and depression when her parents acted as if they didn't want her to play basketball anymore. To help summarize the session, I drew out an illustrated ABC model to clarify her situation, illustrated in Figure 10.2.

Deniz confirmed her understanding of the ABC model and indicated that it was an appropriate summary of what she went through. Key to her experience was an irrational depreciation belief ("If my parents do not approve of me, I am worthless" or, "If I do not get support from my family this means I am not loveable"), since Deniz clearly disturbed herself about her parents' idea that she should quit playing professionally. After I provided psycho-education about emotions according to REBT literature (anxiety, depression, anger, guilt, shame,

Situation: Parents criticizing the decision to continue playing
Adversity: "I'm going to relapse and I won't get into the team. My career will collapse"

Rational Beliefs	Irrational Beliefs
Demand: "I want my parents to approve of me and support me"	**Preference:** "I want my parents to approve of me and support me but I don't absolutely need their approval and support"
Awfulizing: "If I do not get into the team it will be a catastrophe"	**Anti-Awfulizing:** "If I do not get into the team, this will be hard but not catastrophic"
Self-Depreciation: "I am alone, a failure, and worthless"	**Self-Acceptance:** "I am not alone, and not securing their approval does not make me a failure or worthless"
Unhelpful Consequences	**Helpful Consequences**
Emotional: Depression/anxiety	**Emotional:** Sadness/concern
Behavioral: Crying daily Arguing with parents Social isolation Urge to run away	**Behavioral:** Emotional stability Better relationships with parents Socially more engaged

Figure 10.2 ABC formulation regarding perceived criticism

envy, hurt, and jealousy), Deniz and I agreed that her primary disturbing emotion was anxiety, followed by a secondary emotion, depression. She found these two emotions always close to her, but this realization only dawned on her in the session. I ended the session by giving Deniz some reading to complete about REBT.

Session 3

Secondary emotion

Deniz had read the information about REBT given to her the previous week. We briefly talked about what she thought about REBT, the ABC model, the B-C connection, and irrational beliefs. Then, I made another brief presentation about emotions in REBT and why the emotions in REBT are not separated quantitatively, but qualitatively. According to REBT, functional and dysfunctional emotions are qualitatively different, which means that there are two distinct dimensions (the functional and dysfunctional; Digiuseppe et al., 2014). The classical CBT approach usually handles dysfunctional emotions in a single graduated classification. For instance, one CBT therapist may ask a client to specify a number from one to ten, to indicate to what degree they feel anxiety. This is a quantitative approach to identify clients' disturbed emotions. On the other hand, in REBT, we categorize emotions as unhealthy negative and healthy negative emotions and try not to identify them by their intensity; rather, we label them as two different emotions – for instance, sadness or depression, concern or anxiety, regret or guilt. I explained to Deniz that REBT focuses on qualitatively changing emotions, rather than simply reducing emotional intensity, like anxiety or depression.

We started work on her primary (anxiety) and secondary (depressive) emotions. During the session, Deniz said she had depressive feelings and crying moments almost every day, in response to stressful situations, such as being teased by her teammates, her coach yelling at her, or her parents' lack of support. She reported to me that experiencing "heavy sadness", and anxiety, reflected her low self-esteem. According to REBT there are eight unhealthy negative emotions (depression, anxiety, guilt, shame, jealousy, envy, anger, and hurt) that cause disturbance. REBT limits dysfunctional emotions to these eight, and identifies eight more healthy (but still negative) alternatives. Thus, I needed to identify whether her "heavy sadness" was indeed "depression", which would help me find a healthy alternative.

In order to understand whether Deniz's emotions were healthy or unhealthy I needed to look at a number of things. Firstly, was there a physical aspect to her "heavy sadness"? Since Deniz described having stomach aches and pain in her leg the answer was yes. Secondly, was there a dysfunctional behavior that Deniz engaged in while experiencing this emotion? The answer was also in the affirmative. She would cry and socially isolate herself. Finally, was the feeling caused by an irrational belief? Yes, Deniz described herself as "worthless" (depreciation). As a result, I concluded that the "heavy sadness" Deniz reported could indeed be identified as "depression". Another point of interest was how long, how frequently, and how intensely she experienced this emotion. She had been experiencing this emotion, to this degree, for 6 months, such that she wanted to be left alone almost every day and to "leave everything and run away". This further indicated that "depression" was the emotion Deniz experienced.

It is important to note that according to REBT, individuals don't *feel* worthless, but rather *evaluate* themselves to be worthless. I clarified this to Deniz, explaining that "worthlessness" is not an emotion but a "belief". The General Semantics Theory (Korzybski, 1933) used by Albert Ellis in his work states that the individuals are often unable to use words appropriately and relevantly, so they become dysfunctional and confused. Thus, using words improperly negatively affects one's psychological well-being. Deniz understood the importance of making this distinction, and made an effort to describe her emotions and beliefs accurately.

Thus, we formulated Deniz's irrational belief as follows: "I must be loved and approved of by the people around me and those who are important to me. If I am not, I am a worthless and useless person". We agreed to continue to do weekly activities in between sessions, including an ABC record form, where she could document and separate her emotions and beliefs about various activating events during the week.

Session 4

She can't make it into the team!

During our fourth session, Deniz and I examined her ABC activity. She took careful notes on the ABC form, and we went over them together, clarifying the As in a simple way. I pointed out the difference between the inferences and irrational beliefs as we read. After reviewing the homework assignment, I asked whether she had something she wanted to talk about that day. She said that she felt "like a loser", because she spent most of the practice time sitting on the bench, not allowed to play. I asked some follow-up questions in order to clarify Deniz's thought pattern. My aim was to establish the emotion she experienced and the beliefs that led to the emotion. In her mind, not being asked to play meant disapproval and being unloved. She did not see being benched for most of the practice as related to recovering from an injury. She reported having similar emotions when benched prior to her injury, only now they were exacerbated by her depressive state of mind.

REBT strives to establish a B-C link, that is, the link between beliefs and emotions, rather than an A-C link. REBT says that the cause of the problems is "B" rather than "A". Therefore, once we had established that Deniz felt unloved and disapproved of, I could begin to dispute her beliefs about this. My clinical experience says that anxiety and depression are experienced together most of the time, and have many symptoms in common. For example, issues such as getting easily irritated, a decline in self-confidence, physical indications, and emotions of despair often co-occur. Thus, if anxiety is experienced together with "sadness" in some cases, it may lead the "sadness" to turn into depression because of the consequences of increased stress. About 85% of individuals with depression have significant anxiety, and 90% of individuals with an anxiety disorder have depression (Tiller, 2012). According to Dryden, even when they are of low intensity, disturbed emotions are still disturbed (DiGiuseppe et al. 2014). In my opinion, neither anxiety nor depression develop suddenly; it is a gradual process from sadness and concern to depression and anxiety. Frequency, intensity, and duration can make a healthy negative emotion propagate an unhealthy negative emotion. Once I was sure Deniz understood the ABC model, I used a didactic method, followed by an imagery technique:

T: Your current belief is "I must be loved or approved of by people that are important to me otherwise I am a worthless and useless person". This belief may lead to depression. If we substitute a rational belief instead, namely "I would prefer to be loved and approved of by people that are important to me; however, I don't have to be loved and approved of all the time and I still see myself as valuable in those cases", do you think that you can possibly have this kind of belief? Can you do it?

C: I will try. I guess I can do it.

T: Now let's try an imagery technique. I want you to imagine a situation where your coach yelled at you during a basketball match, "I didn't allow you to join this team so you could play like that!" Can you practice thinking about this in two different ways? First, think about the way you do it now – your coach disapproves of you, which means you are a worthless player and a useless person. Notice how this irrational belief is causing you to feel depression and maybe even guilt. Then, after 30 seconds to 1 minute, think of the rational beliefs you can apply here, and feel that you are just sad, but not depressed. Can you do it?

C: I can do it.

For Deniz's next homework, we agreed that when faced with a stressful situation she would ask: "What is the advantage of holding irrational beliefs and rational beliefs in my mind?" and she would take some notes about each option. She would monitor and analyze the impact of her irrational beliefs on emotional, behavioral, and interpersonal relations. She would then categorize these irrational beliefs, and sort their advantages and disadvantages relating to each situation. This would help her become aware about the connection her mind made between the beliefs and thoughts she had about each situation, and begin to adjust her thoughts to healthier patterns. Seeing B-C connections and which type of belief creates emotional disturbances is the first part of the therapy.

Session 5

Rehearsal of rational beliefs

It is important to determine and monitor the goals of therapy in REBT. For Deniz, the goals were to continue playing basketball, to maintain her concentration and performance during games, to avoid being influenced by the negative behaviors of others, to overcome the anxiety stemming from her injury, and to keep her performance high. At the beginning of the fifth session, we reviewed the goals, and examined what Deniz gained or lost due to holding on to her irrational beliefs.

While we discussed Deniz's notes and goals, another issue came up. Once the self-destructive and self-constructive ways of thinking were identified, how would they translate to action? The purpose of REBT is to help us become aware of, and change, our underlying irrational and destructive beliefs to rational and constructive ones (Eisner, 2007). Using this as a starting point, we worked on strengthening Deniz's rational beliefs, and weakening the irrational ones. We used some role-play activities and writing assignments in the session to practice constructing rational beliefs.

In the role-play activity, I took on the role of Deniz's coach, parents, and friends, and we tried to approximate the typical situations that Deniz faced in her daily life. I asked her to repeat the sentence "Being loved and approved by other people is important; however, I don't absolutely have to have love and approval" throughout the role-play activity. This was meant to support the rational belief and to explain why this belief is always the more helpful one. Deniz reported that her crying now occurred less often. She did not feel moved to tears all the time as before, and her voice did not immediately begin to break during these confrontations, as it had done before. She also said that she had become more indifferent to situations in which she had become tearful before. I was not sure if that was functional, or a kind of avoidance behavior in this case. I decided not to address this at the time, as I strongly believed it was indeed related to her adopting rational beliefs. In order to test this in the context of REBT I asked her to give me an example of an event:

C: My trainer yells at me and I cannot say a thing, even though he is not right. That makes me cry.
T: Is this crying out of anger or depression? What do you think?
C: Both. But depression mostly.

After she said that crying is related to depression, I tried to find out what unhealthy anger does to her, in terms of its impact upon her behavior.

T: What about the unhealthy anger? Who is it directed at?
C: Both towards myself and others.
T: Does the anger affect your performance during games as well as exercises?
C: It absolutely does.
T: What is our goal in this therapy?
C: Not to let my performance be influenced by all these events.
T: Then, do you think it would help you to maintain your performance if you can regulate your anger?
C: It may help, of course.
T: Then if I offer you an idea that changing your beliefs about events is not enough but that you could repeat the beliefs until you automatically use them in everyday life, what do you think?
C: I'll try it.
T: In order to feel something different to unhealthy anger, we might train healthy anger by thinking, "I don't want him to yell at me, but even if I do not like it, he can yell at me anyway". And feel the annoyance.
C: Am I going to do this without questioning the belief of "he must not"?
T: Absolutely! Just repeat it to yourself.

I reminded Deniz that REBT suggests that people do not "absolutely" need to be accepted and loved, even though this may seem to be highly desirable (Corey, 2008). We spent the rest of the session working on her irrational beliefs and the B-C link between her beliefs and behavior. I was assured once again that Deniz understood the REBT theory very well. After reverse role-plays she was able to explain the theory and demonstrate its application properly to me. She explained her thoughts, emotions, and experiences according to the ABC model and recognized the four irrational beliefs without my help.

Session 6

A buzzing mosquito over my head!

In the next session, we talked about the anxiety and anger Deniz experienced as a result of her injury. The anger she felt stemmed indirectly from the frustration of being injured. Just an hour before our session, Deniz faced another situation, where her coach told her she would not be allowed to play that week. He also made her play in the substitute team during the practice. We classified this as the activating event (A). Deniz said she had no idea why her coach did this. The inference she made from this was that he did not like her. There was some progress in that Deniz did not tell herself that she was a worthless player. This time, she became healthily angry with her coach instead of directing the emotion at herself. I wanted to examine her anger.

T: What did you do when you got angry? (The purpose of the question was to be sure if the unhealthy negative emotion was really there or not.)
C: Nothing. I kept playing. I was just a little ticked off.
T: What do you mean by ticked off? I mean, did you have any loss of concentration or performance?
C: No, I did not.
T: Then what does it mean to you that your coach told you that he won't give you a chance in the next game?
C: He always tells me that I don't have any self-confidence, but I do have self-confidence. I just cannot shine because he doesn't give me enough time during the games. I know myself, I am a good player but I am just afraid of getting into certain positions when playing due to my injury. On the other hand, his hostile attitudes towards me, or his saying things like: "I won't let you play; I don't know why I even let you into the team", do not mean anything to me at all anymore.
T: Do you find this unbearable?
C: Hmm. No, it's not. I can handle it, I am learning REBT (smiling).
T: So, we can say that it's a kind of disappointment but we can't say that it's genuine anger at that time, right?
C: Yes, I can't call it anger. It's just like a mosquito buzzing over my head!

After checking whether unhealthy anger was present, I concluded that there was no need for disputation.

Session 7

Anti-awfulizing

During this session, we put emphasis on Deniz awfulizing the injury. Deniz had serious concerns regarding her career, stemming from that issue. In her current state at that time, she reported no problems in training or during games. Also, despite admitting that she played well enough to attempt being admitted into a higher league, Deniz still felt afraid that her injury might relapse, in which case she would have to quit playing altogether. She also said that sometimes she could not imagine herself playing in a higher league because of her injury. This potentially demonstrated two main disturbances – awfulizing and demandingness. However, realizing that Deniz's demandingness stemmed also from being a professional athlete and always pushing herself harder, I first tried to dispute awfulizing ideas during this session. Some clients find it easier to understand why derivative beliefs are more irrational than demandingness. Some principles in CBT suggest that if the person has multiple problem areas, they should be realistic, and at first take a relatively new or easier problem (Hughes, et al., 2014). Therefore, Deniz and I took the smallest and easier part of the problem (awfulizing an irrational belief rather than demandingness) and tried to solve it and then stepped up to harder ones. I asked her about the worse-case scenario:

T: Suppose that your injury seriously relapsed and you could never play basketball as a professional again; what would it mean for you?
C: I can't really think of that because I have many years to come, I'm so young, and I can do so much in the sport. It would be really bad.
T: Is this affecting the way you play in your current state?
C: Yes, sometimes when I push myself really hard, I feel this pain in my leg and it scares me. I avoid going into some difficult positions or forcing my leg in a game. And with this kind of anxiety constantly recurring, I get the blues.
T: Can we talk about two emotions then? First, one is your fear of getting injured again, and the second one is the frustration you experience due to your fear of injury.
C: Yes, completely.
T: What do you do when you get scared or get anxious about it?
C: I avoid everything in play; I cannot make any moves.

Having already understood the REBT theory, Deniz was aware of the connection between irrational beliefs, emotions, and behaviors. In this case, it was her anxiety and fear of injury. Since the link was already established, I planned another activity – a *behavioral exposure* assignment. I asked Deniz to animate the movement where her leg felt forced the most. She said the most difficult position was turning on the leg. I asked her to perform the movement in slow motion. As she went through the motions of turning, I applied functional disruption by asking Deniz to keep in mind the idea that irrational beliefs about her injury were not healthy, and would stop her from reaching her full potential as an athlete. Instead, she was to think that getting injured would be very bad – a rational belief – but not the end of her career – awfulizing. Deniz knew that, if she wanted to continue playing, she could not entirely avoid moving in ways that would strain her leg. However, instead of her thinking irrationally about the possibility of injury, I asked her to try and think rationally in order to feel concern. Even if some pain occurred as she moved, it would be cause to move a little more carefully, instead of stopping the movement. We repeated the exercise three times. I told Deniz to use this activity on her own throughout the week, and report back at the next session.

Session 8

Summarization

We had our eighth session two weeks later due to Deniz's intense training schedule. We summarized our earlier sessions, and reviewed the ABC model and how to use disputation techniques, role-plays, and behavioral rehearsal workouts. We also, once again, summarized our therapy goals.

At the end of the session, I asked Deniz to perform another role-play in order to check if she had learned the concept of rational beliefs and healthy emotions as a result. This time, she became the therapist, and I took on the role of the client. I relayed my problems, similar to those Deniz faced, and gave her an opportunity to dispute my irrational beliefs. I even made it harder for her from time to time, to check that she could indeed detect irrational beliefs and substitute them with healthy emotions and rational beliefs. She completed the task with competence. She was able to successfully use the functional dispute ("Does holding this awfulizing belief help you get rid of your problems?") and logical disputation ("Where is it written that 'they must like you' or 'approve' of you?"). She could comprehend the idea of disputation and prepare herself for real events.

Session 9

Results

Three different methods of feedback were relayed in this session. I received the feedback from Deniz and then we conducted the psychometric measurements through pre-test and post-test, after which I jotted down my own observations about her development during sessions.

Verbal feedback from the client:

T: After our short, but intense, sessions lasting 10 weeks I asked: "What are your gains if there are any, and what has changed for you? Have the sessions influenced you in any way?"

C: Yes, first of all, I think that I learned a lot about human psychology and thinking processes. Now, I guess I see things and events around me more clearly. I can understand and explain my behavior better. For instance, if something bad happens to me, I can control myself, and take time to think instead of crying as I used to. For example, when my teammates joke about me in the locker room, I evaluate this, and realize that I have a tendency to over-react to what they are saying.

I noticed that Deniz now talked about her rational belief, namely "they don't have to be nice to me", in a different way. When it comes to REBT, one cannot expect a rational belief to be explained completely and clearly, or in one full sentence. Sometimes, as in Deniz's case, clients express rational or irrational beliefs in their own way.

C: My sense of analysis of events or situations is more enhanced. I don't react to everything happening right away. I analyze the event first before I react.

T: How do you think learning about the four irrational beliefs helped you?

C: It really helped me. I use them when I'm under stress and when they come into my mind. For example, after we lost a match, my coach told me off, saying "you're earning so much, is this how you play in exchange?" and so on. But I didn't cry, or say anything. I just waited and listened to him. I can't always remember all we talked about in the therapy at the moment, however, I see myself getting less and less influenced by these events, especially when I evaluate the event afterwards. My episodes of feeling bad are fewer and will reduce in time.

T: Can we say that you recover from the negative effects more quickly?

C: Yes, definitely. But here's the thing, these types of events are happening less in my life. For example, my teammates' mocking me is gone for good.

T: Just like your fear of injury or feeling unworthy . . .

C: Yes, I feel like the events where I feel that way have started to happen less and less. For example, I have fewer quarrels with my parents. I don't insist on making them accept my ideas about how my future should be. I'm not determined to change their thoughts.

What we see here is that while flexible thoughts are developing, demandingness and irrational beliefs are reduced. I also believe that Deniz's quicker recovery time from negative moods and events is important in terms of the gains made from therapy.

T: Can we say that you have become more realistic?

C: I used to feel the need to depend on people around me. I felt loyalty to an "unnecessary" extent. However, now that I analyze the events and cases first, I automatically get more realistic. I have decided to become a basketball coach, and I am working on getting my certificate for that. I plan to make an agreement with a club, to both play and coach as an assistant coach. I still want to play in the league, and continue my professional sporting life. I want to work for a club where I can play first string. Also, I ultimately want to establish my own sports club.

T: You still want to be a professional athlete?

C: Being a professional athlete is not certain right now. I can't say that I enjoy playing in the same way as I used to, before my injury. I need to keep conditioning my leg, as I still have some pain. I can't get into a team without working hard.

T: What about your leg? Can it take the hard exercises?

C: If I work out, it can. But I read an article the other day, which said that 70% of people with my injury get injured again in the same way. However, I will keep playing. I am not afraid anymore.

It seems that Deniz's goals have changed and may possibly become more exciting. She now plans to be a coach, and establish her own club in the future. She still has some concerns about her injury, but this was now only a concern, and not anxiety.

Psychometric measures

According to the results (Figure 10.3), a decline can be seen in Deniz's irrational beliefs and a large increase can be observed in her rational beliefs. When we examine the State Sport-Confidence Inventory total scores, we can see that Deniz's score increased from 90 to 116. In general we can assume that Deniz's confidence increased significantly after the REBT intervention. For anxiety, a decrease is observed in Deniz's total scores. According to her scores she has increased her rational beliefs, which have provided her with a clear mind to think efficiently about her problems. She says that she now thinks flexibly in stressful events, such as when her coach yells at her in a training session. She says she doesn't care about being yelled at but she stays focused on her play more than in the past. Deniz's results suggest that REBT helped her identify and reduce irrational beliefs and successfully create a B-C link in her thoughts and behaviors. Her thoughts and reactions changed in a way that allowed her to have a more

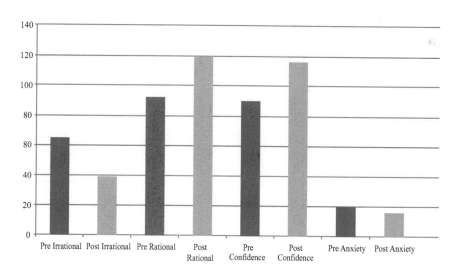

Figure 10.3 Pre- and post-intervention irrational beliefs, rational beliefs, confidence, and anxiety

realistic expectation of herself and her environment, and her outlook on her career prospects and personal relationships improved.

The therapist's observations

When I started working with Deniz, I discovered that she had another issue, unrelated to her injury, which she saw as affecting her performance. She reported that her lack of confidence often interfered with her playing to the best of her ability. This was a problem not directly resulting from Deniz being a professional athlete. Many people, across many spheres of life, struggle with a lack of confidence. However, when I observed Deniz, I concluded that issues with confidence and perceived humiliation directly affected her performance as an athlete. As our sessions progressed, Deniz did not show much improvement on this issue. I wondered if it was because we concentrated primarily on the issues directly relating to her injury. However, this changed during our last session. We had a two-week interval in between our two last sessions, and when I saw Deniz after the break, her personal style had changed. She was confident, crystal clear when she spoke, and had the air of someone who believed she could solve her problems. She appeared to think less about what happened in the past, and to be more decisive. As she talked about her problems, she did not appear hopeless, overwhelmed, or confused, as she had in our previous sessions. She seemed to believe that she would find a solution for every situation in her life. She was more realistic about her goals, and less stressed. She analyzed situations, instead of reacting to them.

Conclusions

According to the psychometric measures taken at the beginning and end of the sessions, as well as both mine and Deniz's own observations, she made significant progress with REBT. She showed outstanding improvement in terms of performance and injury fear. However, the greatest progress she demonstrated was the decrease in her demandingness, which led her to be more flexible and non-dogmatic in her view of her career and relationships. She also demonstrated less emotional disturbance, appeared to value herself more, and had a clear and realistic plan for her future.

One of the primary hypotheses of REBT is that our emotions are the reflection of our own beliefs, evaluations, reactions, and deductions (Corey, 2009). In this case study, we decided that the source of the lack of performance Deniz experienced was the anxiety (A = her injury, B = demandingness and awfulizing beliefs), depression (A = attitude of her parents, coach, and friends towards her, B = demandingness and depreciation beliefs), guilt, and being angry at herself and others (B = demandingness beliefs). I conducted the sessions using Ellis's method, which states that the client does not have to *feel* better after each session. Rather the emphasis is on the process of tuning the client's psychology in a way, which allows him or her to think in a more helpful way about events and people in his or her life. In this method, as well as in Deniz's case, this was achieved by changing the client's beliefs and behaviors and by realizing a "profound philosophical change" (Ellis, 1972a; 1972b; 1979). One of Ellis's ideas, borrowed from Korzybski (1933), was that we need to possess the ability for a more scientific way of thinking in order to live our lives with better and more appropriate emotions. This idea became very pronounced in Deniz's own feedback to her therapy sessions. She reported being able to analyze events and situations, rather than to blindly react to them.

This case also has provided clues that REBT may be useful as a preventative technique, rather than only as therapy for a previously diagnosed psychopathological disorder. This is especially true for certain aspects of REBT, like the ABC model, consolidating the difference between the irrational and rational beliefs, imagination technique, role-play, and assertiveness training. All these can be useful to anyone in their daily life, and can be incorporated as a useful part of any professional training or education. REBT overlaps with the cognitive-behavioral therapies (CBTs) of Aaron Beck (1976), Donald Meichenbaum (1994), and David Barlow (1996). This case is also an example of a CBT intervention. However, the emphasis REBT makes is on hot cognitions (evaluations), instead of cold cognitions (automatic thoughts, inferences) in general. In this case, I concentrated strictly on hot cognitions.

In Deniz's case, REBT has proven to be a useful tool in achieving positive results. I want to thank Deniz for this case study, which I believe will contribute to future psychotherapy studies. I notice that absorbing new effective rational beliefs is a difficult task for clients but at the same time it can lead to permanent changes in clients' psychological health. In REBT, therapists may need to put a lot of effort into sessions and many or all of the following ideas might be utilized: use as many techniques as possible, keep checking the client's recent experience, answer clients' questions about the model, hold the client in this model without allowing them to digress, dispute clients' irrational beliefs, and help rehearsal of rational beliefs.

I worked on irrational beliefs rather than other cognitive structures. One could work on cold cognitions instead of hot cognitions. Irrational beliefs are evaluative cognitive mechanisms and posit rigid, extreme, unrealistic, and illogical appraisals of our cold cognitions such as automatic thoughts (Walen, et al., 1992; Ellis & Dryden, 2007) and inferences, attributions, rules, assumptions, and schemas (Beck, 2011; Leahy, 2003). I choose to work strictly on irrational beliefs as hot cognitions. In my opinion, change from alterations to cold cognitions always tends to be temporary. In order to maintain permanent change, we need to seek philosophical change (primary causal cognitive mechanisms) rather than secondary causal cognitive mechanisms in the development of emotional reactions. At this point I see that we (my client and I) might need additional time to discuss a wider-reaching and more generalizable philosophical change, although ten sessions were not enough in this case. Over time and with practice, REBT skills will hopefully become automatic for her, like making sandwiches or driving a car.

References

Barlow, D. H. (1996). Health care policy, psychotherapy research, and the future of psychotherapy. *American Psychologist, 51*,1050–1058.

Beck, J. S. (2011). *Cognitive behavior therapy: Basics and beyond* (2nd ed.). London: The Guilford Press.

Corey, G. (2009). *Theory and Practice of Counseling and Psychotherapy*. Belmont, CA: Thomson Brooks/Cole.

DiGiuseppe, R. A., Doyle, K. A., Dryden, W., & Backx, W. (2014). *A practitioner's guide to rational emotive behavior therapy* (3rd ed.). New York, NY: Oxford University Press.

DiGiuseppe, R., Leaf, R., Exner, T., & Robin, M. V. (1988). *The development of a measure of rational/irrational thinking*. Paper presented at the World Congress of Behavior Therapy, Edinburgh, Scotland.

Dryden, W., & Branch, R. (2008). *The fundamentals of rational emotive behaviour therapy: A training handbook.* (2nd ed.). Hoboken, NJ: John Wiley & Sons Inc.

Eisner, S. R. (2007). *From destructive to constructive thinking: Techniques of self-therapy for adults with ADD*. Master Thesis. University of North Carolina at Chapel Hill.

Ellis, A. (1972a). Helping people get better: Rather than merely feel better. *Rational Living, 7*(2), 2–9.

Ellis, A. (1972b). *Psychotherapy and the value of a human being*. New York, NY: Institute for Rational-Emotive Therapy.

Ellis, A. (1979). Rejoinder: Elegant and inelegant RET. In A. Ellis & J. M. Whiteley (Eds.), *Theoretical and empirical foundations of rational-emotive therapy*. (pp. 240–267). Monterey, CA: Brooks/Cole.

Ellis, A., & Dryden, W. (2007). *The practice of rational emotive behaviour therapy* (2nd Ed.). New York, NY: Springer Publishing Company.

Hughes, C., Herron, S., & Younge, J. (2014). *CBT For mild to moderate depression and anxiety*. Open University Press. McGraw – Hill Education.

Johnston, L. H., & Carroll, D. (2000). The psychological impact of injury: Effects of prior sport and exercise involvement. *British Journal of Sports Medicine, 34*, 436–439. doi:10.1136/bjsm.34.6.436

Korzybski, A. (1958/1933) *Science and sanity: An introduction to non-Aristotelian systems and general semantics* (4th ed.). Lakeville, CT: The International Non-Aristotelian Library Publishing Co. (now part of the I.G.S., Englewood, NJ).

Lazarus, A. A. (2009). Multimodal behavior therapy. In W. T. O'Donohue & J. E. Fisher (Eds.), *General principles and empirically supported techniques of cognitive behavior therapy* (pp. 440–444). Hoboken, NJ: John Wiley & Sons.

Leahy, R. L. (2003). *Cognitive therapy techniques: A practitioner's guide*. London: The Guilford Press.

Martens, R., Vealey, R. S., Burton, D., Bump, L., & Smith, D. E. (1990). Development and validation of the competitive state anxiety inventory-2. In R. Martens, R. S. Vealey, & D. Burton (Eds.), *Competitive anxiety in sport* (pp. 117–178) Champaign, IL: Human Kinetics.

Meichenbaum, D. (1994) A conversation with M. F. Hoyt at the Institute for Behavioral Healthcare: San Francisco. [On-Line] http://www.behavior.net/column/meichanbaum.

Smith, A. M., Scott S. G., & Wiese D. M. (1990). The psychological effects of sports injuries: Coping. *Sports Medicine, 9*(6), 352–369.

Tiller, J. W. G. (2012). *Depression and anxiety*. MJA Open. University of Melbourne.

Vealey, R. S. (1986). Conceptualization of sport-confidence and competitive orientation: Preliminary investigation and instrument development. *Journal of Sport Psychology*, 8, 221–246.

Wallen, S., DiGiuseppe, R., & Dryden, W. (1992). *A practitioner's guide to rational-emotive therapy*. New York, NY: Oxford Press.

Editors' commentary on Chapter 10: "Rebounding from injury and increasing performance using Rational Emotive Behavior Therapy (REBT)"

At several points within this chapter, Murat makes a clear distinction between inferences at A and evaluations at B. As an example, Deniz noticed pain in her leg (situational A) and inferred that this pain might signal an injury or even the end of her career (inferential A). It might have been tempting to challenge the inference at this juncture, for example, by asking what evidence Deniz had that pain necessarily indicates injury, or that injury predicts the end of her career. This is an option for a practitioner, and it is the option taken by most proponents of Aaron T. Beck's cognitive therapy (Beck, 1976). However, inferential change is not what most proponents of REBT are most interested in. One might construe it as the "silver medal" position. In this chapter, Murat goes for the "gold medal" of philosophical change, or what REBT authors (e.g. DiGiuseppe et al., 2014) refer to as, "the elegant solution" (p. 99). Deniz is encouraged towards adopting a more preferential and accepting philosophy in respect of pain and injury. Our argument is that this kind of change is more helpful in the short-term (it prevented her avoidant behavior during matches) and is more durable in the longer-term (it will still be of use to her when her career actually does come to an end). The central premise of a more functional philosophy, which one might summarize as, "I would prefer adverse things not to happen, but I can accept *that* they do, and I can tolerate them *when* they do", has a wide-ranging quality of durability and resilience about it that goes far beyond changing one's inferences about a specific situation.

Whilst advocating for the elegant solution, it is also important to recognize that the ideal of philosophical change is not always achievable for every individual. Dryden and Branch (2008) argue that one important task for an REBT practitioner is to assess what is achievable in any given context and pitch interventions accordingly. Making a collaborative and realistic decision about whether to pursue inferential or philosophical change is one such decision.

References

Beck, A. T. (1976). *Cognitive therapy and the emotional disorders*. London: Penguin.
DiGuiseppe, R., Doyle, K.A., Dryden, W., & Backx, W. (2014). *A practitioner's guide to rational emotive behaviour therapy* (3rd Ed.). Oxford: Oxford University Press.
Dryden, W., & Branch, R. (2008). *Fundamentals of rational emotive behaviour therapy: A training handbook*. Chichester: Wiley-Blackwell.

11 A Rational Emotive Behavior Therapy (REBT) intervention to improve low frustration tolerance in an elite table tennis player

Gangyan Si and Chun-Qing Zhang

Introduction

The first author of this chapter has been working with national team athletes since 1993. In a broad sense, he adopted the humanistic approach, caring about personal development and the growth of the mind. In his applied practice, he also applied and adopted many principles of Buddhism, for example, life is not always a smooth ride. Athletic life is full of ups and downs and athletes will run into various difficulties at different stages of their sporting lives. Given that Chinese athletes specialize at a very early age, the focus of sport psychology consultation should be on an insight into athletes' social-oriented values instead of individual-oriented values in the context of Whole-Nation System (Chinese sport system). Seeking optimal performance is not always the best option but cultivating rational responses is more workable (Si, 2006). The way to success in sport performance is not to pursue the ideal state but to prepare the athlete in how to cope with adversity in a rational way, specifically through changing their beliefs. The first author's philosophy of sport psychology practice is not to help athletes discover their peak performance state and learn how to recreate it, but rather to help athletes cope more effectively when faced with adversity. This chapter offers a rare opportunity to elaborate and reflect on a published piece of work (Si & Lee, 2008). Here, information beyond the existing report will be presented related to the context, identified issues, needs analysis, structure, and content of the Rational Emotive Behavior Therapy (REBT) intervention, and most importantly the authors' reflections of how to improve the delivery of future REBT interventions.

The adversity coping framework and REBT

Prior to introducing the current REBT intervention case study, we would like to introduce the adversity coping framework developed by Si and colleagues (Si, 2006; Si, et al., 2010). One major idea of developing this framework is to challenge the core idea behind peak performance, which is that athletes will produce perfect performance when they possess an optimal psychological state. Yet, the main difficulty seems to be that even though athletes participate in long periods of mental training, many are still often not sure whether they can reach this

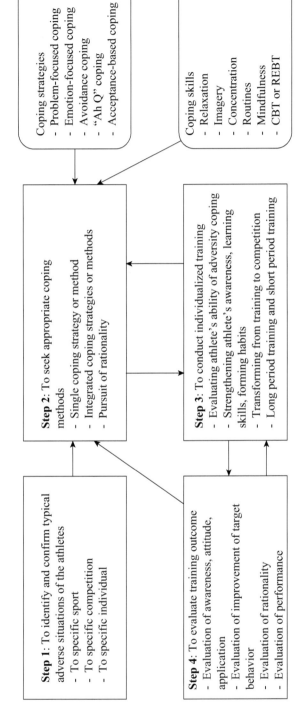

Figure 11.1 Four-stage adversity coping training (adapted from Si, 2006)

"peak" state exactly when they need to reach it. Put simply, it is difficult to find, operationalize, activate, and maintain this elusive and subjective peak state. Having said this, a new definition of peak performance was proposed by Si (2006), namely, successful adversity coping in competitions. To explain, even if athletes do not achieve a "peak" performance state during competition, if they are able to cope reasonably well with most or all adversity, effectively overcome their mistakes, their performance may still be judged as successful. Three elements were included in this new definition: adversity, coping, and rationality. Adversity refers to situations which impede the achievement of competitive goals. Coping refers to the awareness of and methods used to overcome or cope with adversity. Rationality refers to the control of one's own irrational mind and the ability to utilize the opportunity of an opponent's irrational mind, and, following this line of reasoning, peak performance can be defined as a dynamic and continuously adjusted process during competition.

A four-stage adversity coping training framework was developed by Si (2006): (a) to identify and confirm typical adverse situations; (b) to seek appropriate coping methods; (c) to conduct individualized training; and (d) to evaluate training outcomes (see Figure 11.1). This training framework aims to replace "peak" states of athletes with their typical adverse situations, followed by appropriate mental training (e.g., REBT) to enable athletes to cope successfully and rationally with these situations instead of harbouring irrational beliefs along with an obsession with peak or perfect performance. In other words, the adversity coping framework tries to train athletes from "not intentionally learning and accepting adversity" to "intentionally adapting to and transforming adversity". Specifically termed "Ah Q" coping, "Ah Q" is a fictional character in a novel written by Lu Xun, which is famous among Chinese people, and was included as this refers to "spiritual victories" through self-talk and self-deception even when faced with extreme defeat or humiliation. Several of the "Ah Q" coping strategies (which are actually Chinese idioms) read as follows: "Victory and defeat are both common in battle", "The problem will resolve on its own in its own good time", "Allow nature to take its course, for everything is pre-arranged", and "Take a step back and you'll see things from a wider perspective". Among many coping skills and coping strategies, REBT is one of the most effective mental training approaches that has been demonstrated in applied contexts (e.g., Si & Lee, 2008).

Need analysis

The reason why we introduce the adversity coping framework first is because it is in line with the philosophy of REBT, which is that adversity serves as the precedent for irrational beliefs (Turner & Barker, 2013). Another reason is that the framework was used to guide the REBT intervention for the men's doubles table tennis player Leo (pseudonym). Specific adverse situations triggered dysfunctional emotions and behaviors, such as either Leo or his partner making technical or tactical mistakes during competition. As described by Si and Lee (2008), Leo's main irrational belief is that he and his teammate should be consistently perfect during competition and they must make their skills perfect. If this is not achieved his belief is that he is a useless athlete and he and his partner cannot win anything. This leads to his issue of low frustration tolerance (LFT) in that he and his partner could not stand making mistakes during competition. A further assessment of the core components of this irrational and perfectionistic belief related to two technical issues.

Firstly, Leo firmly believed the only way for the pair to beat opponents was to improve their technique in middle- and long-zone, multi-ball confrontations, while both his coach and partner's views were that their advantage and strength was in short-zone or short-ball confrontations. His coach and partner also believed that the truth is that both players were older than their opponents and their technical abilities were stable, therefore, it was unwise to pursue the strengths of other players as mentioned by Leo. A more reasonable strategy should be that they play to their strengths to hide their weaknesses. Yet, Leo did not agree with them and stuck firmly to his beliefs. Secondly, Leo believed that his partner frequently made technical mistakes that could be avoided, which is demonstrated by this quote, "If my partner can train the way I ask, he can live up to my requirements". On the other hand, the coach believed that his partner's skills were quite stable and that this would be difficult to alter. Most importantly, the coach believed that it is quite normal for elite table tennis players to make mistakes during competition under such enormous pressure. The coach also believed that Leo should not be nit picking because his irrational expectations of his partner were beyond any normal level of expectations. The first author didn't use the questionnaire approach because of its lack of ecological validity. In contrast, this triangulation approach of in-depth interview of two players and their coach provided more useful background information.

At one point after a Table Tennis World Championship, the coach said of Leo that, "In terms of table tennis skills, Leo is a phenomenal level athlete, and trains very hard. But, he is obsessed with perfectionism, with many extreme thoughts that are different from normal athletes. He cannot control his temper when encountering adversity. When he loses his temper during competition, he cannot focus on the competition, and this also influences the performance of his partner. Given this reason, he has never achieved any good results in major international games. His partner is an ideal athlete and a good match from technique to personality". His partner commented on him: "In daily life we get along with each other very well, and we work very well in competition when he can control his temper. However, he may suddenly lose his temper, in particular when we have made some mistakes. Sometimes when I didn't play very well, he would be immediately upset. You can feel his bad emotion right away. He sometimes even behaves in such a way as to show how upset he is, which seriously puzzles me".

In total, there were three intervention stages, and one-on-one sessions were the main format of this REBT intervention, which took approximate 75% of the intervention time. The remaining 25% was conducted in a group format together with his coach and partner. In stage 1, a typical method of REBT, psychoeducation was used to enable Leo to become familiar with the concepts of REBT and the ABCDE model. In stage 2, the action/maintenance stage, the first author adopted an integrated approach combining REBT skills (cognitive, emotive, and behavioral interventions) with mental skills training, to facilitate, strengthen, and maintain positive change. In stage 3, the REBT and mental skills continued to be practiced in order to achieve positive intervention effects.

Stage 1: pre-intervention

At this stage, the components of the whole intervention plan were introduced to Leo, and this plan consisted of three aspects: goal, methods, and evaluation.

Goal: To replace previous irrational beliefs with rational beliefs, to allow Leo to calm down and control his emotion (temper).

Methods: (a) to teach Leo cognitive, emotive, and behavioral intervention skills; (b) to teach Leo mental skills and ensure he can use them appropriately, including: deep breathing, imagery, self-talk, and routines; (c) to have Leo read REBT books recommended by the first author; (d) to involve Leo in regular discussions with the first author.

Evaluation: (a) to have Leo conduct self-evaluation; (b) to have the coach and the partner evaluate the progress made by Leo; (c) to evaluate performance in competition.

Stage 2: action/maintenance

Building on the long-term working relationship of the first author with the table tennis team, the REBT intervention started with the verbal consent of Leo, after a team meeting with both Leo, his partner, and their coach. Given that there were several overlaps in the action and maintenance stage, these are described in the same section. Four types of skills were used, including: cognitive, emotive, and behavioral interventions, as well as mental skills training.

Cognitive intervention

In the cognitive intervention, six skills were used, including: empirical disputes, functional disputes, philosophical disputes, cognitive reframing, rational coping statements, and psycho-educational method.

Empirical disputes

The first and most important aspect of the intervention was to deal with Leo's irrational demand on (a) himself and his partner to be perfect on middle- and long-zone multi-ball confrontation and (b) his partner to perform stably. Targeting these two irrational beliefs, formal and informal discussions were conducted over many occasions between the first author, the coach, Leo, and his partner, either during training, after competition, or in the consultation room. The topics of discussions emerged through viewing previous competition videos, in which the coach would point out Leo's dysfunctional verbalizations (e.g., yelling at his partner) and other behaviors (e.g., throwing his towel) when they lost a point during the multi-ball confrontation or when his partner made mistakes. In addition, Leo's partner also shared his feeling when Leo expressed the irrational demands on him to perform perfectly, without making mistakes, as well as to show strengths on their weakness (e.g., to score through middle- and long-zone multi-ball confrontations). After a slow and long-term change process, the first author helped Leo to gradually replace these two irrational beliefs about techniques with more rational beliefs about how he would like to perform stably and turn weakness into strength, but he does not have to. Also, Leo was encouraged to recognize the fact that it is not easy (if not completely impossible) to suddenly turn weakness into strength, when taking their age factors and fixed technique patterns into consideration. In such high-pressure situations, it is the reality that his partner will occasionally make some mistakes. It should be noted that the whole process was not linear and there were several setbacks and fluctuations. Once Leo changed his irrational beliefs he started to talk more with his coach and partner about how to take advantage of their strengths and try to assume joint responsibility, supporting his partner instead of demanding irrational requirements of him.

Functional disputes

The second component of the cognitive aspect of the intervention involved functional disputes, where the first author worked with Leo to question whether his own beliefs were aiding or impeding the attainment of his goal of winning the match. Firstly, the first author repeatedly discussed the extent to which Leo's demand for spotless skill execution and stable performance of his partner was really helpful to them. The first author discussed with Leo whether he thought strict demands with impossibly high standards would immediately lead to perfect results, or cause more negative thoughts (e.g., mistakes being his partner's fault), unhelpful emotions (e.g., unhealthy anger), and uncontrollable behaviors (e.g., throwing his racket or towel). Given the fact that Leo and his partner were veteran athletes, Leo was asked which out of the following two approaches were more functional: (1) fostering strengths and circumventing weaknesses, or (2) overcoming all the weaknesses they have to become perfect athletes. As such, various types of real-life situations were analyzed. Finally, Leo gave up his irrational belief that they need all-round perfect skills, and replaced it with a more rational approach on making better use of their strengths and advantages to help them compete with the world's top-level players.

Philosophical disputes

The aim of the philosophical disputes was to help Leo recognize how his irrational beliefs affected his values, in order to help Leo re-evaluate the meaning of his entire sport career in a rational way. Building on the adversity coping framework (Si, 2006), the first author discussed with Leo the philosophy that adversities and setbacks will always be present in life and in any sporting career. Leo was, therefore, invited to view his sport career and to view the winning or losing of competitions from the perspective that, "life is not always a smooth ride". Gradually, Leo learned to replace his irrational belief that, "we need to be perfect on our skills at all cost" with a new belief/philosophy of, "we want to, but do not need to, be perfect" and was encouraged to "foster strengths and circumvent weaknesses". In addition, Leo used the philosophy of "adversity is normal" as he began to learn to accept the imperfections of techniques and the mistakes in competitions.

Cognitive reframing

The fourth component of the cognitive intervention was cognitive reframing. During the whole intervention, the first author was continually attempting to help Leo reframe the problems that appeared during competition from different angles. The main focus was to assist Leo to be able to view adversity and setbacks as challenges for him to overcome, rather than as threats or signs of bad luck. The process of cognitive reframing was also conducted through discussions, and through a process of building new concepts and viewpoints. Please refer to Figure 11.2 for the REBT ABC formulation.

Activating Event (A)

Situation: Partner of self, making mistakes during competition
Adversity (e.g., the inference drawn about what is most difficult about the situation):
Being imperfect in our (self and/or partner) performance

Irrational Beliefs (iB)	Rational Beliefs (rB)
Demand: "We should be consistently perfect"	**Preference:** "I want to, but do not need to, play perfectly"
Low Frustration Tolerance: "I can't stand not playing perfectly and making mistakes"	**High Frustration Tolerance:** "I can tolerate us not performing perfectly"
Depreciation (Self/Other/Life): "I am useless if we can't play perfectly"	**Acceptance (Self/Other/Life):** "I am not useless if I perform imperfectly"

Unhelpful Consequences (C)	Helpful Consequences (C)
Emotional Consequence: Anger	**Emotional Consequence:** Frustration
Behavioral Consequence: Lose temper Yell at partner Lose focus Perform worse	**Behavioral Consequence:** Control temper Maintain focus Maintain performance
Cognitive Consequence: Self-blame Self-criticism	**Cognitive Consequence:** Greater confidence

---

Figure 11.2 ABC formulation for Leo

Adversity coping statements

Adversity coping statements developed by the first author (Si, 2006) were also used to help Leo (see Figure 11.3 for the 15 adversity coping statements). These statements served the function of reminders, helping Leo to consider whether his beliefs were rational or irrational. The first author discussed the meaning of each statement, and asked Leo to use three of his own examples to illustrate each one. If Leo felt that the statements were meaningful and could link with his own situations, he was encouraged to adapt them using his own words. Several of the statements were repeatedly used by Leo, for example, "life is not always a smooth ride", "Something might be wrong at the critical time", and "Instead of accusing my partner's mistake, what I should do is to encourage him". However, it should be noted that these statements are not technically accurate rational beliefs.

The psycho-educational method

The psycho-educational approach was used throughout the whole action and maintenance stage. This psycho-education was conducted mainly through recommending Leo to read biographies of top-level athletes, philosophical stories

---

Based on the first author's years of applied experience of sport psychology practice, 15 adversity coping statements were developed (Si, 2006). In the current case, these adversity coping statements were used to help Leo better understand his own beliefs.

1. Expect setbacks to be a normal part of competition while smoothness is an exception.
2. Something might be wrong at the critical time.
3. You cannot make sure every key factor works well to guarantee your victory.
4. Even if a strategy looks "stupid", it is not "stupid" any more if it works.
5. When confronting a strong and well-prepared opponent, your pre-set target can never be carried out the exact way you planned.
6. Simple things might be the important things.
7. It might be hard to do the simple things well.
8. You probably have been overly prepared if you think something still needs to be prepared right prior to the competition.
9. If you think that you have studied your opponent from every angle, he or she might have done the same thing.
10. Previous success might never be replicated in the way you expect.
11. Your attention and mood might be influenced by your teammate's mistake rather than your opponent's dangerous attack.
12. Your opponent will never be able to manipulate your mind without your permission.
13. If you try to avoid risks when approaching success you will destroy your own success.
14. A sudden mental collapse might be caused because of the tiny negative thoughts accumulated.
15. You can have an adaptive rationality to the current situation but never expect the perfect rationality to all circumstances.

Figure 11.3 Adversity coping statements

from the Internet on Buddhism and Taoism, REBT-related books, as well as adversity coping books. Through reading and discussing various types of stories, Leo started to discuss with the first author what the rational and irrational beliefs were (e.g., he and his partner don't have to have perfect skills and don't need to have zero mistakes in order to win the competition). This interactive discussion between Leo and the first author helped him form his own rational beliefs. Two months prior to the Olympic Games, the first author prepared a 10,000-word essay and asked Leo to read it and give his opinions. This essay detailed rational ideas in terms of coping with adversities in competition.

Emotive intervention

Three components were included in the emotive aspect of intervention, including: rational emotive imagery, role-play, and social support.

Rational emotive imagery

According to Ellis (1995), there are two aims for using rational emotive imagery: (a) to help individuals find appropriate emotions that he or she wants to experience in the problematic situation; and (b) to help individuals repeatedly experience effective self-talk and other coping skills. To anchor the target for change that was to be focused on through the imagery training sessions, typical situations were identified. For example, after much discussion with Leo, situations (e.g., they had an equal score to the opponents but his partner started to make mistakes causing them to be at a disadvantage) where he became frustrated and lost his temper were used. In the rational emotive imagery, Leo was guided to close his eyes gently, using imagery to help him re-enter the typical situation that frustrated him. When he imagined the situation and experienced the emotions (e.g., anger and frustration), he would raise his hands. At the same time, Leo was required to label the negative emotions. Subsequently, Leo was required to produce new beliefs through discussion or reframing, and to experience the positive emotions that emerged as a result of the new beliefs. Once this transformation was successful, Leo would raise his hands up again. Then, he was asked to return to reality slowly, and open his eyes. The first author questioned his feelings, recorded these feelings, and subsequently enquired about how Leo managed to transform his emotions and with the recorded details. Once again, the importance of the beliefs that helped Leo transform his emotions was discussed. This rational emotive imagery was practiced regularly in the consulting room under the supervision of the first author and Leo also completed regular imagery homework after daily training at his apartment in the sports institute.

Role-play

In order to help Leo to better experience and understand his own dysfunctional behaviors, the first author proposed a role-play in a group meeting and the coach, Leo, and his partner agreed. Two types of role-play were conducted through two separate scenarios. That is, Leo played the role of his partner and also his coach in a real and in an imagined situation. The reality role-play was conducted at the training venue, in which his partner lost his temper with Leo in order to allow Leo to experience the feelings associated with this type of situation. Leo also exchanged roles with his coach, to experience how the coach may have thought or felt when Leo lost temper under pressure or when facing adversity. Role-play was also conducted through imagery and discussion. That is, Leo was asked to imagine how his partner and his coach would expect Leo to behave; his partner and coach also commented on this imagined role-play. The durations of the role-play were usually short, with the main purpose being to allow Leo to experience new beliefs and feelings. Using role-play as an intervention means that irrational beliefs can be discussed, and discussions through which cognitive reframing would be possible could be practiced. Through this process, Leo experienced engaging interactions with his partner and his coach and was therefore able to co-develop an atmosphere of mutual understanding.

Social support

Social support, in particular, emotional support, plays a stress-buffering effect via modifying the cognitive appraisal of the situation when perceiving the availability of support (Wethington & Kessler, 1986). In the current case study, the emotional support was provided by Leo's coach and partner beyond the professional relationship with the first author. Leo became more actively involved with changing his beliefs due to the development of positive rapport and social support from his partner and coach throughout the whole intervention period. The first author had developed a three-way agreement during the preparation stage to encourage and support Leo to make the necessary changes. Each month, after a major competition, the first author, Leo, his coach, and his partner came together to evaluate the progress that had been made during that stage, and to proactively encourage and support Leo. During competitions, the coach also encouraged Leo when he demonstrated positive emotional control; when Leo failed to do so or had ups and downs, the coach and partner supported Leo by showing full acceptance and offered positive comments and suggestions.

Behavioral intervention and mental skills training

To evaluate the behavioral intervention, self-evaluation was conducted by Leo with the Goal Attainment Scale (GAS; Kiresuk & Sherman, 1968; Martin, et al., 1998). In addition, written and verbal feedback on Leo was collected from his coach and partner, and performance evaluation on Leo was conducted through video observation (see Si & Lee, 2008 for details).

In the mental skills training component, deep abdominal breathing and self-talk were integrated with the imagery training to form routines (see Si & Lee, 2008 for details). Specifically, the practice of all four mental skills was conducted during the action and maintenance stage, whereas the routines were mainly conducted during the stability stage, when Leo had become familiar with the use of the mental skills. The mental skills were integrated into the REBT to help him gain better understanding and control of his cognitions and emotions. Leo could use the rational belief words to replace the irrational belief words in his self-talk, and could imagine coping with a situation in a rational way.

Stage 3: stability

At this stage, no major relapses occurred and Leo's emotions progressed towards greater stability. Several of the rational statements on adversity and acceptance of imperfection (e.g., it is acceptable for him and his partner to make mistakes during competition and it is normal that their skills are imperfect as long as they are able to take most advantage of their strengths) had become effective, with Leo identifying these statements as part of his own new belief system. In the stability stage, Leo's coach and his partner continued to provide their unconditional support. Leo had demonstrated significant improvement in his overall ability to control his emotions and to deal with adversity through his developed coping ability. See Figure 11.4 for the cognitive, emotive, behavioral, and mental skills that had been used across three time points.

Evaluation

Given that the evaluation of the target behavior change has been reported elsewhere (Si & Lee, 2008), the current chapter focuses predominantly on the change in Leo's irrational beliefs of perfection on skills and performance during

Stage	Cognitive Skills	Emotive Skills	Behavioral Skills	Mental Skills
Pre-Intervention	–	–	–	–
Action/ Maintenance	Debates: (a) Empirical debates; (b) Functional debates; (c) Philosophical debates Cognitive reconstruction Rules of rational coping Psycho-education	Emotive imagery skills Role-play Social support (coaches and partner)	Enforcement (self-evaluation, other evaluation, and video evaluation)	Imagery and deep breathing Self-suggested behavioral routine
Stability	Rational coping	Social support (coaches and partner)	Enforcement	Behavioral routine

Note: – represents no interventions were conducted.

Figure 11.4 Cognitive, emotive, behavioral, and mental skills that have been used at three periods of time

competition. It was considered that the primary cause of Leo's behavioral change was through the way he had cognitively reframed his beliefs. The core component of Leo's irrational belief was the demand for perfection that was related to his skills. This perfectionistic tendency required that not only did he have to perform without fault, but also, so did his partner. There are some differences in the mental processes and emotional reactions between his skill-related perfectionism and partner-related perfectionism. The mental process of the skill-related perfectionistic idea was directed towards himself, therefore self-accusation, emotional impatience, and anxiety might emerge, and self-esteem might be lowered (Cozzarelli & Major, 1990). In contrast, the mental process of the partner-related perfectionism was directed towards others, and accusing his partner resulted in Leo venting his anger towards him, producing irritable emotions. To overcome these two types of irrational belief, different cognitive reframing methods were adopted. In addition, no matter whether the rational beliefs were toward Leo or his partner, the more fundamental core belief that developed was "adversities and setbacks are normal in competition", which could facilitate the understanding that "if I am calm, I will perform better next time".

The first author repeatedly double-checked whether Leo's belief system had been changed. Firstly, after each major competition, the first author had discussions with Leo about the problems that were still present and the progress that had been made. Feedback from the coach was also considered in order to give an overall evaluation of Leo's belief system. Specifically, based on the mistakes made by Leo and his partner, the targeted behavioral evaluation (see Si & Lee, 2008) was combined to examine the change of rational beliefs. During the action and maintenance stage, the first author joined Leo, his coach, and his partner to watch the competition videos repeatedly and discussed opinions with Leo. With the help of the coach, the change in Leo's beliefs was a gradual process over the whole cognitive intervention. In the Olympic qualification stage, Leo was no longer stuck to his belief related to "perfect skills" (i.e., demanding himself to be perfect all-round and that his partner absolutely must not make any mistakes). Leo would still suddenly lose his temper due to his own and his partner's performance, reacting with self-criticism and blame. However, he could consciously challenge himself, and react with more rational beliefs. To quote Leo's own words, "Let go of the mistakes, only require myself and my partner to play to our strengths". After the competition, Leo summarized that if he could stick to his rational beliefs, he was able to control his temper, and then he was able to pay full attention to the competition. In doing so, his self-confidence was not jeopardized, and the tacit understanding with his partner was maintained. During a subsequent competition, Leo used the rational beliefs to challenge himself when required. When he made a mistake, he was able to tell himself, "It doesn't matter; just focus on the next ball"; and when his partner made a mistake, Leo chose to assume joint responsibility of not being able to push their opponents, and provided positive comments about their skills. The comment given by Leo was, "the key is belief, I need to find a good reason (rational beliefs) to persuade myself". Finally, when it came to the Olympic Games, Leo had already fully adopted the rational belief that "adversities and setbacks are normal and not awful" and used this to guide his behaviors. He could clearly describe how he coped rationally in the debriefing session after each game during the group stage. For example, in the semi-final game, Leo and his partner were sitting with a 2:2 draw in the fifth and sixth sets; he was able to calmly deal with this situation by being confident in himself and encouraging his partner. The result was that the pair finally won the competition. The degree to which the rational beliefs were used and developed over time to guide behaviors was clear and this newfound strength was repeatedly tested with adversity and setbacks.

Secondly, verbal feedback and progress summaries at different stages from Leo, his coach, and his partner were evaluated; and again, Leo was invited to participate in the discussions to confirm if it had been the changes in his beliefs that had led to the changes during competition. Within the summary of the action and maintenance stage, Leo thought that his beliefs had been greatly improved by turning them from irrational into rational beliefs, whereas his coach thought that Leo still had some "strange thoughts". However, the basic concept to "foster strengths and circumvent weaknesses" had been established without sticking to Leo's demand for "perfection". On the other hand, his partner believed that they had reached a consensus about the belief that "adversity is normal". Leo commented, "Actually, in every important major competition there are mistakes and setbacks. Previously I thought this should not happen, and I could not deal with it, then I would lose my cool. However, now the beliefs have been changed, I understand adversity, and think rationally, so that I can control myself". His coach and partner also thought that it was the change in Leo's beliefs that had led to the improvement of his ability to control himself.

In the stabilization stage, Leo commented that his non-awfulizing belief that "adversities and setbacks are normal" was solid, and that he had developed stability in using rational beliefs to deal with adversity. In other words, he believed that this had helped him to develop better control in dealing with "mistakes and setbacks". The coach also commented on Leo with his summary that the rational beliefs that Leo had in competition were now stable. The coach also believed that this change was the key for Leo and his partner, and that it impacted positively on performance. Leo's partner believed that due to the stabilization of Leo's thoughts and emotions, the "Olympic Games is the best competition we have ever completed".

The aforementioned discussion can be summarized as:

(a) Leo's beliefs had been reframed as a result of the cognitive intervention. The changes in Leo's belief system during competition and the related performance effects have been confirmed through follow-up evaluations
(b) Leo's change in beliefs about competition had caused the change in his behaviors.

Under the guidance of his rational beliefs, Leo demonstrated calm, control, trust, and encouragement towards his partner, even in the face of adversity. In all, this demonstrates a significant improvement in Leo's performance and that of his partner.

Reflection

One key reason for the successful application of this REBT intervention is the high level of trust that had been established prior to the Olympic Games that gradually made Leo recognize and learn to manage his problem with demanding perfection and not being able to tolerate imperfection. In the pre-intervention stage, the key issue to tackle was Leo's suspicion of the effectiveness of REBT, which is common in the Chinese athletes we have worked with. Building on the pre-established rapport with Leo, the first author used many examples of cases where an REBT intervention had been used in competition in order to familiarize him with the intervention plan.

In the action and maintenance stage, the main purpose was to implement the intervention and facilitate Leo's change process, and at the same time to strengthen the changes that Leo had already made. In this stage, there were two key problems to tackle:

(a) Leo's awareness of his irrational beliefs and the use of rational beliefs to replace them
(b) The use of different types of mental skills to help Leo establish the right behavioral reactions

Regarding the first problem, with the help of coach and partner, the first author used competition videos and stroke analysis, and the irrational beliefs related to Leo's sport-specific skills were explored. This was important to help Leo develop a deeper understanding of his irrational beliefs and to search for more rational beliefs. At the same time, discussions were used to help Leo reframe his beliefs about his values and to re-evaluate the influence of his existing values on his entire sporting career and his life. During the process of discussions and cognitive reframing, improvement in the irrational beliefs was a gradual process, with occasional setbacks. In Leo's case the change in his irrational beliefs about technical skills generalized to improvement in other parts of his irrational belief system. In terms of the second problem, the mental skills training worked well in combination with the REBT skills, and this training offered Leo a concrete and operational set of skills when he needed to control his behaviors, and subsequently, Leo used these mental skills to good effect during competition.

In the stability stage, the main purpose was to strengthen the established positive intervention effects. The main issue in the last stage was to prevent a relapse into unhelpful behaviors. During the two months prior to the Olympic Games, cognitive skills and rational coping statements had been internalized by Leo, and the mental skills routines had been well mastered which made an important contribution to the stabilization of Leo's emotions and behaviors.

Overall, both the first author and Leo believed that the combination of the REBT and the mental skills provided an effective training method. Specifically, Leo mentioned two points that were of particular importance to his behavioral control during competition: (a) focusing on rational beliefs at critical moments (e.g., when Leo and his partner were lagging behind their components, when his partner made mistakes) during competition; and (b) having operational skills that could be used was clearly important for him to be able to control his behavior during the competition.

There are several limitations in this case that could be improved for future interventions. Firstly, the emotive intervention was weak compared to the cognitive intervention. The depth and frequency of the rational emotive imagery and role-play were insufficient, and were difficult to evaluate. Secondly, the rational emotive imagery skills in REBT and the imagery skill used in mental skills training (action/maintenance stage) were difficult to keep consistent and productive, which resulted in Leo sometimes feeling confused. On the other hand, the imagery in mental skills is clearly defined (internal imagery requires athletes to image from the perspective of self to complete specific sport skills; external imagery refers to athletes imaging the completion of sport skills from the perspective of others). Together with the kinesiology of skills, this type of imagery focuses on controlling skills. Thus, it was viewed that the imagery skills from mental skills training could be integrated into the rational emotive imagery skill in REBT.

From the perspective of the first author, two things are important. Firstly, the first author was, at that time, a full-time staff member based at a sports institute, which allowed him to continuously follow up throughout the whole intervention. The intervention was a multiple-site, multiple-situation, and continuous intervention. In addition to regularly interacting with Leo at the training base, the first author could travel with Leo to overseas training and competitions. This made it very convenient for the first author to take advantage of the different types of situations and get first-hand information and quality interaction with the athletes. The best moment to implement the intervention is always as the problem arises. Normally, with the help of the coach and Leo's partner, the most complete and thorough discussions with Leo happened at hotels and restaurants when problems had appeared during the competitions. Secondly, cooperation from the coach was important. For Leo, his coach was a coping resource but also a stressor. Therefore, it was important to include the coach in the whole intervention plan, as the interactions with Leo required the coach's understanding and cooperation. Actually, the coach played a crucial role in this intervention, from being involved in discussions about Leo's irrational beliefs, monitoring Leo's irrational behaviors, providing comments and evaluations, and providing time and financial support. The intervention may not have been completed without the support of the coach.

Although we were quite confident that it was the intervention that led to the reduction of demandingness and low frustration tolerance, the external validity of the intervention should be considered. In future, mixed method designs should be used. In other words, applied practitioners should focus on more advanced data analysis methods in single-case studies. Additionally, to help athletes become more aware of their irrational beliefs, mindfulness skills can be practiced, although the mindfulness approach focuses on accepting irrational ideas rather than replacing or changing them (Gardner & Moore, 2007; Si, et al., 2016). Recently, the two authors have become interested in an acceptance and mindfulness-based approach, which has potential to be integrated into REBT (Ellis, 2005). Acceptance and Commitment Therapy (ACT) and REBT significantly overlap in their theory and practice. This provides a promising avenue for future applied practitioners and researchers to integrate these two approaches – for example, using cognitive defusion techniques and reliance on direct experience to replace disputation (Hayes, 2005). Moreover, when conducting REBT interventions, the local culture or theoretical framework should be considered. For example, the adversity coping framework (Si, 2006) was used in the current intervention.

References

Cozzarelli, C., & Major, B. (1990). Exploring the validity of the impostor phenomenon. *Journal of Social and Clinical Psychology*, 9, 401–417.

Ellis, A. (1995). Changing Rational-Emotive Therapy (RET) to Rational Emotive Behavior Therapy (REBT). *Journal of Rational-Emotive & Cognitive-Behavior Therapy*, 13(2), 85–89.

Ellis, A. (2005). Can Rational-Emotive Behavior Therapy (REBT) and acceptance and commitment therapy (act) resolve their differences and be integrated? *Journal of Rational-Emotive and Cognitive-Behavior Therapy*, 23, 153–168.

Gardner, F.L., & Moore, Z.E. (2007). *The psychology of enhancing human performance: The mindfulness-acceptance-commitment approach*. New York, NY: Springer.

Hayes, S. C. (2005). Stability and change in Cognitive Behavior Therapy: Considering the implications of ACT and RFT. *Journal of Rational-Emotive and Cognitive-Behavior Therapy*, 23, 131–151.

Kiresuk, T. J., & Sherman, R. E. (1968). Goal attainment scaling: A general method for evaluating comprehensive community mental health programs. *Community Health Journal*, 4, 443–453.

Martin, S. B., Thompson, C. L., & McKnight, J. (1998). An integrative psychoeducational approach to sport psychology consulting: A case study. *International Journal of Sport Psychology*, 29, 170–186.

Si, G. (2006). Pursuing "ideal" or emphasizing "coping": The new definition of "peak performance" and transformation of mental training pattern. *Sport Science*, 26, 43–48. (in Chinese)

Si, G., & Lee, H. C. (2008). Is it so hard to change? The case of a Hong Kong Olympic silver medallist. *International Journal of Sport and Exercise Psychology*, 6, 319–330.

Si, G. Y., Lee, H. C., & Lonsdale, C. (2010). Sport psychology research and its application in China. In M. H. Bond (Ed.), *The oxford handbook of Chinese psychology* (pp. 641–656). Hong Kong: Oxford University Press.

Si, G., Lo, C.-H., & Zhang, C.-Q. (2016). Mindfulness training program for Chinese athletes and its effectiveness. In A. Baltzell (Ed.), *Mindfulness and performance* (pp. 235–267). New York, NY: Cambridge University Press.

Turner, M., & Barker, J. B. (2013). Examining the efficacy of rational-emotive behavior therapy (REBT) on irrational beliefs and anxiety in elite youth cricketers. *Journal of Applied Sport Psychology, 25,* 131–147.

Wethington, E., & Kessler, R. C. (1986). Perceived support, received support, and adjustment to stressful life events. *Journal of Health and Social behavior, 27,* 78–89.

Editors' commentary on Chapter 11: "A Rational Emotive Behavior Therapy (REBT) intervention to improve low frustration tolerance in an elite table tennis player"

This chapter gives us a rare opportunity to dig deeper into the interpersonal issues within a table tennis partnership. In this case, it is the interpersonal issues and details that stood out to us as something that we rarely see in literature. Emotional support provided by the client's partner and coach are instrumental in helping the client to overcome his behavioral issues, and of course helping the client to endorse rational beliefs. It is easy to forget the importance of the athlete's support network when working with REBT on a one-to-one level. But with regards to helping athletes deal with the demands of performance, social support is very important. Indeed, research dating back to the 80s recognized that social support can help an individual to see that they have coping abilities adequate to cope with stressors, or induce the perception that if a need to cope arises, others will help (Cohen & McKay, 1984). As such, social support can serve as a buffer to stress (House, 1981), and in the context of REBT, can include teammates and support staff providing guidance and information to help the client implement REBT in training and competition.

Of course, in the chapter Si and Zhang are careful to set this up properly, in part by obtaining a three-way agreement to involve the partner and the coach in the client's change process. This arrangement extended to group evaluation of the client's progress post-competition, and to support the client further in his behavioral goals. This aspect of the intervention obviously relies on the openness of all parties, and the skill of the practitioner in bringing together this group in the support of the athlete in question, in a safe, supportive, and effective manner. In our work, teammates and support staff are vital in aiding the progress of the client through REBT, and research should focus on this more often.

References

Cohen, S., & McKay, G. (1984). Social support, stress, and the buffering hypothesis: A theoretical analysis. In A. Baum., S. E. Taylor., & J. E. Singer (Eds.), *Handbook of psychology and health.* Hillsdale, NJ: Erlbaum.

House, J. S. (1981). *Work stress and social support.* Reading, MA: Addison-Wesley.

12 Applying Rational Emotive Behavior Therapy (REBT) resilience "credos" with a South-East Asian elite squash player

Saqib Deen

Introduction

At the time of my work with Adam (pseudonym), I was an MSc student studying Sport and Exercise Psychology and was introduced to REBT by my tutors. I enrolled on the Primary Practicum in Rational Emotive Behavior Therapy at the Centre for REBT and the training opened my eyes to how REBT can be used, and it made a lasting impact on my approach and philosophy to working with clients.

My approach to working with athletes is humanistic, as I consider athlete well-being to be more important than performance as an athlete will always be a human first, and an athlete second. REBT provides a sound theory and explanation of psychological dysfunction, in that the ABC model is relatively simple and easy to use, and my personality is well-suited to using it as REBT is active-directive (Dryden & Branch, 2008). REBT involves some collaboration between the client and practitioner (Dryden, 2009), with the practitioner acting as a guide to therapeutic change within the client, and I like to empower clients by educating them in the REBT process and my goal is for clients to be able to use REBT independently. This is so clients need not be entirely reliant on a practitioner to understand and remediate their own psychological dysfunction, in this sense being able to wean off from the therapist (and the therapy) over time.

This chapter presents an REBT intervention with Adam, a South-East Asian squash player, who at the time of this work was 19 years old. In this chapter, I will cover the structure of REBT that I adopted, and the use of credos as a tool in REBT. I will also reflect on using REBT in foreign settings.

Context

Following my studies in sport psychology, and training in REBT, I was a frustrated bank manager who wanted to gain further experience working in sport settings, and specifically as a sport psychology consultant. I managed to secure an internship at a national sporting institute in South-East Asia for six months, and left my job so that I could carry this out. This institute provided an array of sport science support for athletes, which included psychological support, and I arrived as an intern based in the psychology department. Prior to my arrival, I had only made some brief contact with my internship supervisor and I was wary about how I was going to cope in a new country for half a year. However, I quickly felt at home as my new colleagues were so welcoming and helpful.

I had official tasks in my schedule upon my arrival to the institute, and I was required to network with coaches and staff so that I could observe training sessions, shadow other psychologists, attend local competitions, and take part in workshops and lectures. Even though most of my psychology colleagues spoke a high level of English, not everyone in the national sporting complex did, including support staff from other departments, coaches, athletes, and administrators. Staff members who did speak English were typically well versed in at least two languages, and this was how they managed to communicate with everyone efficiently. Upon realizing how many people did not speak fluent English I took the challenge upon myself to learn at least the local language by any means, so I purchased a dual-language dictionary, downloaded phone apps, and spoke with as many people as I could so that I could gain practice, being unafraid to make mistakes.

This attitude is important to mention because my efforts to learn the local language paid off and I became a figure of interest in the sports complex, eventually gaining access to many sports teams. It was a real joy as a sports fan to see such a wide range of sports in action first-hand, such as wushu, bowling, badminton, gymnastics, track and field, football, and many more. Through these experiences, I learnt a vast amount about the culture that I was in, and gained a basic understanding of the organizational structure. A colleague of mine had introduced me to one of the national squash coaches, who was also from the UK, to see if there were any opportunities for me to gain experience of conducting applied work. I explained to the coach that I was pursuing Chartership with the British Psychological Society (BPS) and had just received formal training in REBT. The coach felt positively towards sport psychology and allowed me access to his athletes. Several young athletes were referred to me, one of whom was Adam, and this was the context in which I first encountered him.

My six months as an intern dictated the circumstances of my work with Adam, and therefore the work I conducted was very different from that which full-time applied psychologists might typically do. Had I been employed as a resident psychologist in the same institute, I would have had more time to develop lasting relationships with athletes and coaches alike and would have a set number of athletes under my charge. I would have potentially travelled with them to competitions and been with them for a significant chunk of their careers, as opposed to a relatively short stint as an intern from abroad. In short, the context in which I delivered REBT was potentially very different to how it is typically applied.

Presenting issue

I had briefly explained REBT to the coach, and he liked the idea of his athletes gaining an understanding of psychological dysfunction, learning about their own belief systems and behavioral patterns, and achieving some level of rationality by working with me. It was not difficult to sell to the coach that a more rational athlete is an athlete who has greater potential well-being, and that this may indeed result in greater performance attainment (Turner, 2016b). I explained that it would be exciting to use REBT with the athletes as it was not widely reported in sport at the time, and it would be a unique opportunity for the athletes to have sessions with a trained practitioner. The coach felt that Adam would greatly benefit from REBT, and the coach informed me that Adam had struggled in the past to manage his emotions, particularly when performing. In a typical working setting, a practitioner may only choose to use REBT after conducting a needs analysis and preliminary interview with an athlete (Marlow, 2009; Turner & Barker, 2014).

The coach arranged for me to meet with Adam as an introduction, and this initial meeting lasted 20 minutes. My first meeting was relatively pleasant. Adam wasn't that much younger than me and we developed good rapport as I used to play squash for several years in my youth, but now focused on badminton. Adam also took an interest in this fact about me, and he knew a lot about badminton as it is very popular in South-East Asia.

Adam reported that his recent performances were highly inconsistent and he blamed his emotional temperament in the court. If he was facing opponents who were ranked lower than him, or players who were younger than him, he felt that he "should" be beating them every time, and at this point irrational beliefs began to present themselves in his speech. During his matches, he struggled to close games in which he was leading and would often "throw away" games by making numerous unforced errors and having small outbursts on court. Adam worried that highly inconsistent performances may place him in a potential firing line to be dropped from the squad in the future, which could mean a quick end to a short professional career. He was also far away from his hometown and he reported a low frustration tolerance belief that he "couldn't bear being away from home for long periods of time".

Adam elaborated that being a full-time athlete was tough for him, and that suffering defeats, being mistreated by his peers, and performing poorly in training sessions would leave him frustrated for long periods of time. Further to my initial interpretations, I asked Adam about how being away from his family affected him on a day-to-day basis and at this point he explained that because he missed his family, "small things" tended to make him feel angry often. He reported that he wanted to reduce his level of anger, as this was impacting on his relationships with those around him. At this point, it was also clear to see that Adam was creating an A-C link (events directly cause emotions), and I used all this information to plan an REBT intervention with Adam. I informed Adam about REBT and what I planned to do, following a practitioner-led model, which is suitable for cognitive-behavioral therapies (Keegan, 2016). I highlighted the importance of between-session tasks that Adam would be required to carry out at this initial stage to instil the importance of such tasks in an REBT intervention, and to prepare Adam to undertake independent work, as task completion would be essential to his success. The between-session tasks were pivotal in this case study given the structure of REBT I used with him.

Needs analysis

Adam had completed the irrational Performance Beliefs Inventory (iPBI; Turner et al., 2016) prior to the intervention. The iPBI is to be used in performance environments (such as military, business, sport), and measures four core irrational beliefs (demands, low frustration tolerance [LFT], awfulizing, and depreciation). An example item for the primary irrational beliefs is "Decisions that affect me must be justified" (demands), and example items for the three secondary irrational beliefs are "I can't stand not reaching my goals" (LFT), "It is appalling if others do not give me chances" (awfulizing), and "If my position in my team was not secure, then it would show I am worthless" (depreciation). A composite score of all these beliefs was calculated for Adam, and he scored 28.5 out of a possible maximum of 35. This high score indicated that he had a high amount of irrational beliefs, which further meant that he was susceptible to undesirable maladaptive responses in the face of adversities. Adam scored particularly highly on the LFT subscale (33 out of 35), which was consistent with what I felt in the first meeting. From what Adam had told me, he was unable to tolerate everyday acute stressors and I thus decided to observe another psychological construct at this point. In the REBT literature, the construct of resilience is linked very closely to rationality. Dryden (2011) states that, "Resilience comprises a set of flexible cognitive, behavioral and emotional responses to acute or chronic adversities that can be unusual or commonplace. These responses can be learned and are within the grasp of everyone. While many factors affect the development of resilience, the most important one is the belief the person holds about the adversity. Therefore, belief is at the heart of resilience" (p134).

A large part of resilience is about adapting well in the face of adversity. Education in challenging appraisals and meta-reflection strategies can include minimizing catastrophic thinking, challenging counterproductive beliefs, and encouraging cognitive restructuring (Fletcher & Sarkar, 2012); which are all central tenets of REBT. In REBT, a rational philosophy is to be strived for in order to achieve high resilience (Dryden, 2007; Dryden, 2011; Neenan & Dryden, 2011) Turner, 2016a), which leads to adaptive responses when facing acute and chronic adversity. I surmised that measuring resilience levels in Adam prior to the intervention would be advantageous given the number of stressors he reported and the maladaptive responses he was frequently exhibiting.

Adam completed the Connor-Davidson Resilience Scale-10 (CD-RISC-10; Connor & Davidson, 2003), which is a useful, short questionnaire that measures resilient qualities using ten items, and has been used in past sport psychology literature (for example, see Gucciardi et al., 2011). Higher scores in the CD-RISC-10 reflect higher levels of resilient qualities. Adam scored 15 out of a maximum of 40, which is relatively low. These initial scores provided initial guidance for me as there was substantive data I could use to support my initial assumptions. It would be around a month before I could start working with Adam due to our schedules. Adam agreed to complete six more measures of the iPBI and the CD-RISC-10 (two times a week for three weeks), and we continued this pattern throughout the work we did together. This meant that when I did get to work with Adam I could observe changes in his results after the sessions started and compare these changes in the data from pre- to post-REBT phases (for more details on similar data collection methods, see Ottenbacher 1986). To simplify the data collection, I had compiled the two questionnaires online and gave the URL to Adam, which he could then access via his smartphone. Adam could complete the questionnaire anytime and anywhere if he had an Internet connection. The average composite irrational beliefs score was 27.86, and for resilient qualities it was 19.86, for these seven pre-REBT data points (see Figures 12.4 and 12.5 later in the chapter).

The intervention

Figure 12.1 shows the structure of REBT that I used with Adam, including five sessions each with a one-hour duration. We had one session per week and there were four with varying cognitive and behavioral between-session assignments set. I had followed guidelines set for using REBT and credos with athletes (see Turner & Barker, 2014; Turner, 2016a). The flow for the sessions and the between-session assignments complemented each other and it was important to keep the intervention in a logical order. I created worksheets for the first four sessions (for guidelines, see Ellis & Dryden, 1997), which I then used to support the work I was doing with Adam.

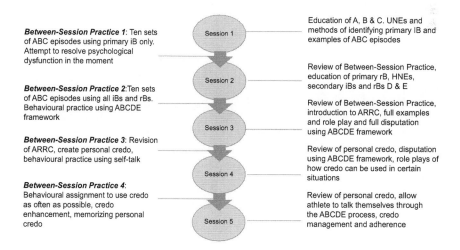

Between-Session Practice 1: Ten sets of ABC episodes using primary iB only. Attempt to resolve psychological dysfunction in the moment

Session 1 — Education of A, B & C. UNEs and methods of identifying primary IB and examples of ABC episodes

Session 2 — Review of Between-Session Practice, education of primary rB, HNEs, secondary iBs and rBs D & E

Between-Session Practice 2: Ten sets of ABC episodes using all iBs and rBs. Behavioural practice using ABCDE framework

Session 3 — Review of Between-Session Practice, introduction to ARRC, full examples and role play and full disputation using ABCDE framework

Between-Session Practice 3: Revision of ARRC, create personal credo, behavioural practice using self-talk

Session 4 — Review of personal credo, disputation using ABCDE framework, role plays of how credo can be used in certain situations

Between-Session Practice 4: Behavioural assignment to use credo as often as possible, credo enhancement, memorizing personal credo

Session 5 — Review of personal credo, allow athlete to talk themselves through the ABCDE process, credo management and adherence

Figure 12.1 Structure of REBT used with Adam

Session 1

I began with an overview of what the goals were for the session and what we would hope to achieve in the next hour. I gave Adam a folder in which he could keep his worksheets and gave him new sheets to work on as the sessions went along, and this folder would eventually contain all written work conducted in the intervention. The worksheets were used in the sessions to guide the process of REBT and were not the sole focus of the sessions. I then briefly explained the meanings behind the Stoic maxim, "people are disturbed not by things, but by the view which they take of them" (Ellis, 1989, p. 6), as this embodies the core philosophy of REBT.

I presented Adam with a list of emotions (unhealthy and healthy negative emotions: see Dryden, 2009) and asked Adam when he had last felt one of the emotions (C), what it felt like (physiological consequence), what he did when he had that feeling (behavioral consequence), and what he was thinking (cognitive consequence). Adam reported that he had felt anger (C) recently during and after a team talk, and described this emotion in detail. We then progressed to find the adversity (A) that was linked to this emotion. As there are many potential As in a client's perceptual field (Dryden & Branch, 2008), it took some skill to educate Adam on finding the "critical A". I used a simple questioning technique, which is effective in finding the critical A (Dryden & Branch, 2008). I asked Adam to imagine the scenario in which he felt anger, and to pretend that he could not change anything about this situation at all. I asked him to stick with that scenario for a moment. I would then ask Adam to pretend that I had given him the magical power to amend just one, and *only one*, element of this scenario/situation which would make him feel better instantly. I then asked, "what is the *one thing* that you would change so that you will feel better instantly?" With this questioning technique, it becomes simple to understand which part of the situation (A) is the most critical and important part.

Adam said that, "if the coach spoke positively about me in the team talk, I would feel better". To get the critical A from this situation (the team talk), all we have to do is use whatever is the opposite of the client's answer. In this instance, the opposite of Adam's answer is "the coach spoke negatively about me in the team talk", and this is the critical A. Once the critical A was found, we began our search for the irrational beliefs (B) between the A and C. I strongly emphasized the B-C connection by educating Adam as to how primary irrational beliefs can present themselves, and sensitized him to "musts, needs, oughts, and shoulds". I used a whiteboard to write down his ABCs throughout our work (see Figure 12.2).

I elaborated on Figure 12.2 to make sure we covered each part of the A, B, and C in as much detail as possible. Adam was clearly learning a lot about himself and I saw that this process encouraged him. Collaboratively, we identified that when he is angry, his behavioral response is that he immediately seeks to be alone so that he might cool down and attempt to arrange his thoughts. He construed this as taking a long time to "sulk like a kid". Although it could have been quite

Activating Event (A)

Situation: My coach's attitude towards me

Adversity: Not being able to return to my hometown because my coach won't allow me to

Irrational Beliefs (iB)	Rational Beliefs (rB)
Demand: "I want to go home so I must be allowed to return home when I want to"	**Preference:** "I want to go home, but that doesn't mean that I have to go now"
Awfulizing: "It is so terrible that I am not allowed to go home and see my family"	**Non-Awfulizing:** "It isn't so bad that I can't go home at the moment"
Low Frustration Tolerance: "I cannot handle being denied my rights to go home"	**High Frustration Tolerance:** "I can handle not going home this time"
Other-Depreciation: "I hate my coach and I cannot accept such harsh and pointless decisions"	**Other-Acceptance:** "I understand that sometimes my coach will make decisions that I really don't like, and I can accept that he's a fallible human being who won't always say what I want to hear"

Unhelpful Consequences (C)	Helpful Consequences (E)
Emotional: Depressed, angry	**Emotional:** Sad, disappointed
Behavioral: Withdrawal	**Behavioral:** Remaining included, willing to express emotions in a healthy manner
Cognitive: "I just want to go home, I hate my coach"	**Cognitive:** "It's okay, I can still keep in touch with my family and I will get to go home soon enough"
Physiological: Tears, increased heart rate, restlessness, hot around the collar	**Physiological:** No tears, more stable heart rate, less restlessness

Figure 12.2 ABC formulation

a heavy and negative session, Adam began to find his behavioral responses particularly amusing once he had seen them written on a whiteboard. It may have been his age, or the way in which I had explained the ABC combinations, that made him laugh. I used humour by just being myself so that both of us would feel comfortable and I felt that with Adam, this worked and allowed him to take more interest in what we were discussing, so I decided to continue to use humour for the course of the intervention. Between sessions 1 and 2, I requested Adam complete ten sets of these ABC combinations and I highlighted that I would be marking these at the beginning of the second session before any other further REBT education was to be completed. I also gave Adam free reign when completing the Cs, for example, he could write "lower confidence", "distracted", or "annoyance", so that he could use his own words to describe best what he felt, as opposed to just using UNEs (see Dryden, 2009).

Session 2

I adopted a didactic approach and marked Adam's between-session work at the beginning of the session, providing ticks, crosses, and feedback on the worksheets that he had written on. He had successfully understood all that was covered in the first session, and had reported his C as "anger" on numerous occasions. I used this as the platform for the session by enquiring about these scenarios. Even though Adam was a full-time athlete, he was of course a human being first – a teenage boy, who was not too unlike myself when I was his age. I explained to Adam that I had overcome similar adversities, which had eventually made me a better and wiser person, and in this sense portrayed myself as a role model of rationality and resilience which would encourage the therapeutic process (Dryden & Branch, 2008). I set out the goals for the session in that I would teach Adam the further secondary levels of his irrational beliefs and how to successfully dispute these and replace them with rational, healthier, flexible, logical, and non-extreme rational beliefs.

I used the whiteboard again, and split it into two sections by drawing a line down the middle. On the left, I had the same ABC format from the work before with the words "must", "should", "need", and "have/has" written in bold. On the right, I wrote the same ABC format, but with the words "wish", "want", "would like", "hope", and "desire" to represent the core of counterpart primary rational beliefs. Using primary preferences, however, in an "asserted" fashion is only the first part of a true rational belief, as it can be ultimately made irrational. For example, "I wish to do well in this tournament, and therefore I must". In this example, the belief starts with a flexible non-dogmatic preference and becomes an extreme and rigid demand. To stop this from happening, I used the word "BUT" to conjoin the initial "asserted preference" of "I wish to do well in this tournament" to its counterpart known as a "negated demand", to form the full rational belief that, "I wish to do well in this tournament, BUT I do not have to". We rationalized each of his prevalent irrational beliefs at the primary and secondary levels for each specific scenario.

I used a pop-quiz style to assess Adam's current understanding of the primary and secondary rigid and flexible beliefs as there was a lot covered in the second session. His between-session work was then based on a behavioral practice in which he was to attempt to manage his emotions in the moment by reminding himself of the primary rational beliefs through the practice of self-talk, as self-talk is considered the key to cognitive control (Zinsser, et al., 2010).

Sessions 3, 4, and 5

Adam had reported that he felt he was able to control his emotions better than before, which helped him in training by improving his focus and feeling less uneasy about being away from home. His between-session work included a wide variety of sporting and personal scenarios for which he was successfully able to identify the irrational and rational beliefs. Adam seemed to have a clear grasp of the ABC framework, and at an intellectual level, he was able to recognize both irrational and rational beliefs.

Prior to REBT, Adam's levels of resilience were inconsistent, and in those seven pre-REBT data points he scored 15 out of 40, then 22, 20, 20, 12, 25, and 25, meaning that the range average (the largest score of 25 minus the smallest score 12) was 13. After two sessions, his scores had increased and had become more stable (23, 22, 24, and then 27), with the range now being only 4, showing that there was far less variability when compared to the pre-REBT scores. I now felt that it was appropriate to introduce Adam to the Athlete Rational Resilience Credo (ARRC: Turner, 2016a), which became the central focus of the subsequent work done in sessions 3, 4, and 5. Credos are defined as "a set of beliefs, which expresses a particular opinion and influences the way you live" (Dryden, 2007, p. 219). The ARRC comprises five paragraphs, one for each of the primary and secondary rational beliefs, and one promoting adherence to the credo itself (for a full version of the ARRC, please see Turner, 2016a).

Adam had made great strides in his written between-session tasks, so I had no doubt that he would take well to the credo, as it is a lengthy written text. I explained to Adam that the ARRC:

(a) . . . was a guide that would help him further internalize a rational philosophy.
(b) . . . would serve Adam even after the five sessions we had together were eventually completed.
(c) . . . is a specific tool for athletes and therefore relevant to him.
(d) . . . provides a motivational target for an ideal level of rationality and resilience.
(e) . . . could be personally adapted to suit his needs should he feel that he could produce something more powerful than what was presented.

Coaching using the credos

First, Adam was tasked with annotating each section of the ARRC with a highlighter and pen, focusing on parts he found interesting or didn't understand. Then, an open discussion around each paragraph was held to briefly explain what it meant. This did not take long as Adam had a good understanding of the ABCDE framework. Following that, I provided examples where specific sections could be used in certain scenarios, referring to previous between-session task sheets. Then, we discussed how sections of the credos can be used, suggesting implementation with other mental skills training such as self-talk, imagery, pre-performance routines, and breathing techniques. Adam was asked to further adapt the credo in a behavioral assignment, so that he may create his own version of the ARRC. I felt that a personal version would be more potent, powerful, meaningful, and significant if it was written in his own words and style (cognitive task). I then set targets for how often the credo would be used and which sections (e.g., the HFT paragraph twice a day as this was highly specific to Adam). I reviewed the personal credo to ensure that it was still consistent with REBT principles, and

My name is Adam and I am a normal human being. As a human being, I naturally have both positive and negative thinking. Having negative emotions can lead to a negative life, which can be very stressful. I also know, that negative thinking and rigid beliefs are the foundation of unhealthy negative emotions. But now I know how to be positive every single time when I'm having a bad day, and with the help of my psychologist I can try to be flexible.

I am a human being, and as a human I am also not perfect. Every single human makes mistakes in their lives but whether they make the effort to make a change on their own is the important thing. There's always times that you will have to deal with some shitty situation, and this will always be true, but it's okay because that is life. Everyone has some issue at some point, it's never just me. Life is being fair to all of us, and the task we have is to try and handle what life throws at us. My goals are sincere and if I don't achieve my goals, it doesn't mean my life is over. There's always something I can do, and I will try my best to be as flexible as I can.

When I look back at the adversities I have faced and have overcome positively, I realise that is done in a healthy way. I realise that it was because I eventually placed adversities in perspective. I would always think, "why do people do this to me? . . . is it because they are having some bad day? Are they just like that all the time?" But now when people hurt me, I can look at myself and realise there are times when I have done the same to others too. And when I really think on it, actually, people hurting me isn't even that sad after all. Whatever I'm suffering probably isn't as bad as I can make it out to be and doesn't compare to what they have gone through, or what others go through all the time around the world. I can think of my Dad and how he was back in the days when he used to finish work so late at night and came back carrying all the stress, but his behavior and mood was always flexible and that's how he dealt with it. He used to tell me that "this is life, you can't always get what you want". Every day I look at him as my hero as he just kept on getting stronger when he was faced with problems. When I think about my Dad, I ask myself too, "how can he be so positive with his thinking when there are so many obstacles in his way?" If he can do it, then I know I can do it too.

When I am faced with life adversities, I will tell myself to accept it. For example, after I lose a squash match. I will tell myself to work harder so that when I face that opponent again I can get my revenge by winning. I know it will be tough to follow this credo but I will always practice it and read my credo every single day. I will use certain parts of the credo to remind myself of what I have learnt. If I catch myself being rigid I will use my credo to be flexible as I can. Even if it doesn't work straight away, I can accept being rigid sometimes and give myself sometime to be flexible.

I've learnt a lot in my psychology sessions and I gain confidence with what I have learnt. Even if I fail in the national squash programme, it doesn't mean my life is over. I can still find other ways to have a life. When adversities happen, I will try to keep their size and proportion into perspective so that I won't be negative, and so that I can think clearly in pressure situations and stay focused on my goals and what I want to achieve in life.

Figure 12.3 Adam's credo

reminded Adam to continually update the credo, removing parts which were no longer effective and adding and substituting content (cognitive task), as this would ensure that the credo was as strong as possible. I encouraged Adam to place small copies of the credo in his wallet, racket bag, fridge, phone cover, and drawer so that it was easily accessible and to serve as a reminder so that he could use certain parts in specific situations (behavioral task). Finally, I encouraged Adam to also memorize specific sections so that he could use them in the moment to functionally influence his emotions, cognitions, and behaviors (behavioral task).

As can be seen from the previous discussion, the ARRC was used in both cognitive and behavioral between-session assignments, in which Adam could reflect on the credo, and use parts of it when he felt it could be beneficial or as part of a routine. By the time the sessions were finished, Adam had remarked that he could visualize adversities as challenges and as opportunities to grow as a person, and this rendered him less fearful of facing adversities and he saw the benefits of overcoming adversities in an adaptive fashion. Figure 12.3 shows the credo that Adam had written and sent to me via email.

The credo work took three sessions. It was important to apply the ARRC fully and meaningfully, rather than to introduce it as merely an additional element of REBT. I felt that the ARRC would help Adam to imbed REBT into his life, and by the end of the fifth session, I was fully confident that Adam could use REBT effectively on himself and that he understood the best practices with regards for using the credo. I assessed this by allowing him to talk himself through the ABC(DE) process from start to finish several times using a mix of hypothetical scenarios, and he successfully implemented the credo into the DE stages of the framework.

Outcome analysis

The data collected over the course of the REBT work is shown in Figures 12.4 and 12.5. After the work had finished, Adam was to continue completing questionnaires for a further three weeks and then to take a one-month break in which he wouldn't submit any data, and then just to submit one final data point, as this would show post-intervention effects as I was interested in how his irrational beliefs and resilience might change after our work had finished.

As can be seen in Figures 12.4 and 12.5, Adam's irrational beliefs decreased and his levels of resilience increased. After the intervention was completed, these effects were maintained, and this may have been due to Adam rehearsing the credo repetitively again and again. For descriptive statistics, Adam's composite irrational beliefs mean score dropped from 27.86 (out of 35) to 14.34 at post-intervention. Furthermore, his mean resilience score increased from 19.86 (out of 40) to 30.81 post-intervention.

I arranged for a third party, who was a fellow psychologist known to Adam, to interview Adam after the fifth session to ask him some questions regarding the intervention. The interview focused on three specific areas, which were (a) the social significance of the goals of the intervention, (b) the appropriateness of the procedures, and (c) participant satisfaction with the results of the intervention (Wolf,

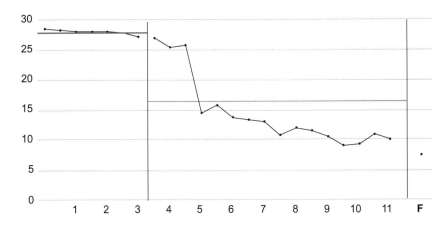

Figure 12.4 Composite irrational beliefs across the REBT intervention

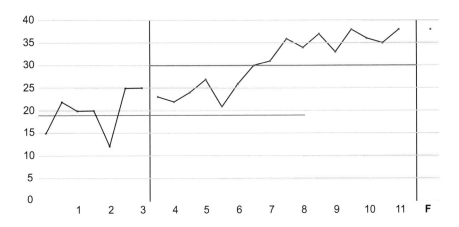

Figure 12.5 Resilient qualities across the REBT intervention

1978; Page & Thelwell, 2013). Adam explained that his levels of well-being and emotional control had increased, his unhealthy anger had reduced, and he was able to handle adversities more effectively than before. Adam felt lucky to have received the REBT intervention, reporting that it was useful and unique, and that he never imagined that he could learn something like this from a sport psychologist. He felt confident with using the credo, stating that, "if you're facing an adversity, and you read that credo . . . you won't feel so bad. Yeah, you will feel much better". Additionally, Adam rated the entire intervention with a score of 8 out of 10.

Recent correspondence between myself and Adam via text message confirmed that he still uses the credo and that it always works for him, however, there have been times where he has found it more difficult to use than others. Adam has progressed approximately 100 places in world ranking, and he attributes at least

50% of his success to the work we did in those five sessions and on-going usage of the credo. Adam is doubtful as to whether he would have gained so much from the REBT intervention in the long-term had he not taken ownership of his credo and kept it with him for usage.

Critical reflections

This work was beneficial to Adam. In REBT, resilience is the result of holding rational beliefs, and observing resilience as well as rationality over the course of the intervention helped to indicate how effective REBT was. Taking data scores before working with Adam helped to ascertain what his baseline temperament was like, and this was vital because I did not know Adam prior to my work with him. Allowing a trend to be observed in a time-series helped me to understand more about Adam. Some may consider it unethical to delay an intervention that might benefit an individual, in order to collect multiple baseline data points, but our schedules did not allow us to start the work immediately. Adam liked that he could fill in the questionnaire online, and I encourage fellow practitioners to take advantage of technological advances and progress with them. Regarding the pre-intervention baseline, I would have liked to use fewer quantitative measures and make more use of the coach's feedback and observations similar to Si and Lee (2008). Had the circumstances allowed me, I could have observed Adam in training and competition and recorded maladaptive responses or undesired behaviors (such as outbursts in the court).

At the time of the work described in this chapter, I was fresh from the REBT training course and although I was confident using REBT, I sometimes felt nervous about the idea that the session may not go as well as I hoped. During my work with Adam, I was also working with other athletes and I faced some unexpected situations in those sessions. This led me to question myself as to whether I could have avoided these difficulties by doing things a different way, however, I have to recognize that I was a new practitioner then and it is to be expected. To keep track in sessions, I devised my own worksheets, which helped me to structure my sessions especially when I first started practicing. Secondly, I decided to focus on feedback I received in my training, in which I was commended for my "soft skills" in engaging clients, such as the judicious use of humour. Therefore, I made an utmost effort to smile and be welcoming, to create a level of understanding through humour, and to really focus on the client-practitioner relationship. Even though it is not essential that the practitioner be liked by the client to successfully use REBT, it is helpful to remember as practitioners that our clients are people, that people can be vulnerable, and therefore must be treated with care and nurtured through the therapeutic process. I would suggest that practitioners do not present themselves as all-knowing gurus, coming across as arrogant or bluntly direct or even flippant, as from my own experiences this type of behavior was not well accepted within the culture I was working in. Practitioners must understand that having a "buy-in" from a client to use such a therapy is important, and gaining their trust by being a likeable human being is essential from this aspect. Therefore, in my view, one reason that this case study was a success was due to my rapport-building skills, making Adam feel comfortable using humour, and my own use of relevant and limited personal disclosure, in which I presented myself as humbly as I could.

In terms of working with diversity, learning the local language and fully immersing myself in the culture worked in my favour. I also did this by frequenting local areas and main attractions in the city, getting to know as many people as I could, keeping up to date with local news, gaining access to a variety of sport settings, and using my colleagues as valuable sources of information. Adam found me a person of interest due to this and there were times in the sessions when we would be conversing in two languages. Understanding cultural norms and the uniqueness of cultures is considered an essential counselling competency (Weinberg & Williams, 2010), and it can help practitioners to be sensitive to sociocultural systems, religion, spirituality, and language use (Hanrahan, 2011; Sarkar, et al., 2014). As sport psychologists, we will often learn more about our client's sport when we begin working with them. I actively encourage practitioners to take such education further by learning more about their clients' backgrounds (considering factors such as family, religion, ethnicity, nationality, social status, etc.) and be wary of such important demographic information, whether they are working domestically or abroad.

I would suggest that using credos with athletes be done in a way that suits the athlete. For example, an athlete could easily record credos on a mobile phone or voice recorder as opposed to writing them down. On a similar note regarding individuality, I update my own credo frequently (once every two months), and there is one section that always remains entirely unchanged as so far it has always been effective.

References

Connor, K. M., & Davidson, J. R. T. (2003). Development of a new resilience scale: The 7 Connor-Davidson resilience scale (CD-RISC). *Depression and Anxiety, 18*, 76–82.

Dryden, W. (2007). Resilience and Rationality. *Journal of Rational-Emotive & Cognitive-Behavior Therapy, 25*(3), 213–226. doi:10.1007/s10942-006-0050-1.

Dryden, W. (2009). *How to think and intervene like an REBT therapist.* London: Routledge.

Dryden, W. (2011). *Understanding psychological health: The REBT perspective.* New York, NY: Taylor & Francis.

Dryden, W., & Branch, R. (2008). *The fundamentals of rational-emotive behavior therapy.* Chichester: Wiley.

Ellis, A. (1989). The History of Cognition in Psychotherapy. In A. Freeman, K. Simon, L. Beutler, & H. Arkowitz (Eds.), *Comprehensive Handbook of Cognitive Therapy.* New York: Plenum Press.

Ellis, A., & Dryden, W. (1997). *The practice of rational-emotive behavior therapy.* New York, NY: Springer.

Fletcher, D., & Sarkar, M. (2012). A grounded theory of psychological resilience in Olympic champions. *Psychology of Sport and Exercise, 13*, 669–678.

Gucciardi, D. F., Jackson, B., Coulter, T. J., & Mallett, C. J. (2011). The Connor-Davidson resilience scale (CD-RISC): Dimensionality and age-related measurement invariance with Australian cricketers. *Psychology of Sport and Exercise, 12*, 423–433.

Hanrahan, S. J. (2011). Sport psychology services are multicultural encounters: Differences as strengths in therapeutic relationships. In Gilbourne, D., & M. B. Andersen (Eds.), *Critical essays in applied sport psychology* (pp. 145–156). Leeds: Human Kinetics.

Keegan, R. (2016). *Being a sport psychologist*. London: Palgrave.

Marlow, C. (2009). Creating positive performance beliefs: The case of a tenpin bowler. In B. Hemmings & T. Holder (Eds.), *Applied sport psychology* (pp. 65–87). London: Wiley.

Neenan, M., & Dryden, W. (2011). Understanding and developing resilience. In Neenan, M. & S. Palmer (Eds.), *Cognitive behavioural coaching in practice: An evidence based approach* (pp. 133–152). London: Routledge.

Ottenbacher, K. J. (1986). *Evaluating clinical change: Strategies for occupational and physical therapists*. Baltimore: Williams & Wilkins.

Page, J., & Thelwell, R. (2013). The value of social validation in single-case methods in sport and exercise psychology. *Journal of Applied Sport Psychology, 25*(1), 61–71.

Sarkar, M., Hill, D. M., & Parker, A. (2014). Working with religious and spiritual athletes: Ethical considerations for sport psychologists. *Psychology of Sport and Exercise, 15,* 580–587.

Si, G., & Lee, H. (2008). Is it so hard to change? The case of a Hong Kong Olympic silver medallist. *International Journal of Sport and Exercise Psychology, 6,* 319–330.

Turner, M. J. (2016a). Proposing a rational resilience credo for use with athletes. Journal of Sport Psychology in Action, 7(3), 170–181.

Turner, M. J. (2016b). Rational Emotive Behavior Therapy (REBT), irrational and rational beliefs, and the mental health of athletes. *Frontiers: Movement Science and Sport Psychology, 7,* 1423.

Turner, M. J., Allen, M., Slater, M. J., Barker, J. B., Woodcock, C., Harwood, C. G., & McFadyen, K. (2016). The development and initial validation of the irrational performance beliefs inventory (iPBI). *European Journal of Psychological Assessment.* doi:10.1027/1015-5759/a000314.

Turner, M. J., & Barker, J. B. (2014). Using Rational-Emotive Behavior Therapy with Athletes. *The Sport Psychologist, 28,* 75–90.

Weinberg, R. S., & Williams, J.M. (2010). Integrating and implementing a psychological skills training program. In J. M. Williams (Ed), *Applied sport psychology: Personal growth to peak performance* (6th Ed.) (pp. 361–391). London: McGraw-Hill.

Wolf, M. W. (1978). Social validity: The case for subjective measurement or how applied behavior analysis is finding its heart. *Journal of Applied Behavior Analysis, 11,* 203–214.

Zinsser, N., Bunker, L., & Williams, J. M. (2010). Cognitive techniques for building confidence and enhancing performance. In J. M. Williams (Ed.), *Applied sport psychology: Personal growth to peak performance* (6th Ed.) (pp. 305–335). London: McGraw-Hill.

Editors' commentary on Chapter 12: "Applying Rational Emotive Behavior Therapy (REBT) resilience 'credos' with a South-East Asian elite squash player"

Within this volume, the reader can learn about a variety of different strategies for intervention, each delivered within the context of REBT. Saqib's chapter provides a notable example of this technical eclecticism in his use of a Rational Resilience Credo. This is a lesser-known technique and not something that would be widely taught on REBT training programmes. However, one can clearly see how it is utilized here to develop and reinforce a more functional philosophy. Within the extended ABC(DE) framework, the credo is predominantly working at E, although it could be argued that it contains aspects that support Adam's learning at each stage of the model. The chapter refers to certain limitations around the delivery of REBT in this case. These limitations perhaps fuelled a more creative approach, with the credo and the ABC quizzes exemplifying this.

Whilst the ABC formulation is a consistent feature of the work of REBT practitioners, the model is flexible enough to accommodate a range of interventions and one is likely to see overlap with other psychotherapeutic models (e.g., with Cognitive Therapy in the use of graded exposure, or with Acceptance and Commitment Therapy in the use of self-acceptance metaphors). What is key for practitioners to hold in mind is that whilst technical eclecticism is valued in REBT, theoretical integrity is of greater importance. Whatever technique is employed should (that is a *should* in the recommendation sense of the word and not the demanding sense!) be delivered in such a way that maintains coherence with the fundamental tenets of the model. Before employing any technique outside of the classical options such as disputation or rational emotive imagery (REI), practitioners would do well to ask themselves what it is they are trying to achieve in using it. Will it undermine irrational beliefs? Will it promote a more functional behavioral repertoire? A second opinion is always useful in terms of keeping faith with the model, and so we would always recommend on-going REBT as a means of promoting adherence.

13 Delivering Rational Emotive Behavior Therapy (REBT) education in youth rugby union

Aaron Phelps-Naqvi and Jonathan Katz

Presenting issue

I (lead author) was contacted by the assistant coach of a youth rugby union team about a 'performance dip' that was attributed to psychological factors. Specifically, the coach highlighted that perceived negative discourse, a lack of belief amongst the squad, and demotivated body language were indicators that the team had been struggling psychologically with performance demands. Individual intake interviews (Andersen, 2005) with the team captain and head coach were undertaken to gain background information and explore their views related to the 'psychological well-being' of the squad. The captain disclosed his perspective on the difficulties that he and the team were facing, which heavily suggested the existence of a lack of confidence, and dysfunctional thinking and behaviors. Such findings were in line with the feedback from the head coach who stated:

> They don't seem to realize that I just want them to enjoy themselves, because when they do, they play well as a team . . . at the moment confidence is so low. They think they have to do everything right all of the time . . . it doesn't work like that.

These interviews provided an opportunity to devise a needs analysis to inform the chosen psychological support approach (Hemmings & Holder, 2009).

Context

I was made aware that the coaching staff was very keen to utilize sport psychology and I was offered full use of the facilities (the seminar room at the rugby club and on the training pitch) to deliver support provision. This allowed for use of indoor learning materials and amenities (laptops, projectors, TVs, shelter, tables, and chairs) and also outdoor space in order for me to offer practical learning opportunities. In addition, I was made aware that the team were only together twice per week, so it was important to integrate group-based educational workshops and practical exercises (Ellis, 2004; Harrington, 2005) into the existing training sessions and match days.

Needs analysis

Following the intake interviews, behavioral observations were conducted across two training sessions and one match day. The existence of negative dialogue ("this is absolutely poor!", "I can't do this"), behaviors indicative of low frustration tolerance (head in hands, hitting the ground), and awfulizing comments ("you are terrible") were noted. These observations corroborated the information obtained from the intake interviews. Following behavioral observations, an introductory workshop and team meeting discussed how the group viewed the current issues. The group meeting also provided an opportunity to feedback the outcome from the behavioral observations (Andersen, 2000). Within this meeting, key counselling skills such as active listening were adopted as a way of initiating a working alliance (Katz & Hemmings, 2009), and Socratic questioning (Paul & Elder, 2006) to encourage the athletes to reflect on the factors that they believed contributed to their recent poor performances. Utilizing such techniques also helped to explore observed findings surrounding dysfunctional emotions and behaviors with the team.

During discussion and 1:1 conversations, 100% of the athletes disclosed that they felt a high degree of anxiety before and during games and were low in confidence and motivation on match days. In addition, an athlete described performing poorly and, "Thinking about it for days after" due to, "Too much pressure on me because I take all the kicks. . . . They look to me to win the game all the time". This led to rumination on the potentially negative consequences of not performing to his best. Such discourse suggested some potential irrational thinking about his performances. Further discussions with the group uncovered a variety of dysfunctional thoughts (e.g., "if the boss sees me playing like this, I'm off, I hope he rates me well today") and dysfunctional behaviors (e.g., mood swings and being physically aggressive with team mates), which may have been contributing to anxiety and loss of confidence.

The observational data, interviews, and team meeting data prompted a group assessment by administering the Shortened General Attitudes and Beliefs Scale (SGABS; Lindner, Kirkby, Wertheim, & Birch, 1999) with each player in order to assess the prevalence of irrational beliefs and agree upon a suitable support approach (Neenan & Dryden, 2001). The SGABS provided a valid and reliable measure of irrational beliefs, and has been used with athletes in the past (Turner & Barker, 2014). It was important to consider the scores from the SGABS alongside observations and discussions with the athletes and support staff to determine whether the use of REBT was justified. I was required to carefully present the need and value of using this psychometric, as squad members were reluctant to engage with completing a questionnaire. Once the purpose and value to them was understood and accepted, the squad agreed to complete the SGABS.

The SGABS information was important in tailoring REBT to the athletes' specific irrational beliefs. For example, their pre-intervention scores (see Figure 13.1) indicated high need for achievement, approval, and fairness, which suggested that they might benefit from adopting a more rational approach, underpinned by preferences instead of demands (Palmer, 2000). The triangulation of

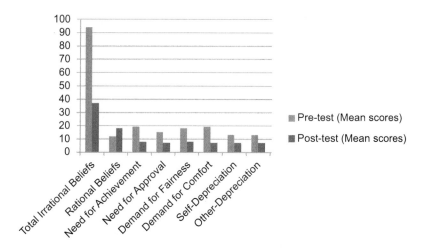

Figure 13.1 Pre- and post-REBT self-report data for the athletes

data from observations, athlete and support staff discussions, and data from the SGABS inventories confirmed that REBT was a suitable approach.

In addition, to measure the effectiveness of session delivery a qualitative pre-designed social validation questionnaire was provided to athletes after each session to identify their perceptions of the delivery and efficacy of the intervention (Page & Thelwell, 2013). This consisted of both Likert-scale and open-ended questions comprising the perceived importance, usefulness, and impact of the workshop on the athletes' thoughts and behaviors and on-going sporting performance (Macavei & McMahon, 2010). This provided a valuable 'real time' insight into how the group was engaging with the programme, allowing for adaptations to the delivery of the intervention to meet the collective needs of the team over time, and to gain a further insight into individual views and opinions on their progress.

It seemed to me that the team's recent poor form was contributing to, and impacted upon, a negative outlook on their ability. For example, the team were reported to offer negative forms of communication with each other (e.g., pass blame and shame others) during training and on match days, which was believed to limit self and collective belief. The specific dialogue that was noted during observations and discussions, and in the data from the SGABS, indicated a prevalence of irrational beliefs, dysfunctional cognitions, emotions, and behaviors, within the team. As a result, I decided to implement a REBT-based education programme with the team to help uncover and challenge individual and collective beliefs. REBT was also chosen as it could provide a logical and flexible structure with practical application that is simple for athletes to follow and complemented the need to deliver the support programme within the existing team's time constraints. Additionally, due to high mean scores of total irrational beliefs on the SGABS (M = 94/120), REBT aimed to educate the athletes and raise awareness of different types of beliefs and their impacts on performance whilst offering a workable standard of evaluation to dispute irrational beliefs and understand functional emotions and behaviors. The decision to use an REBT approach was shared with the group, which was accepted as a way of raising the team's awareness of dysfunctional thinking and how changing this could positively impact on both individual and team performance (Turner & Barker, 2013).

Based on the needs analysis, the aims of support were to (a) outline the use of REBT in an easily understandable way and (b) educate the team in how to identify and manage performance issues rooted in rigid beliefs. Furthermore, the delivery of REBT was underpinned by specific training (Primary Practicum in REBT) and informed by previous literature (Gonzalez, et al., 2004; Turner et al., 2014; Turner & Barker, 2014).

The REBT programme

The REBT programme consisted of educational workshops, group discussions, and practical exercises broken down into the following phases. The programme focused on the REBT ABCDE model and took place across seven forty-minute interactive workshops and group discussions. Sessions 1 and 2 comprised fundamentals of the model and techniques advocated in research (Dryden, 2009; Ellis & Dryden, 1997). Specific reference was made to the ABCDE model in each session with sport specific examples to ensure athlete understanding of the REBT model.

Sessions 3, 4, and 5 focused on understanding the different core irrational and rational beliefs and how to dispute and re-evaluate irrational performance beliefs. Specifically, the group discussed rational beliefs as flexible, non-extreme, and logical, and contrasted them with irrational beliefs (rigid, extreme, and illogical). Once an understanding of this distinction had been confirmed the group-explored beliefs in more detail, exploring the four core rational and irrational beliefs. This phase consisted of using a worksheet and a flipchart to present how the beliefs can be broken down and understood. In addition, the team were split into groups to identify and discuss their own beliefs in addition to common irrational beliefs to the squad that they experienced during competitive play. This was then shared with the full group for discussion and to explore the players' understanding of the role and function behind why these 'group beliefs' were held. Sessions 6 and 7 focused on applying what had been learned in different scenarios via role-playing. For example, the team was split into smaller working groups on the training pitch and asked to recreate pre-determined scenarios that would provoke an irrational thought or response. This was an excellent way for the athletes to utilize the knowledge gained from educational sessions in rugby specific situations by applying the agreed preferred 'belief' and behavioral responses in the scenarios.

The REBT process

A large part of the work done with the team included the ABCs of REBT. Here, I detail this particular element. Initially, I explained the ABCs of REBT to the team, highlighting the notion that when facing adversity, a challenging situation, or an activating event (A), it is the belief(s) (B) about the adversity that determines the emotional and behavioral consequences and associated responses (C). This reinforced the view that it is the perception and appraisal of events and not the event itself that produce the emotional and behavioral consequences. For example, the pressure caused by others (A) is unlikely to cause anxiety (C) alone without irrational beliefs (B). This served to challenge the validity of statements such as "this much pressure makes me anxious", which suggests the erroneous link between the adversity (A; pressure) and the emotional consequence (C; anxiety). Here, the team was split into smaller groups to identify and discuss common irrational beliefs that they held during competitive play and training across a range of situations. It was vital at this stage that the athletes realized that it was their belief(s) that were leading to feelings of anxiety and a lack of confidence, and that they could develop their ability to control such beliefs, and thus control emotional and behavioral responses. On demonstrating their understanding of the fundamental REBT process, via verbal and written feedback and progress in sport specific role-play (Macavei & McMahon, 2010), we proceeded to identify common ABCs (Dryden, 2012).

Identifying the relationship between beliefs, emotions, and behaviors

To provide the group with an underpinning understanding of emotional and behavioral responses an introductory sport psychology workshop was delivered. This enabled the athletes to understand that 'feeling anxious' and 'underperforming' were emotional and behavioral (Cs), resulting from experiencing irrational beliefs in association with a challenging situation or event (A). Additionally, the athletes were made aware that anxiety can be viewed as unhealthy because of its association with behaviors that are incongruent with achieving the desired or stated performance goal. Concern was suggested as a healthy alternative as it is associated with behaviors consistent with achieving preferred goals (Ellis & Harper, 1997). The group initially struggled to understand the subtle differences between healthy and unhealthy emotions such as concern versus anxiety. The support delivery focused on providing opportunities for discussion and group activities demonstrating the difference between the two, using sport specific scenarios to provide relevant contextual appreciation. Group members began to grasp the significance of how the quality of cognitions, rational and irrational beliefs, impacted associated emotional and behavioral Cs. Once this was understood, the athletes were able to evaluate their beliefs, and challenge them to generate healthier alternatives.

Finding the adversity (A)

REBT emphasizes the importance of identifying the specific features or aspects of a situation that create discomfort – the activating event. In the current programme, therefore, it was essential to find the team's common critical adversities (A) because one or more A's can trigger, or activate, irrational beliefs. To identify the critical adversity, we utilized a technique called inference chaining (Ellis et al., 1997) to facilitate the discovery of underlying inferences that represented common core beliefs surrounding important matches. I used a flip chart to demonstrate inference chaining as a way of demonstrating the chain from start to finish, raising awareness of the consequences of how faulty thinking can change one's views. The most significant inference chain identified was used before matches, which led players to feelings of anxiety.

Inference chaining

SEP (Psychologist):	What makes you guys anxious when going into an important match?
P1 (Player 1):	If you play bad, everyone will think you're a poor player and show no respect.
SEP:	Why is that an issue?
P1:	Everyone will think you're not good enough.
SEP:	Why would that be bad?
P2 (Player 2):	The coach might think you're not good enough and won't recommend you to bigger clubs and you would probably struggle to get a contract.
SEP:	Why is this so bad?
P1:	You won't get your big chance to play at the highest level. Even though it's a long shot.
SEP:	Okay, let's assume that's true, if you have a bad game and you get dropped. Why would that be such a bad thing?
P2:	If you get dropped, you'll never become a professional . . . just a failure and others won't respect you anymore.

As an outcome of this inference chaining, the athletes indicated that never reaching professional status was a central concern. For example, important matches were found to provoke excessive anxiety, rather than concern, partly due to the perception by some players that the coach's pre-game evaluation and judgment were particularly intense. Thus, failure in these situations would be viewed as detrimental to goal attainment (becoming a professional). Furthermore, common critical adversities were identified including: importance of performing well, not being respected by others, others performing better, not deserving to play, and not being able to compete with the opposition. Each one was explored via inference chaining. Importantly, these critical adversities were generated by the athletes and provided them with an opportunity to become more self-aware, which was viewed as helpful by the group (see Figure 13.2 for an example of an ABC formulation of one such critical adversity).

Identifying irrational beliefs (IBs)

The fundamental therapeutic purpose of REBT is to change irrational beliefs to rational beliefs and therefore identifying common irrational beliefs was a key

---

Activating Event (A)

Situation: Playing in a competitive match against a rival
Adversity: "Playing poorly means I'll never become a professional player"

Irrational Beliefs (IB)	Rational Beliefs (RB)
Demand: "I want to play well and I have to do so in every game"	**Preference**: "I want to play well but I realize I don't absolutely have to every single time I play"
Awfulizing: "It will be the worst thing if I play poorly today"	**Anti-Awfulizing**: "It would not be the worst thing ever if I underperformed; it would be a bad experience that is a common part of playing sport"
Low Frustration Tolerance: "I can't hack playing poorly"	**High Frustration Tolerance**: "I can manage playing below my best; I am a fallible human being"
Self-Depreciation: "If I play poorly, I'll be a complete failure"	**Self-Acceptance**: "It is acceptable to have an off day because I know I can play better; I will get another chance; I'm not a complete failure"

Unhelpful Consequences (C)	Helpful Consequences (C)
Emotional Consequence: Feeling anxious and down	**Emotional Consequence:** Feeling concerned but ready
Behavioral Consequence: Avoiding game situations Feigning injuries	**Behavioral Consequence:** Approaching game situations to challenge your beliefs
Cognitive Consequence: Telling yourself what you shouldn't be doing (negative self-talk)	**Cognitive Consequence:** Positively reinforcing self-belief
Physiological Consequence: Feeling sick	**Physiological Consequence:** Feeling prepared

---

Figure 13.2 Example of ABC analysis

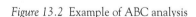

focus within the programme (Turner & Barker, 2014). Using a critical adversity (A), I used Socratic questioning in small groups of five, to locate primary irrational beliefs, as this methodology was systematic, encouraged player reflection, and allowed me to check athlete understanding. For example, I posed questions such as, "What are you saying to yourself about A that is causing the emotional and behavioral response (C)?" Specifically, a number of primary irrational beliefs emerged such as, "I must always give, and play, my best", "I just have to win", and "The coach has to see me doing my best". Key words such as "have to" or "must" were noted in an absolute sense and were challenged by asking, "must you?" and "do you really have to?" as a way of encouraging the athletes to think about their beliefs. I believe that these challenges were influential towards the quality of athlete reflection, which was essential in changing irrational beliefs. By having these (irrational) statements challenged the athletes were able to vocalize their beliefs and become increasingly (self) aware of how 'irrational they sound' especially when related to more serious life events such as a broken limb. Importantly, challenging statements brought resistance and defensiveness from some athletes. For instance, when I questioned their responses, some athletes were abrupt and dismissive: "of course I have to . . . what kind of question is that?" It is noteworthy that intellectual insight on its own can be insufficient to produce the desired change from irrational beliefs to more rational beliefs. Recognizing the need for patience is important as change is gradual and it is possible that a player may be invested in maintaining an irrational belief despite knowing that it is unhelpful.

Next, we revisited the inference chaining exercise to provide a useful insight into the secondary irrational beliefs (Dryden, 2012) related to influencing anxiety, a lack of motivation, and low confidence. Of particular note were comments referring to the adversity as 'terrible' or 'shocking'. Each word was explored to understand the meaning and to establish the secondary irrational beliefs, which clarified their meaning and raised awareness of how these beliefs can negatively impact on thoughts, emotions, and behaviors. Understanding the meaning that specific words (shocking) represented for an athlete was important as they can elicit a range of emotions, and highlighted the importance of clarity, especially when aiming for a collective understanding.

With the primary and secondary beliefs now identified, it was possible to construct a set of full irrational beliefs with each group. For example, "I must always play well and win the approval of others, otherwise it would be terrible" or "I have to be able to compete against them". Eliciting and constructing these statements, explicitly, was essential in raising awareness of how these beliefs could induce anxiety, lower confidence, and impede motivation. For example, it was stated by one athlete, "Wow, when I say it out loud I can actually feel myself getting nervous", which indicated that in the face of adversity, it is the individual who controls his or her unhealthy emotions by holding irrational beliefs, and it is not caused by the adversity. It was viewed as important for the athletes to remain focused on the connection between beliefs (B) and emotional and behavioral responses (C) to improve understanding.

To assist in this, weekly 'mental training' tasks were set consisting of cognitive and behavioral exercises to guide the identification, awareness, and disputation of irrational beliefs. Initially, the majority of athletes did not complete the tasks set, reportedly due to time constraints and a lack of organization. On reflection, it is possible that I was expecting too much from the athletes when providing them with between-session practice. However, between-session activities have been suggested as good practice for reinforcing understanding, aiding identification of beliefs, and producing cognitive change (Dryden, 2012). Further, it is possible that the athletes did not value these tasks enough to prioritize them away from the learning environment so they were transferred and practiced in the physical environment as a way of enhancing understanding and adherence with utilizing the REBT model.

Disputation phase

The final phase of education was learning how to dispute irrational beliefs and strengthen rational beliefs (Dryden, 2012). This phase took place across three forty-minute workshops. Here, the aim was to help the athletes to dispute commonly held 'group irrational beliefs' as a strategy to aid desired performance. Attention was placed on the effort required to get the best out of the sessions, how to effectively dispute irrational beliefs, by applying the knowledge gained during the programme to date. Outlining these expectations, alongside my enthusiasm for the positive outcomes they could gain from practice, may have aided group compliance to subsequent between-session practice.

The first step was to highlight that adversities can be viewed in different ways, which recognize the importance of performing well, without being demanding or inflexible. Here, the link between rigid demands ("I must") and dysfunctional emotions (e.g., anxiety), contrasted with flexible preferences ("I would prefer to") and functional emotions (e.g., concern), was reinforced. Suggestions were offered and discussed for replacing the rigid (irrational) beliefs with more flexible (rational) beliefs. For example, "although I want to do my best all of the time, I don't have to; it is unrealistic for even the best players in the world".

To aid understanding, a rugby specific scenario was provided to highlight how different beliefs can lead to different emotions and behaviors before attempting to dispute them. Here, athletes were encouraged to imagine they had converted ten penalties or made ten clean tackles, with the belief that they would prefer to have converted or tackled eleven times, and it would be bad if they didn't, but it wouldn't be terrible. Then, they were asked how they would feel, stating that they "would be a bit annoyed, but could cope". Then, athletes were asked to imagine the same situation but this time with the belief that they absolutely 'must' score or tackle eleven times, and it would be horrible if they achieved less. This exercise illustrated how rigid demands can cause dysfunctional emotions and that by changing a rigid demand to a flexible preference, functional emotions can be promoted (Opris & Macavei, 2005). For example, it is possible that an athlete can still care about winning and losing without being irrational.

After the athletes gained an awareness of common irrational beliefs and their accompanying emotional and behavioral consequences (C), the disputation phase aimed to motivate the athletes to change irrational beliefs and promote healthier emotional alternatives. Here, the adversities are assumed to be true and are not disputed, since the inferences (A; the coach's evaluation) are not under scrutiny, but instead the irrational beliefs prompted by, and held about, the A are challenged and disputed (David, et al., 2010). By assuming that adversities are true the athletes were able to highlight and compare their severity (minor) against other more serious life events, put them into perspective, and dispute them.

Here I provide some examples of disputation of primary irrational beliefs (demands); disputation of secondary irrational beliefs can be found in the extant literature (Turner & Barker, 2014). Following REBT guidelines, common irrational beliefs were disputed using three strategies (evidence, logic, and pragmatics) which were explored systematically and comprehensively to standardize the process (Ellis & Harper, 1997). For evidential disputation, the athletes were asked to provide evidence of where it is written that their demands are true. For example, where does it state that they 'must' always perform well, and how can they prove that they 'must' always perform well. This assertive tactic was helpful in encouraging them to keep thoughts in perspective, using evidence from previous successes. Further to this, the athletes were encouraged to empirically question IBs at moments of poor performance to highlight that irrational demands do not always hold true. This was utilized during training sessions to aid understanding and trigger a rational thought and/or response.

For logical disputation, the athletes were encouraged to consider the notion "just because you want to perform well all the time, it does not mean it must happen", to which a few players responded that they were confused by this statement because they believed that they 'must' always perform well if they want to become professional rugby players. However, after I further challenged and provided current examples of professional athletes' performance level, or form, using statistics (completed passes/kicks), the group appeared to demonstrate an understanding and resonance with thinking logically about the issue. That is, they could see that even the best players make mistakes and underperform at times.

For pragmatic disputation, I aimed to raise awareness of how strongly held and frequently used irrational beliefs are not helpful and may actually be contributing to negative emotions and poor performances. Athletes were asked pragmatic questions such as "how is this irrational belief helpful to you?" This stage was met by some challenges from athletes, which was possibly due to a lack of awareness of their currently held irrational beliefs and "how just assuming that something is not helpful makes things any easier". As mentioned previously, some athletes may be invested in maintaining irrational beliefs, so a single challenge in isolation may not be strong enough to facilitate change. With further pragmatic questioning, the athletes began to understand that holding such irrational beliefs was dysfunctional and realized that it was not the coach, others, or the important match causing anxiety or loss of confidence, but more likely a consequence of rigidly held belief.

Whilst disputing, I did face some challenges from the athletes. For example, some athletes commented, "this is easier said than done", and "have you ever experienced this? You don't play rugby, so how would you know?" The athletes were of course correct in their opinions, however, it was important to reiterate that the model can be transferred to different scenarios and situations, thus it matters little whether or not the practitioner has experienced the exact adversity in question. Additionally, it was key for me to express that my lack of experience of playing rugby was not an important factor in being able to teach athletes how to identify, dispute, and re-evaluate beliefs as I had undergone training in REBT and had extensive experience of working within the sport of rugby. Lastly, a critical element when faced with such challenges was gaining empathic under-standing of what encouraged them to challenge the REBT process, which aided me to evaluate the content and delivery of REBT education.

Between-session practice

It was important to refer to assignments as 'between-session practice' because words such as homework have educational connotations (Turner et al., 2014) and by avoiding such terminology I believed that adherence may increase. Impor-tantly, I was able to gain some support from the coaching staff to supervise athlete behavior in sessions and reinforce the importance of completing between-session practice.

Assignments were set between sessions to accompany the content discussed and placed focus on cognitive and behavioral tasks. This was an aid to reinforce the ABCD process and development of rational (E) beliefs (Dryden, 2009), and was sport specific to increase engagement and relevance. These assignments were viewed as important because it provided each individual athlete with the opportunity to engage with the content of the session in their own way, away from their team mates. For example, different cultural norms within group environments (e.g., a knowledgeable athlete being judged by others for demonstrating understanding) can inhibit athletes from clarifying their understanding within a group setting and if necessary improving and reinforcing it. Importantly, I found that with these ath-letes, it was more useful to encourage them to complete cognitive and behavioral assignments that had a physical element that they could transfer into their own practice on their field of play rather than exclusively a written exercise or task.

Cognitive assignments involved working through the ABCDE process on a self-help worksheet similar to that illustrated in Ellis and Dryden (1997, p. 52–54). A reading assignment was also utilized by distributing workshop slides to the athletes to offer further information to support learning, and advice on how to maintain and enhance their understanding and ability to be rational. Specifically, this assignment was set to reinforce learned material, to aid understanding of how to use the REBT process, and to encourage them to start identifying and chang-ing their own irrational beliefs when they occur. The athletes were encouraged to write down a list of irrational beliefs that they had identified and to produce a healthy alternative for each. Following this they were expected to repeat the healthy alternatives (verbally) to encourage them to regularly dispute an unhelp-ful belief and assume the rational belief to be true. I believe that the structure provided by the between-session practice made it possible for the athletes to learn and understand the process of changing irrational beliefs and to become empow-ered by their success.

In addition to cognitive tasks, behavioral assignments involved producing behaviors that were congruent with the new rational belief. Initially, the athletes were encouraged to buy-into and act 'as if' they already strongly believed their E belief. For example, they were encouraged to project confident facial expressions (smiling, keeping their heads up) and a confident posture (standing upright with shoulders back) whilst communicating positively ("it's okay", "that's okay"). Acting in this manner was intended to strengthen their conviction in the rational (E) belief when faced with adversities, as the athletes recognized helpful consequences in response to the preferred behavior.

Further to this, I set a behavioral assignment involving exposure (Froggatt, 2005) to directly challenge the avoidant tendencies associated with anxiety or a lack of confidence, – for example, by encouraging the athletes to consider situations that provoke negative thoughts and feelings and approach them in order to build a tolerance or resilience to stressful situations. During these situations, athletes were encouraged to reinforce their new E belief. For example, if anxiety became uncontrollable, they were encouraged to recall the ABCDE process and to remember that they are in control of their reactions through their beliefs and not the adversity. Feedback from athletes such as "it all seems easy to believe when you repeat it" and "repeating the negative stuff before obviously made it hard for me to be positive and rational" suggested that this task was helpful in raising awareness of how to identify and dispute irrational beliefs.

Effective new rational belief (E) phase

This final part of the REBT process (Dryden, 2009) took place over two sessions. This was due to the importance of revisiting the disputation process in relation to the specific irrational beliefs and to pick up from where the disputation phase ended. To be precise, we explicitly and collaboratively worked towards creating and promoting effective new rational beliefs. This consisted of reflecting on changing irrational beliefs to something that would be congruent with our previous disputations. Here, the athletes started by negating each adversity to a more balanced perspective, for example, "Although I'd like to play my best all of the time, I don't have to play my best all of the time", "Even though I want to be better than everyone else, I don't absolutely have to be", and "It is true that I would like the coach to always see me doing my best, but he doesn't have to". As expected, these statements were challenged by a number of athletes, with responses such as, "None of them feel true" and "They are not realistic to us becoming professional players". However, a number of other athletes took the lead to dispute these challenges by explaining the importance of flexible beliefs over rigid demands and how these impact on thoughts, feelings, and behaviors. The group dynamic appeared to be an aid to the collective learning and understanding as some players acted as positive role models in relation to applying and adhering to the ABCDE process. As a consequence, I approached these individuals to encourage their efforts in supporting others.

Next, the rational belief statements were disputed in the same manner as the irrational beliefs using a table with the irrational beliefs and the rational beliefs (E) labelled at the top of each column. Then, the athletes were asked to tick the column with the appropriate response to a series of questions that were asked: "Which one of these statements is true?"; "Which is logical?"; "Which one is helpful?"; and "Which ones do you want to strengthen?" The E belief statements received all ticks and each was discussed to ensure that the athletes' reasons were empirical, logical, and pragmatic. At the end of this phase, a rational belief statement was formulated, for example, "I want to be the best, although I don't have to be the best to enjoy my sport. I would prefer to enjoy playing than worry about underachieving or being the best".

Evaluation of effectiveness

Quantitative

Data were collected at the baseline phase (pre-REBT) and after the intervention (post-REBT) to assess beliefs across the irrationality dimensions (see Figure 13.1). The data collected suggested reductions in irrational beliefs after REBT was administered. As can be seen in Figure 13.1, the mean data of athletes' responses reported reductions in total irrational beliefs from pre-intervention (94) to post-intervention (37), but most notable is the decrease in the subscale variables representative of need for achievement (pre = 19, post = 8) and need for approval (pre = 15, post = 7). The marked decrease in these variables suggests that the content of the sessions may have influenced the self-report data. As previously noted, the athletes' demands for performing well (need for achievement) and coach approval (need for approval) were disputed and rational preferences were adopted. Similarly, the need for comfort (pre = 19, post = 7) and fairness (pre = 18, post = 8) content areas decreased, suggesting that the education and disputation phase was effective at challenging irrational beliefs. To explain, two sessions focused on irrational beliefs related to low frustration tolerance indicated by the athletes' commonly reporting not being able to manage or tolerate certain behaviors of others ("I can't stand it when the coach ignores me"). These sessions encouraged the athletes to accept that at times others act unfavourably, but this does not mean that they are bad people (other-acceptance), and that they are able to tolerate being treated unfairly (high frustration tolerance).

Qualitative

To conclude each session, I administered a social validation questionnaire to identify the team's perceptions of the delivery and efficacy of the intervention (Page & Thelwell, 2013). The questionnaire consisted of a Likert-scale and open-ended questions about perceived changes in irrational beliefs, the intervention process, and their performance. This provided valuable information about how the athletes received REBT, and how I delivered to meet their collective needs. For example, a number of athletes commented that REBT had helped them to, "keep sport in perspective". The athletes' data also suggested that the intervention was helpful in reducing feelings of anxiety, and being more emotionally controlled. Data also suggested that REBT had changed the way performance outcomes were viewed. For example, it was noted by more than half of the athletes that an intentional change in their beliefs, via keeping things in perspective, was helpful in decreasing the pressure felt. This suggested that most athletes understood and utilized the B-C connection of the model, due to the realization that they were contributing to their own perception of pressure. However, on occasion, answers were vague, which was a limitation for me in gaining a level of certainty of their understanding.

Critical reflections

My approach to delivering REBT education was systematic, efficient, and collaborative in an attempt to meet the collective needs of the athletes. I arrived at sessions with a structured agenda to retain focus on the important aspects and exercises whilst being mindful of demonstrating core conditions (warmth, empathy, and unconditional positive regard) to encourage a safe and open learning environment (Addis & Bernard, 2002). Although sessions were structured, there were times when it was necessary to be flexible and adapt my teaching to aid understanding. Here, my understanding of the REBT model and the sport of rugby was a key component in my ability to adapt my consultancy style to provide information and demonstrate ideas to meet different learning styles.

The existence of irrational beliefs and their impact on performance were comprehensively explored via group discussions, behavioral observations, and SGABS data before I decided to use the REBT framework. The data highlighted that REBT was a suitable strategy for assisting the team. Had the group not agreed to proceed with this approach, we may have focused on a different form of education, such as Psychological Skills Techniques due to their efficient and practical application in sports settings (Fifer, et al., 2008). Importantly, SGABS data collected at the end of the education programme indicate support for the use of the model (see Figure 13.1) as irrational beliefs were reduced from pre- to post-intervention.

I believe that the effectiveness of the REBT education programme was due, in part, to a collaborative group effort and the willingness of the group to engage in education and tasks from the start (Tod & Andersen, 2012). In reflecting on my delivery, I believe that there is also a more implicit aspect that may have promoted positive change in REBT aside from its efficacy in changing irrational beliefs. For example, my existing relationship with the squad, an understanding of the model, and my optimism and enthusiasm for the approach may have contributed to a placebo effect, potentially contributing to the compliance and faith in REBT. This notion has been supported via the data retrieved, suggesting that my conviction in REBT and a collaborative effort may have been influential in the success of the programme. Additionally, the outcome may have been different had I adopted a more authoritative manner as it may have inhibited self-discovery and autonomy.

The use of SGABS inventories and social validation questionnaires was central to informing my delivery style and effect of the education and techniques used. However, it is possible that some questions were answered dishonestly potentially due to a dislike for completing paperwork and/or in an attempt to appease the questions with idealistic responses.

Practitioner reflections

When promoting the use of REBT with the team there were a number of concerns. For example, the players were young athletes who had a basic understanding of sport psychology and little or no knowledge of REBT. For this reason, it was important to keep educational sessions simple, short, and practical. The delivery of REBT education had an integrated focus due to the needs of the team. To explain, due to the sporting environment and the expectation of practical and sport specific learning, REBT was delivered in classroom-based sessions as a collective, in small groups of four to five athletes, and on the training pitch. Each form of learning included different tasks and scenarios in an attempt to improve understanding and engage the audience. I believe that the mixture of learning opportunities was an essential factor to the high level of compliance and understanding shown by the group. Deviating from the ideal delivery methodology resulted in the support process to be less individualized and personal, however, it appeared appropriate and suitable for engaging and educating a large audience.

Gaining the engagement of the team, when exploring a new approach and encouraging them to complete inventories, may have been influenced by my existing relationship with them. Specifically, I believe that if I had not worked successfully with the team in the past and if I had not outlined a set of rules when engaged in learning, the impact of the programme may have been smaller. A higher rate of group engagement may have been achieved had the support staff offered more assistance to encourage engagement and buy-in during sessions. However, it would have been important to clarify the staff's understanding of the content of sessions before they could assist others, thus using valuable time that was for the athletes. Although gaining the assistance of support staff was not greatly achieved I still encouraged them to be present during educational sessions to show their support to the group and me. Unfortunately, there were times when the staff projected emotions and behaviors that suggested that they were disinterested (using their phones, looking out of the window), which caused me concern as I was expecting them to reinforce the information in my absence. For this reason, I asked each member of staff to join a group of athletes during sessions, as I believed that the athletes had developed a better understanding of the model.

Demonstrating confidence in REBT and 'modeling the model' when teaching were essential to the impact that I aimed to have upon my audience. For example, at moments when I felt that some athletes were bored and being disruptive I had to be mindful that it was not personal as everyone has different attention spans and although I wanted everyone to engage with the content of my workshops, 'they did not absolutely have to'. This was helpful to my feelings of confidence and competence which I have had difficulty with in previous consultancy as I have allowed my audience's responses to affect my thoughts, feelings, and behaviors negatively.

Limitations

This case study promotes REBT as a potentially valuable support approach for helping athletes to deal with dysfunctional emotions and unhelpful behaviors. It does, though, have limitations. Firstly, for long-term change, REBT research (Turner et al., 2014) advocates using one-to-one sessions of varying length for varying durations across a season depending on the rate of progression through the process. This is due to findings that suggest that group REBT support has a short-term influence on irrational beliefs, with irrational beliefs returning to pre-REBT levels following the educational period (Turner et al., 2014). Unfortunately, due to time constraints and availability of the athletes I was unable to conduct one-to-one sessions or deliver the programme throughout the season.

I believe that the time allocated to educating the athletes about the ABC phase was influential in the need to dedicate less time to disputation and develop E beliefs. Additionally, all athletes were made aware of the option of one-to-one support should they have needed it. It is important to note that although group education was adopted to aid efficiency, individual learning opportunities were set to aid further understanding. Further to this, due to the team's availability, I was unable to re-assess their beliefs post-intervention. Doing so may have provided me with an understanding of whether they were actively using REBT and if the intervention was having any long-term effect on their beliefs (Addis & Bernard, 2002). It is important to note that data were collected via a measure not validated with athletes and are not a measure of sport specific beliefs. One such measure has recently been developed, though (irrational Performance Beliefs Inventory; Turner et al., 2016).

Although utilized successfully with the rugby team in question, REBT may not be the most suitable strategy to use with young athletes in all problematic situations as it does not offer a quick fix solution and may not serve the athletes' immediate needs. For example, an athlete seeking help for performance anxiety before an important tournament is more likely to benefit from more palliative strategies such as relaxation techniques that in the short-term alleviate unpleasant symptoms rather than addressing the underlying cognitive determinants such as irrational beliefs. For this reason, it is important to conduct a thorough needs analysis and agree upon the most suitable approach. For this particular case study, the needs analysis was relatively comprehensive and indicative of irrationality amongst the team, which was consistent with REBT tenets and educational approach to support. However, due to being newly educated and enthusiastic about the delivery of REBT it is possible that I 'sought out' links to irrationality amongst the group. This may have had a slight impact but it is important to mention that the results from the needs analysis suggested that an REBT approach would be a suitable approach and yielded positive outcomes that may not have been achieved via the use of another approach.

As a final point, should my future consultancy experiences provide a new opportunity to educate and support athletes using REBT, I would encourage the clients to allow for more time and one-to-one opportunities. Explicitly, learning to recognize and dispute self-depreciating beliefs towards adopting an unconditional self-acceptance perspective is no easy task and requires quality and purposeful repetition. For this reason, I would be keen to provide one-to-one opportunities and explore new ways of 'selling the model' to young athletes as a way of gaining their full engagement, and to promote purposeful practice and understanding. In addition to this, gaining more support from coaching staff, in terms of reinforcing learning in my absence, and identifying an electronic form of administering SGABS and social validation questionnaires could have aided efficiency for data gathering and afforded more time to learning.

References

Addis, J., & Bernard, M. E. (2002). Marital adjustment and irrational beliefs. *Journal of Rational Emotive & Cognitive Behavior Therapy, 2*(1), 3–13.

Andersen, M. B. (2000). *Doing sport psychology.* Champaign, IL: Human Kinetics.

Andersen, M. B. (2005). *Sport psychology in practice.* Champaign, IL: Human Kinetics.

David, D., Lynn, S. J., & Ellis, A. (Eds.). (2010). *Rational and irrational beliefs: Research, theory, and clinical practice.* New York, NY: Oxford.

Dryden, W. (2009). *How to Think and Intervene Like an REBT Therapist.* London: Routledge.

Dryden, W. (2012). The 'ABCs' of REBT I: A preliminary study of errors and confusions in counselling and psychotherapy textbooks. *Journal of Rational-Emotive & Cognitive-Behaviour Therapy, 30,* 133–172.

Ellis, A. (2004). Why Rational Emotive Behaviour Therapy Is the Most Comprehensive and Effective Form of Behaviour Therapy. *Journal of Rational-Emotive & Cognitive-Behaviour Therapy, 22*(2), 85–92.

Ellis, A., & Dryden, W. (1997). *The practice of rational-emotive behaviour therapy.* New York, NY: Springer.

Ellis, A., Gordon, J., Neenan, M., & Palmer, S. (1997). *Stress counselling: A rational emotive behavior approach.* London: Cassell.

Ellis, A., & Harper, R. (1997). *A guide to rational living* (3rd Ed.). Hollywood, CA: Wilshire Book Company.

Fifer, A., Henschen, K., Gould, D., & Ravizza, K. (2008). What works when working with Athletes. *The Sport Psychologist, 22,* 356–377.

Froggatt, W. (2005). *A brief introduction to rational emotive behavior therapy.* Retrieved from www.rational.org.nz/prof-docs/Intro-REBT.pdf.

Gonzalez, J. E., Nelson, J. R., Gutkin, T. B., Saunders, A., Galloway, A., & Shwery, C. S. (2004). Rational Emotive Therapy with children and adolescents: A meta-Analysis. *Journal of Emotional and Behavioral Disorders, 12,* 222–235. doi:10.1177/10634266040 120040301.

Harrington, N. (2005). Dimensions of frustration intolerance and their relationship to self-control problems. *Journal of Rational Emotive & Cognitive Behaviour Therapy, 5*(1), 120.

Hemmings, B. & Holder, T. (2009). *Applied Sport Psychology: A Cased-Based Approach.* Chichester: Wiley-Blackwell.

Katz, J., & Hemmings, B. (2009). *Counselling skills handbook for the sport psychologist.* Leicester: The British Psychological Society.

Lindner, H., Kirkby, R., Wertheim, E., & Birch, P. (1999). A Brief Assessment of Irrational Thinking: The Shortened General Attitude and Belief Scale. *Cognitive Therapy and Research, 23*(6), 651–663.

Macavei, B., & McMahon, J. (2010). The assessment of rational and irrational beliefs. In D. David, S. J. Lynn, & A. Ellis (Eds.), *Rational and irrational beliefs: Research, theory, and clinical practice* (pp. 115–147). New York, NY: Oxford.

Neenan, M., & Dryden, W. (2001). *Learning from errors in rational emotive behavior Therapy*. London: Whurr.

Opris, D., & Macavei, B. (2005). The distinction between functional and dysfunctional negative emotions: An empirical analysis. *Journal of Cognitive and Behavioural Psychotherapies*, 5, 181–195.

Page, J., & Thelwell, R. (2013). The value of social validation in single-case methods in sport and exercise psychology. *Journal of Applied Sport Psychology*, 25(1), 61–71.

Palmer, S. (2000). The future of REBT in the New Millennium. *The Rational Emotive Behavior Therapist*, 8(1), 3–4.

Paul, R. & Elder, L. (2006). *The Art of Socratic Questioning*. Dillon Beach, CA: Foundation for Critical Thinking.

Tod, D., & Andersen, M.B. (2012). Practitioner-client relationships in applied sport psychology practice In S. Hanton & S.D. Mellalieu (Eds.), *Professional practice in sport psychology* (pp. 273–306). London: Routledge.

Turner, M. J. (2016). Rational Emotive Behavior Therapy (REBT), irrational and rational beliefs, and the mental health of Athletes. *Frontiers in Psychology*, 7, 1–16. doi. org/10.3389/fpsyg.2016.01423.

Turner, M. J., Allen, M. S., Slater, M. J., Barker, J. B., Woodcock, C., Harwood, C. G., & McFayden, K. (2016). The development and initial validation of the irrational performance beliefs inventory (iPBI). *European Journal of Psychological Assessment*, 1–7. doi:10.1027/1015-5759/a000314.

Turner, M. J., & Barker, J. B. (2013). Examining the efficacy of Rational-Emotive Behaviour Therapy (REBT) on irrational beliefs and anxiety in elite youth cricketers. *Journal of Applied Sport Psychology*, 25(1), 131–147.

Turner, M. J., & Barker, J. B. (2014). Using Rational-Emotive Behaviour Therapy with Athletes. *The Sport Psychologist*, 28(1), 75–90.

Turner, M.J., Slater, M.J., & Barker, J.B. (2014). Not the end of the world: The effects of rational-emotive behaviour therapy on the irrational beliefs of elite academy athletes. *Journal of Applied Sport Psychology*, 26(2), 144–156.

Editors' commentary on Chapter 13: "Delivering Rational Emotive Behavior Therapy (REBT) education in youth rugby union"

We connected with Aaron and Jonathan's chapter a lot. The application of REBT within a team environment, delivered to groups, has its own challenges that the authors reflect on valuably for the reader. Because of the structure of REBT, group sessions driven towards the exploration of the ABCDE framework can be really vibrant and powerful for all involved. For a practitioner, it's exciting to see the theory come alive with energetic and inquisitive athletes. Athletes benefit from the sharing of thoughts and beliefs too. They have to figure out how to put their thoughts into words, but also have to interpret others' contributions in interactive tasks, helping them to apply what they have learned about REBT. This type of work certainly rests on the practitioner's ability to construct and deliver practical activities with the group. A one-hour lecture on REBT won't be appealing to many athletes. Aaron and Jonathan share with us some great practical activities that can engage athletes in REBT without being too didactic.

The key reflection for us was the remark about a lack of engagement from staff in the sessions. It still surprises us when we don't get full backing from support staff, especially because we are all there for a common purpose: to help the athletes fulfil their potential. In addition, the people around an athlete are vital for the installation and maintenance of good performance habits, whether that's rational beliefs, or pre-performance nutrition. In many cases, the practitioner is in contact with the athlete much less than other support staff, and much less than the parents (in young athletes). Thus, we would always recommend separate education sessions with support staff and parents around *their* irrational beliefs, so that they can experience the benefits, thus potentially garnering greater engagement and involvement from them in the athlete sessions.

14 "Is it really that bad?"

A case study applying Rational Emotive Behavior Therapy (REBT) with an elite youth tennis player

Andrew Wood and Charlotte Woodcock

Introduction

My (first author) decision to become a sport and exercise psychologist was conceived during the final year of a degree in sport and exercise science, a pursuit that combined my passion for sport and human behavior. From a young age I became frustrated with the disparity in performance between training and competition that I experienced. When starting as a 'neophyte' practitioner I was armed with a toolbox of psychological skills ready to improve an athlete's performance and life for the better. Such a utopic state was short-lived, and soon I had told myself that I was clearly no good. Indeed it was an irrational and unhealthy story I had unwittingly concocted, but also a common experience reported by trainee sport psychologists (Tammen, 2000). It was only when a fellow trainee commented on the pressure I had been placing on myself, a belief that I had to provide the cure-all solution, did my irrational bubble burst. Two and a half years later I find myself nearing the end of a PhD that explores the effects of Rational Emotive Behavior Therapy (REBT) on performance, as well as continuing my training to become a chartered sport and exercise psychologist. During this period I have been immersed within REBT and share a rational philosophy towards life that inherently underpins my applied practice. These 'core conditions' include: empathy towards others, unconditional acceptance (i.e., viewing humans to be fallible and too complicated to be globally evaluated), genuineness, and humour (Dryden & Branch, 2008). Over time I have felt a weight of expectation lift, hereby experiencing greater freedom, enjoyment, and, dare I say, success as a practitioner, a response that has been mirrored by many athletes I have applied REBT with.

Context

Using the following case, we provide a detailed account into the application of REBT with a nationally ranked youth tennis player. We also detail changes in the player's ability to self-regulate over the course of the intervention. REBT is traditionally a psychotherapeutic model (David, et al., 2005), and in sport it occupies a chasm between therapy and cognitive behavioral coaching. Acknowledging the boundaries of our professional competence, we describe its application as mental skills training, empowering the athlete with an approach to enhance performance and pro-actively reinforce an athlete's mental health. Both authors were involved in the initial consultation with the client, whereby a collective approach provided us with an adequate view of the client's problems and resulting solutions (Pitt et al., 2015). The first author delivered the entirety of the intervention and provides the narrative of the case. The second author examined changes in self-regulation strategies prior to and after the intervention.

Presenting issue

Tom (pseudonym) was brought to our attention by his father who had requested sport psychology support. Accordingly, we arranged an introductory consultation session. Whilst drawing heavily upon cognitive behavioral techniques within our practice (i.e., the what) within this initial consultation we utilized a client-centered humanistic approach (i.e., the how) to glean important contextual information, whilst building a strong therapeutic alliance (Turner & Barker, 2014).

Tom was a nationally ranked, 17-year-old tennis player who was deciding whether to pursue a career as a professional tennis player, and like with many other sports, the amateur ranks were financially demanding. Subsequently, he had given himself one year to make it onto the ATP world-ranking list. Tom was ambitious and presented an unyielding, outcome-focused goal for the upcoming season. Accordingly, this seemed to exacerbate the demanding and unhelpful pressure he was placing upon himself to be successful. By his own admission, Tom was struggling to perform consistently and was frustrated about not fulfilling his potential. When playing tennis, he would be pre-occupied with what significant others were thinking and anxious about underperforming, in the belief that it would reflect badly on him as a player and person. Tom felt he had little control over his emotions, leading to unhelpful anxiety and angry outbursts during crucial moments of a game (i.e., losing the first set, break points, and umpire's decisions). He was unable to effectively self-regulate his performance. He mentioned, "When things are going well it's great, but when they are not you can definitely tell".

Needs analysis

Tom's pre-occupation with others' thoughts, his experience of distressing emotions (e.g., extreme nervousness and anger), maladaptive behaviors (e.g., shouting, poor body language), and a rigid outcome goal suggested that he was harbouring irrational beliefs. The irrational Performance Beliefs Inventory (iPBI; Turner et al., 2016) was used to quantify Tom's irrational beliefs. In comparison to normative values, Tom reported high scores on composite irrational beliefs (normative value = 20.93, Tom time-point 1 = 24.50) and low frustration tolerance (normative value = 23.05, Tom time-point 1 = 28.50), a combination of which is commonly associated with increased unhealthy anger expression (Jones &

Trower, 2004). Typically, practitioners have utilized the canon of psychological skills (Andersen, 2009), such as self-talk, pre-performance routines, relaxation, and imagery, to enhance performance in tennis players (Mamassis & Doganis, 2004). Albeit a valuable cornerstone of applied sport psychology, such techniques may be unable to challenge the underlying beliefs that may hinder a player's ability to overcome challenges in the pursuit of their respective goals (Turner, 2016a). Tom wanted to enhance his control over his emotions and better regulate his actions on court, prior to and during tennis matches, ultimately ensuring he was able to perform closer to his potential on a more consistent basis.

The intervention

We predicted that the adoption of a new rational philosophy would offer a long-term solution to the disruptive performance issues he was currently experiencing. We also predicted that this would cement the foundations upon which skills could be taught to further manage symptoms that were having a debilitative effect on his performances. The context of Tom's case also afforded an extended period in which to work. Tom's competition life meant he lived a somewhat nomadic lifestyle, often competing at national and international tournaments for several days at a time, thus contact between us would be limited and sporadic.

The notion of working towards redundancy as a sport psychologist presents a poor business model, that is, not being a crutch for the athlete who becomes overly reliant on the support and guidance of the practitioner. Nevertheless, we firmly believe that effective sport psychologists can present athletes with greater awareness, enhanced perceived control over their emotions, and greater clarity regarding the mental aspects of their sport. Indeed, effective REBT might allow Tom to autonomously manage and respond adaptively to challenges across varying contexts. The intervention was delivered over nine sessions, spanning 6-months, with each session lasting for 60-minutes. Using the ABC(DE) framework (Ellis & Dryden, 1997), sessions 1 to 7 were focused on REBT and were separated into education, disputation, and reinforcement phases (Turner & Barker, 2014). Sessions 8 and 9 consisted of developing Tom's ability to employ psychological skills that would help him manage difficult symptoms prior to and/ or during competition.

Sessions 1 and 2: building the foundations

The education phase was conducted across two sessions. The aim was to help Tom understand that it was his beliefs (B) that determined his emotional and behavioral consequences (C), rather than the adversity alone (A) (Dryden & Branch, 2008). It was important to ensure Tom developed a strong foundation around the ABC(DE) framework that would provide the building blocks for subsequent phases. REBT is traditionally associated with an active and directive approach (Dryden & Neenan, 2015), however, practitioners might flexibly shift between that and a client-centered approach. In particular, I have found the adoption of Motivational Interviewing (MI; Miller & Rollnick, 2012) techniques an invaluable way to better educate, understand, and elicit the client's beliefs, which can be difficult to access and change.

To begin, I asked Tom to describe a challenging situation that he had recently encountered (A) and how he then responded (e.g., thoughts, feelings, and actions). Tom spoke of having very negative thoughts, which led to angry outbursts (i.e., shouting and throwing his racquet) (C) when he was losing to an opponent who he thought he should have been beating (A). As a between-session practice I asked Tom to complete an A-C diary of his week. This task encouraged Tom to reaffirm the content of the previous session, as well as serving as a method to gauge his engagement in the REBT process. At the beginning of the second session, we initially reviewed Tom's A-C diary. Following this, I encouraged Tom to pick the most poignant A-C example and consider how he would want to feel if this situation was to arise again. Tom highlighted that he wanted to feel annoyed but not extremely angry, to not berate himself and/or his opponents for his performance, to focus on tennis specific processes, to maintain confident body language, and to uphold an energetic tempo that was characteristic of his game (see Figure 14.1). This process elegantly emphasized to Tom the unhelpful vs. helpful distinction in how individuals respond to adversity, as well as setting clear emotional, cognitive, and behavioral goals in respect of what he wanted to achieve.

Session 3: taking control

Following session 1 and 2, we began exploring and eliciting his beliefs about the adversity (A) and the consequences (C). Here, an emphasis was placed on ownership and control over his response to adversity. This realization was met with the surprise that he alone was able to decide, rather than being dictated to by the situation.

Although a simple concept, from Tom's perspective, it was not something that he had previously considered. To begin exploring his beliefs, I asked Tom what he was telling himself about the situation (A) and how he then responded (C). Because irrational beliefs are often held implicitly, athletes will commonly offer cognitive consequences (i.e., "what is the point", "this isn't going well") rather than their irrational beliefs. I reminded Tom of this and offered suggestions as to what I judged the core beliefs to be. After some discussion, the poignant beliefs were welcomed with a smile of realization (see Figure 14.1, left column). Once the initial set of irrational beliefs had been established it became clear for Tom that he had been placing much greater pressure upon himself, in comparison to the pressure that the situation alone afforded. When using terminology such as irrational and rational it is important to normalize, rather than stigmatize, beliefs as being 'abnormal'. Alternatively, terms such as helpful and unhelpful or illogical and logical beliefs could have been used interchangeably. For Tom, this served to quell unhelpful meta-cognitions about being anxious, normalizing the ubiquity of human fallibility.

Activating Event (A)

Situational: Losing to an opponent
Adversity: "I know that I am a better player than my opponent"

Irrational Beliefs (iB)	Rational Beliefs (rB)
Demand: "I would like to beat opponents who I know am better than, therefore I absolutely must"	**Preference:** "I would like to beat opponents who I know am better than, but I do not absolutely have to"
Awfulizing: "If I do not win then it would be awful"	**Anti-Awfulizing:** "It would be bad but certainly not terrible if I did not win"
Low Frustration Tolerance: "It would be unbearable if I lost"	**High Frustration Tolerance:** "Losing would be uncomfortable, but not impossible to tolerate"
Depreciation (Self): "Losing would make me a complete failure"	**Acceptance (Self):** "Losing does not make me a complete failure. I cannot be defined by the outcome of a single match"

Unhelpful Consequences (C)	Helpful Consequences (E)
Emotional Consequence: Unhealthy anger	**Emotional Consequence:** Annoyed
Behavioral Consequence: Aggressive behaviors (e.g., throwing racket, shouting at opponents)	**Behavioral Consequence:** Strong and confident body language. Maintained energy and effort throughout the game
Cognitive Consequence: Negative self-talk and losing match focus	**Cognitive Consequence:** Helpful self-talk (i.e., focus on processes)
Performance Consequence: Struggle to regain momentum and then lose consecutive points and/or games	**Performance Consequence:** Minimize/ nullify a dip in performance and regain match momentum

---

Figure 14.1 Example of Tom's first schematic representation of the ABC model

Sessions 4 and 5: disputing and replacing irrational beliefs

When applying REBT, one aims to match the pace and content of the sessions with the client, and in Tom's case he was verbalizing a strong understanding of the ABC model. Nevertheless, the education phase merely provides the building blocks for the next and most important phase within the REBT intervention process. Disputation (D) can sometimes be a challenging process, however, my experience suggests younger athletes are more open to abandoning their irrational beliefs and adopting new rational beliefs. I highlighted with Tom that we would not dispute his inference of the adversity (A), and instead would accept that it was true. Often in tennis, players will encounter situations outside of their control (e.g., strong opponents or umpires making 'bad' decisions) and REBT promotes a shift to a focus on what they can control (e.g., their own thoughts, feelings, and actions) to help them attain their goal, which is often winning. To systematically dispute each irrational belief three main strategies were adopted, namely empirical, logical, and pragmatic disputation. I first disputed the demand (see Figure 14.1). The following section illustrates some of the questions that were used for each rational argument:

Empirical disputation

"Where is the evidence to say that you must beat your opponent?", "Is there a law of the universe which states that you must?", and "Where is it written that just because you really want to, that you really must beat your opponent?"

Logical disputation

"Does it logically follow that because you want something, that you absolutely must have it?", "Just because I want a Ferrari does that mean I must be given one?", and "Where is the logic in your demand?"

Pragmatic disputation

"How helpful has this belief been so far for you?", "Where has this rigid demand you have been placing on yourself got you so far?", and "How do you feel and behave when you tell yourself that you must?"

During the disputation phase a combination of didactic and Socratic approaches was used to ensure a focused and collaborative process (Dryden & Branch, 2008). REBT poses philosophical questions, and giving Tom time and space to cogitate over these questions was important to ensure that he did not feel overloaded. It was during these moments when the fundamental shifts in Tom's philosophy began. When disputing irrational beliefs I often encounter conditional musts, which are both empirically and logically rational. It is helpful if these are made distinct from the core irrational demands to avoid confusion for the athlete. For example, if Tom needed to proceed to the next round of a tournament, he would 'have to' beat his opponent. This disputation process was repeated with Tom's awfulizing, low frustration tolerance, and self-depreciation beliefs (see Figure 14.1 – left column). Helping Tom to realize that there is no evidence for these beliefs, we worked through creating rational alternatives for each belief. Importantly, the three main strategies used to dispute irrational beliefs were also used to reaffirm the new rational beliefs.

In Tom's case he largely agreed with the disputation process, however, it is not uncommon for athletes to propose their irrational beliefs have/are helpful for their performances. To negate what can become a philosophically difficult conversation I will ask athletes to reflect on several key questions. For example, asking, "Would it be fair to assume that these irrational beliefs have been helpful for you?", "Is there any evidence to suggest that you cannot be successful with rational beliefs?", and "What might the benefits be of holding rational beliefs, not only in performance but also in day-to-day life?" Quite often this resistance is down to a misconception that rational beliefs create indifference.

Here practitioners might articulate that rational beliefs change the quality of the motivation rather than reducing its intensity. Indeed, researchers (Turner, 2016a) have drawn comparisons between irrational demands such as 'ought to' and 'have to' with internalized external regulations, where the perception that one should or ought to engage in an activity is considered a hallmark of introjected regulation (e.g., Gillison, et al., 2009). The disputation process was then repeated with different adversities that were not restricted to sport.

Sessions 6 and 7: reinforcing a new rational philosophy

The main reinforcement phase was conducted over two sessions and incorporated cognitive, emotional, and behavioral techniques (Dryden & Branch, 2008).

Rational credo

Tom's newly established rational beliefs were adapted into a shortened mantra that he would re-read prior to and during matches. Rational credos are commonly used in REBT practice to help reaffirm a rational philosophy (Dryden, 2007) and are only recently being used with athletes (e.g., Turner, 2016b).

Big I and Little I

To dispute and reinforce Tom's irrational beliefs around self-depreciation, I used the *Big I and Little I* technique. Tom was asked to draw a large 'I' and within this draw little Is, labelling each aspect of his life that contributed to defining who he was. These included being a tennis player, a brother, a son, and a loyal friend to name a few. This exercise allowed Tom to visually comprehend that he could not wholly rate his being based on a single aspect. Indeed, together we discussed how humans are not all good or bad, but contain varying aspects of each.

Badness scale

When Tom rated losing as terrible it would be imply there was nothing in this world that was worse than losing, exaggerating the ramifications of failure more than the situation warranted. Prior to a match, the prospect of losing was awful, in turn elevating Tom's fear of failure and causing him to feel extremely anxious. The *badness scale* provided an effective and engaging way of challenging his awfulizing beliefs (Turner & Barker, 2014). Firstly, Tom was asked to place a series of adversities unrelated to sport on a scale of 0–100% in badness (e.g., getting a cold). I then asked him to place a series of tennis-related adversities on the same continuum (e.g., dropping two break points during a final). Expectedly, he placed these adversities much higher on the badness scale. Finally, I then asked Tom to place a series of major adversities (e.g., losing a loved one) on the badness scale. It was at this point Tom expressed a chuckle of realization, recognizing his awfulizing beliefs were irrational and that losing a match was not the end of the world. Ultimately, the badness scale enhanced Tom's ability to take perspective. Tom kept the badness scale in his tennis bag and referred to it whenever he started to feel overwhelmed by a situation.

The use of metaphor

During our sessions together, Tom referred to his earlier self as a landmine. Here I used this metaphor to reinforce distinctions between a helpful and unhelpful consequence. Consequently, Tom suggested that he wanted to be more like a homing missile: calculated, efficient, and smart, yet able to inflict damage on his opponent (metaphorically). The use of metaphor directly informs the athlete's internal dialogue (e.g., Lindsay, Thomas, & Douglas, 2010), and provides a clear image of the desired state Tom wanted to achieve.

Behavioral strategies

The one-to-one sessions were conducted in a relaxed space away from tennis; nevertheless irrational beliefs can become primed during stressful and challenging situations (David, 2003). Therefore, over the sessions I introduced behavioral tasks to help Tom reaffirm his new rational beliefs. Firstly, I asked Tom to actively seek challenging situations (i.e., major tournaments), commonly known as in-vivo exposure (Froggat, 2005). This experiential process aimed to test the validity of his fears (e.g., losing makes him a complete failure), de-awfulize his belief that underperforming was terrible, and negate his avoidant behavior through falsifying his irrational beliefs. I also asked Tom to act against his irrational beliefs and take greater risks during moments of a game that he perceived to be crucial (e.g., break points, first game, set points) with the aim of interrupting his irrational self-talk when he felt notably anxious.

Sessions 8 and 9: psychological skills

By the end of the reinforcement phase Tom appeared to be making good progress, articulating his understanding of the ABC(DE) model, reporting reductions in irrational beliefs, and reflecting on between-session practices. After consulting with Tom, I decided to introduce specific psychological skills that would further provide him with the ability to manage symptoms that may hinder his ability to perform. I have found the application of REBT with psychological skills a fruitful combination, whereby the effects of the latter become amplified after experiencing a fundamental shift towards a rational philosophy. Firstly, 'trigger' terms generated by Tom were used as a focusing strategy at pre-determined scenarios prior and during a match. These included: 'explosive', 'risk', and 'never give in'. These were further supplemented with 'be smart', 'aggressive', and 'tactical'. To reduce Tom's uncertainty, we reviewed both controllable (e.g., preparation, thoughts) and uncontrollable (e.g., opponent, outcome) factors. Finally, I introduced rapid relaxation techniques that would reduce the somatic symptoms of anxiety that he frequently encountered prior to important matches. Following session 9 Tom noted that he felt sufficiently equipped, mentally stronger, and more independent in his approach to tennis. We agreed to end our regular one-to-one sessions at this point, whilst maintaining regular drop-in sessions to monitor his progress.

Outcome analysis

Irrational beliefs

Over the course of the intervention, Tom reported decreases in composite irrational beliefs as well as reductions in the core beliefs of low frustration tolerance and demand, both commonly associated with anger expression (Jones & Trower, 2004; see Figure 14.2). The adoption of a rational philosophy is not simply characterized by the frequency and endorsement of self-reported irrational beliefs, but also expressed by the presence of emotions and behaviors that facilitate goal achievement. Considering this, less is understood about the effects on behavior (Szentagotai & Jones, 2010) and athletic performance (Turner, 2016a). The context of elite tennis afforded a fitting medium to investigate the effects of REBT on Tom's ability to self-regulate.

Self-regulation: pre-intervention

Irrational beliefs are likely to undermine attempts for adaptive regulation, such as setting and striving for controllable process goals, functional use of psychological

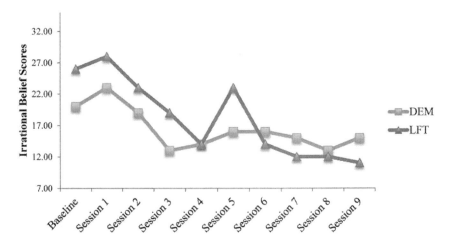

Figure 14.2 Tom's self-reported irrational beliefs scores on a session-by-session basis

skills to focus on the task, monitoring goal progress, as well as fair performance appraisals (Zimmerman, 2000). An increase in Tom's emotional control and rational beliefs was argued as a likely outcome of better self-regulation, and formed an important component of intervention evaluation. Tom's on-court behaviors and his ability to self-regulate were monitored through two semi-structured interviews prior to the onset of the intervention and following programme completion. An interview schedule, drawing on Zimmerman's (2000) three-phase cyclical model of self-regulation, targeted Tom's tournament goals (forethought phase), performance strategies (performance phase), and evaluation and reaction (self-reflection phase).

Tournament goals

Tom had identified process (improve his backhand) and outcome (win the match) tournament goals. Clearly defined strategies were identified for mastering his backhand, as Tom described, "Technically looking to accelerate my left arm more and drop the racket more". Conversely, Tom did not seem to have any pre-planned strategies for determining match results, as he explained, "I don't really have a say [in] how I'm going to win the match, or how I'm going to go about it, it is pretty much compete in the match and play your game".

Performance strategies

During the tournament, Tom's outcome goal took precedence over his process goal. Tom stated, "I got caught up in the tournament and focused more on my result than my backhand". Focusing on his outcome goal meant Tom reacted to match situations rather than pro-actively utilizing controllable strategies for goal attainment. Part of this reaction manifested in Tom's emotions, motivational drive, and confidence levels, which seemed to co-vary with the momentum of the match. Tom commented, "the score helped when I was leading. . . . I felt a little bit more confidence" and when Tom was behind, he told himself, "I need to get going . . . putting a little bit of pressure on myself". A tendency to prioritize outcome goals is often seen in athletes who are still developing adaptive self-regulatory processes.

Evaluation and reaction

Tom's outcome focus led to a performance evaluation based on the result: "If I won the match it was a success, but if I didn't that was bad". Although Tom lost the match, he felt he played well. Tom could recognize several performance-based goals, which he could take forward, including "higher percentage first serves" and "to be more aggressive". A pre-occupation with outcomes can undermine athletes' subsequent motivation, however, Tom showed more adaptive forms of self-regulation in identifying potential improvements based on less than desirable performance outcomes (Zimmerman & Kitsantas, 1997).

Self-regulation: post-intervention

Tournament goals

Following the REBT intervention, Tom's tournament goals centered on performance and process. Tom described his match aims to be "aggressive and enjoy myself" and "play the best I can". Pre-planned controllable strategies enabled Tom to direct his efforts towards achieving these goals and included, "Doing what I did before, adhering to routines, making sure I warm up . . . make sure my body is warm . . . and be aware that I'm going to play a match". Although outcome goals are not inevitably detrimental to performance, Tom's preference towards process and performance goals enabled him to focus on key strategies he pre-planned for success.

Performance strategies

Consistent with his goals, Tom consistently used his strategies throughout the match, displaying a more controlled and less reactionary approach compared to pre-intervention. Although Tom remained aware of the score, it did not influence his emotions. Tom stated, "I wasn't really getting angry, the guy was making a lot of balls but I wasn't getting angry" and "I'm just so calm and I'm not letting anything affect me". This more consistent approach may be viewed as inflexible and unable to adapt to the dynamic challenges athletes face during performance. However, this did not seem to be the case for Tom, whose calmness reflected reduced anxiety over outcomes. This allowed for an adaptive analysis of his game: "Instead of worrying about the shot, or the result, I'm worrying on what I can do to make myself better and win matches".

Evaluation and reaction

Like pre-intervention, performance evaluation was based on goal progress. Tom's process and performance goals meant goal attainment was not dependent on factors beyond his control. Tom reflected on his achievement and stated, "I know that I have achieved the things I wanted to coming into the match", and "things I wanted to do I did, and I know that was trying my hardest". Evaluations based on controllable strategies lead to higher levels of self-satisfaction and reflect higher quality self-regulation processes.

In summary, Tom increased the quality of self-regulation processes from pre-intervention to post-intervention. He progressed from being merely reactive to the challenges faced on court, to relying on a more pro-active approach, implementing pre-planned strategies to achieve controllable self-set goals. Tom attributed these positive changes to the REBT work he engaged with. In summarizing the impact of REBT, Tom stated:

> My beliefs have changed. . . . I've just rationalized everything – is it that bad if I lose a tennis match? And that's really helped me. It's put me in a better

frame of mind going into matches and leaving matches, and I think that helps me to just not get angry on court. I feel pretty calm which obviously allows me to perform better.

Being able to rationalize his beliefs meant that Tom could set and strive towards adaptive goals. Adopting a more rational outlook enabled Tom to effectively employ routines and psychological skills without unhelpful reactions to an unfavourable adversity becoming a barrier.

Critical reflections

The intervention with Tom was received positively, however, time between sessions was often sporadic and on some occasions the momentum from the previous session would often be lost. Here I felt as though I was unable to provide an engaging and impactful tool that Tom could use away from our sessions together to further reaffirm his rational philosophy. Practitioners would be wise to give equal attention to both face-to-face and between-session practice tasks and to keep sessions close together. Furthermore, the use of technology (i.e., smartphones) may offer a platform for practitioners to reaffirm the rational principles acquired during the intervention.

Sport psychology support is rarely a perfect science and this case offers no exception to this rule. REBT is seemingly logical within its application, however, it can also be a challenging and nuanced endeavour that requires continuous reflection and development. For example, practitioners may slightly misinterpret the theory of REBT, fail to clarify semantics surrounding REBT terminology, or mismanage the balance between directive and client-centered methods during the disputation phase. These are just some examples that I have encountered that may lead to ineffective application. To this end, whilst I may never offer the perfect intervention it is important that those who practice REBT are aware of and able to evaluate bad practice. Ultimately, for sport psychologists who are looking to adopt REBT, it would be prudent to accumulate a strong theoretical grounding in REBT as well as completing practitioner qualifications.

References

Andersen, M. B. (2009). The "canon" of psychological skills training for enhancing performance. In K. F. Hays (Ed.), *Performance psychology in action: A casebook for working with athletes, performing artists, business leaders, and professionals in high-risk occupations* (pp. 11–34). Washington, DC: American Psychological Association.

David, D. (2003). Rational Emotive Behavior Therapy (REBT): The view of a cognitive psychologist. In W. Dryden (Ed.), *Rational emotive behaviour therapy: Theoretical developments* (pp. 130 159). New York, NY: Brunner Routledge.

David, D., Szentagotai, A., Eva, K., & Macavei, B. (2005). A synopsis of Rational-Emotive Behavior Therapy (REBT): Fundamental and applied research. *Journal of Rational-Emotive & Cognitive-Behavior Therapy, 23*, 175–221. doi:10.1007/s10942-005-0011-0.

Dryden, W. (2007). Resilience and rationality. *Journal of Rational-Emotive & Cognitive-Behavior Therapy, 25,* 213–226. doi:10.1007/s10942-006-0050-1.

Dryden, W., & Branch, R. (2008). *The fundamentals of rational emotive behavior therapy* (2nd ed.). Chichester: John Wiley & Sons, Ltd.

Dryden, W., & Neenan, M. (2015). *Rational Emotive Behaviour Therapy: 100 key points and techniques.* Hove: Routledge.

Ellis, A., & Dryden, W. (1997). *The practice of rational-emotive behavior therapy.* New York, NY: Springer.

Froggatt, W. (2005). *A brief introduction to rational emotive behavior therapy* (3rd Ed.). New Zealand, Stortford Lodge: Hastings. Retrieved from www.rational.org.nz/prof-docs/Intro-REBT.pdf.

Gillison, F., Osborn, M., Skevington, S., & Standage, M. (2009). Exploring the experience of introjected regulation for exercise across gender in adolescence. *Psychology of Sport and Exercise, 10*(3), 309–319.

Jones, J., & Trower, P. (2004). Irrational and evaluative beliefs in individuals with anger disorders. *Journal of Rational – Emotive and Cognitive – Behavior Therapy, 22,* 153–169. doi:10.1023/B:JORE.0000047305.52149.a1.

Lindsay, P., Thomas, O., & Douglas, G. (2010). A framework to explore and transform client-generated metaphors in applied sport psychology. *Sport Psychologist, 24,* 97–112. doi:10.1207/s15324834basp0701_2.

Mamassis, G., & Doganis, G. (2004). The effects of a mental training program on juniors pre-competitive anxiety, self-confidence, and Tennis performance. *Journal of Applied Sport Psychology, 16,* 118–137. doi:10.1080/10413200490437903.

Miller, W. R., & Rollnick, S. (2012). *Motivational interviewing: Helping people change.* New York, NY: Guilford Press.

Pitt, T., Lindsay, P., Thomas, O., Bawden, M., Goodwill, S., & Hanton, S. (2015). A perspective on consultancy teams and technology in applied sport psychology. *Psychology of Sport and Exercise, 16,* 36–44. doi:10.1016/j.psychsport.2014.07.002.

Szentagotai, A., & Jones, J. (2010). The behavioral consequences of irrational beliefs. In D. David, S. J. Lynn, & A. Ellis (Eds.), *Rational and irrational beliefs in human functioning and disturbances* (pp. 75–98). Oxford: Oxford University Press.

Tammen, V. V. (2000). First internship experiences or, what I did on holiday. In M. B. Anderson (Ed.), *Doing sport psychology* (pp. 181–192). Champaign, IL: Human Kinetics.

Turner, M. J. (2016a). Rational Emotive Behavior Therapy (REBT), irrational and rational beliefs, and the mental health of Athletes. *Frontiers in Psychology, 7,* 1423. doi:10.3389/fpsyg.2016.01423.

Turner, M. J. (2016b). Proposing a rational resilience credo for athletes. *Journal of Sport Psychology in Action, 7*(3), 170–181. doi:10.1080/21520704.2016.1236051.

Turner, M. J., Allen, M., Slater, M. J., Barker, J. B., Woodcock, C., Harwood, C. G., & McFadyen, K. (2016). The development and initial validation of the irrational performance beliefs inventory (iPBI). *European Journal of Psychological Assessment.* doi:10.1027/1015-5759/a000314.

Turner, M. J., & Barker, J. B. (2014). Using Rational Emotive Behavior Therapy with athletes. *The Sport Psychologist, 28,* 75–90. doi:10.1123/tsp.2013–0012.

Zimmerman, B. J. (2000). Attaining self-regulation: A social cognitive perspective. In M. Boekaerts, P. R. Pintrick, & M. Zeidner (Eds.), *Handbook of self-regulation* (pp. 13–35). London, UK: Elsevier Academic Press.

Zimmerman, B. J., & Kitsantas, A. (1997). Developmental phases in self-regulation: Shifting from process goals to outcome goals. *Journal of Educational Psychology, 89,* 29–36. doi:10.1037/0022–0663.89.1.29.

Editors' commentary on Chapter 14: "'Is it really that bad?': a case study applying Rational Emotive Behavior Therapy (REBT) with an elite youth tennis player"

This chapter makes several useful technical and conceptual points regarding the application of REBT. Andrew and Charlotte illustrate many of the challenges that a neophyte practitioner might face when attempting to translate a theoretical understanding of the model into a workable intervention. The precise nature of beliefs is one such challenge. Whilst this book contains numerous figures illustrating ABC formulations, it is highly unlikely that the athletes in the chapters verbalized them so elegantly, at least not straight away. Irrational beliefs take a lot of eliciting and shaping before the process of disputation can begin. In this chapter, the authors make reference to 'suggesting' irrational beliefs. Whilst this may not be very Socratic, it can be a very efficient way of working. For example, imagine a scenario in which an athlete reports anxiety (C) about an upcoming match (A). If in response to a prompt for an irrational belief (B), an athlete says something like, "I just want to win", the practitioner can attempt to clarify the rational/irrational nature of this belief by 'suggesting' the following: "In that moment when you really feel that anxiety about the upcoming match, do you think you believe that you would prefer to win and that it is not the end of the world that you do not, or do you believe that you have to win and that not winning would be an absolute disaster? Which of those options best represents your belief?" This approach is undoubtedly leading the individual somewhat, but it is also clearly theory-driven and will help both parties clarify the nature of the beliefs in question. It is important not to assume that distress is always the product of irrational beliefs, since with the concept of healthy negative emotions Ellis made clear his view that some emotions are adaptive, even if they are uncomfortable. Part of the practitioner's task with an individual is assessing suitability for intervention and clearly discriminating helpful and unhelpful beliefs is a key aspect of this. Suggesting beliefs, in the service of this discrimination, can be a very productive strategy.

15 "It's the end of the world as we know it (and I feel fine)"

The use of Rational Emotive Behavior Therapy (REBT) to increase function and reduce irrational beliefs of an injured athlete

Robert Morris, David Tod, and Martin Eubank

Context and presenting issue

I (first author) was first approached to work with Andrew when he was in his early 20s and competing as a professional rugby player. Andrew approached me directly via links that I had with his professional rugby club and the University I worked at. In the initial instance, Andrew asked if I would help him with his performance, including how to control his anxiety levels when competing, as he had become overawed in major games. He also reported some personal issues he wanted assistance with, specifically in how to overcome challenges in his personal relationships with his girlfriend and young family. In addition to being a professional rugby player, Andrew was also studying for an undergraduate degree in Law. We also worked together on Andrew's lifestyle, to ensure he was able to manage and balance his life demands, which were varied and plentiful. I worked with Andrew for an initial period of 9-months and had developed a strong working relationship with him, with the focus of our sessions together aiming to ensure that Andrew was in peak mental condition when competing in matches and that he had high levels of psychological wellbeing.

One day, I had four missed phone calls from Andrew, with a voicemail message that insisted I call him back as soon as possible. I phoned him back as soon as I could, and heard in his voice almost immediately that something was wrong – Andrew had suffered a major knee injury while competing and was going to require knee surgery. He was going to be out for a minimum of 7-months and he was clearly highly distressed. Despite being considered one of the best players in the team by teammates and coaches, during this phone call Andrew outlined that he had quickly become uncertain about everything he had accomplished as a professional athlete and viewed the injury as "the worst thing that could happen" to him. Due to the severity of the injury and the way Andrew was responding emotionally and cognitively, we quickly agreed to meet up to speak in more detail and outline his likely recovery path. We also identified how we could work together to ensure that he was psychologically prepared for, firstly, what he was about to undergo during rehab, and secondly, what he may have to overcome to become a successful professional rugby player again.

It was clear from the first time that Andrew and I met after his injury that he was experiencing several strong negative psychological reactions, and these were also having an impact upon his personal life. He continually talked about how rugby was the "most important part" of his life, how he felt useless because he could not do much prior to having surgery due to the pain he was in, and that he was continually "falling out" with his partner because she "didn't understand" what he was going through. In essence, Andrew was experiencing heightened anxiety and stress as a result of his injury and was unable to cope effectively with the challenges this presented. From a humanistic perspective (this was the framework I had always adopted with Andrew) I helped him to understand how he perceived the event and how it may influence his capability to achieve self-fulfilment and satisfaction in life (Rogers, 1959). As a model of practice, the approach draws on optimism and outlines that humans have the capacity to overcome hardship, pain, and despair (Rogers, 1959), something with which Andrew and I were both congruent. Working with Andrew within this framework, I was able to help him to better manage the psychological distress he was experiencing prior to his operation, which was one of the immediate issues with which he presented. The plan was that Andrew would have his operation, after which we would work together with staff at the club to determine a rehabilitation strategy, incorporating physiotherapy, medical support, and psychological assistance.

Having put this plan in place, the physiological and psychological recovery subsequently appeared to be progressing well. Two months post-operation, I received a phone call from the physiotherapist at the club. Andrew had just been reinjured in training and was about to head to hospital. I was informed that it was likely that his first operation had been unsuccessful and Andrew may require more extensive surgery to find out the root cause of his re-injury. At that time, I was uncertain how to react – Andrew had been progressing well psychologically, but I knew from the fact that the job of phoning me had been given to the physiotherapist that he did not want to talk, and that he would see the re-injury as a major blow.

Andrew required a second major operation on his knee, which this time involved major reconstructive work. Andrew felt devastated, was highly anxious and worried about what was to come – he thought he had been progressing well with his recovery and now he was being told that his knee was so severely damaged that he would be out for a year and could potentially never play again. To Andrew, it was, as he put it, the "end of the world". I continued to work with Andrew using the same humanistic approach before and after his second operation. I expected that, after a period of working with Andrew from a humanistic perspective, he would start to show signs of improved mental wellbeing. However, there was no clear sign of progress, with Andrew still showing signs of being highly anxious and worried about his situation. To contextualize, Andrew still believed that the injury was devastating and the worst thing that could have happened to him. At this point, I started to challenge whether my humanistic model of practice, while previously helpful to Andrew, was enough. The approach I used did not help to contextualize to Andrew the importance of his injury and his recovery when compared to other aspects of his life. Consequently, I started to consider other methods I may use to support Andrew in his recovery.

Needs analysis

During my training as a sport and exercise psychologist and in my subsequent readings on interventions to support athletes who were experiencing injury, I often wondered how I would choose to work with athletes who had deeply rooted issues because of their injury. Acknowledging my own doubts about the lack of progress I had made using my humanistic approach with Andrew, I knew I needed to return to the literature to consider other models of approach and congruent interventions that had empirical support for their effectiveness that could be applicable in helping Andrew. It was during this period that I came across the work of Turner and Barker (2014), who were writing about the application of REBT as a way of increasing athletes' functioning and reducing irrational beliefs. Although not focused on injury, Turner and Barker (2014) outlined the principle of irrational beliefs and how this could negatively impact an athlete's mental health and wellbeing. I started to read more of the literature associated with REBT, including some of the original works by Ellis (1957) and some of the more recent works where REBT was applied to sport (e.g., Turner & Barker, 2013), and attending workshops around its application in sport. It became clear to me that the thoughts and feelings Andrew had could be categorized as irrational, especially when he was outlining to me that the injury he was experiencing was the "end of the world" and the "worst thing that could have happened". Previous literature (e.g., Tripp, et al., 2007) has highlighted that a fear of re-injury, negative affect, and catastrophizing were all significantly correlated with athletes' confidence in their ability to return to their sport. It is, therefore, important that there is a conscious reduction in catastrophizing in order that athletes who are injured may be able to confidently recuperate and perform to an optimal level post-recovery. As a consequence of Andrew's current needs, the REBT evidence base, and the literature associated with sports injury rehabilitation, my case formulation led me to incorporate REBT into my support for Andrew as he moved through his recovery period, drawing on the framework of Turner and Barker (2014).

The REBT intervention

My needs analysis with Andrew had identified that he was experiencing a significant emotional reaction to his second injury that needed to be overcome to increase his functioning as a human and athlete. To increase and improve his functioning and mental wellbeing would take a lengthy period of time. Initially, and in the shorter term, there was also a need to start getting Andrew to think more rationally about his injury and how important this was in the broader spectrum of his life.

Education phase

When I was working with Andrew, the main focus of the education phase was to, firstly, outline the ABC process of REBT (e.g., Dryden, 2009; Turner, et al., 2014) and, secondly, explain what ABC meant in the context of his situation (Turner & Barker, 2014). Outlining that when facing the adversity (A), it was his belief (B) that determined his emotional and behavioral responses (C), and not the injury itself, was the first step in helping Andrew recover. This outline involved me explaining to Andrew, via a presentation on these concepts, what he could and could not control in this process – he could not control his injury, but he could control his belief that it was the "end of the world" and consequently his emotional and behavioral responses to this belief. The ABC assessment table below (Figure 15.1) provides a summary of the main activating event, irrational beliefs, and unhelpful consequences and highlights more clearly why REBT was an appropriate intervention to help Andrew with his situation.

Emotional and behavioral responses (C)

In order to advance the intervention, I started to identify the main emotional and behavioral reactions Andrew had in response to the injury. To identify these, I first asked Andrew how he felt and what actions he carried out when he found

---

Activating Event (A)

Situation: Second stage long-term knee injury, which required reconstructive surgery, with an anticipated 12-month period out of rugby

Adversity: Rugby is all Andrew bases his worth upon and having a long-term period out of the game is something he would find very difficult to overcome. From Andrew's point of view, rugby is everything

Irrational Beliefs (iB)

Demand: "I must recover as I absolutely must play rugby again"

Awfulizing: "If I cannot play again, it is the end of the world and this is the worst thing that could have happened to me"

Depreciation: "If I cannot play again, I am no use"

Unhelpful Consequences (C)

Emotional Consequences:
Increased anxiety and anger about the recovery process and subsequent performances after the recovery

Behavioral Consequences:
Avoidance coping
Withdrawal

Figure 15.1 ABC assessment table for Andrew

out about the severity of his injury. Andrew identified that he immediately felt anxious and angry when he knew he was injured.

Finding the adversity (A)

The next stage of the REBT framework was to identify with Andrew the critical adversity that had triggered the irrational beliefs he was experiencing. In this instance, I used "inference chaining" (Ellis, et al., 1997), a technique in which Andrew was continually asked why his experience was a problem, in order to establish whether or not the injury itself was the underpinning adversity or merely the trigger point for other, more central inferences about it. Inference chaining enabled me to identify that it was not the injury itself that was the adversity, but the potential outcomes and consequences of not being able to recover and play rugby again, including self-depreciation and questioning of worth.

Irrational beliefs (B)

After establishing the critical adversity, I explored with Andrew the main irrational beliefs he held, primarily through the use of questions such as "What are you saying to yourself about the adversity that is causing the emotional and behavioral response?" When I asked this question, Andrew took some time to consider his response, before identifying that, to him, rugby was his "life" and that he had to recover because playing it "is an absolute must", otherwise he is "no use". Andrew also continually "awfulized" throughout our conversations – "If I cannot play again, it is the end of the world and this is the worst thing that could have happened to me". He did not consider that there was anything maladaptive with any of these beliefs, but after I reflected them back to him, he started to understand why such beliefs might be unrealistic and unhealthy. He also started to identify that it could be these thoughts that had resulted in him experiencing increased anxiety and anger about the recovery process.

Disputation (D)

Within this phase, the main area of focus during the work I carried out with Andrew was around understanding the pragmatics of his beliefs and how they were contributing to his actions and behaviors. Initially, to dispute Andrew's beliefs, I used the "badness scale" technique, outlined by Ellis et al. (1997). I gave Andrew a range of adversities that he may encounter throughout his life, both within his sport and outside of it. I initially asked him to rate on a scale of 0% (not bad at all) to 100% (the worst thing that could ever happen) where he would rate his current injury situation. Andrew initially identified his injury situation as one of the worst things that could ever happen at "85% bad". Subsequent to this phase, I then asked Andrew to identify on the scale where he would put aspects such as stubbing his toe, being paralyzed, contracting an incurable disease, never playing rugby again, losing a loved one, losing an important match, or being relegated.

Andrew started to appreciate two things. Firstly, he started to realize that, regardless of how bad any situation may become, it was never awful or insurmountable. Andrew had identified that losing a loved one, in particular his girlfriend, was the worst thing that could happen to him, but that he could recover from even that situation. He rated this event at "95% bad", which was below awful, or "101% bad" (Ellis et al., 1997). Andrew also started to understand that the situation he was in with his injuries was not as bad as he had considered it to be when he was first asked to put this on the scale. When we were working through the other events that may be considered adverse in a person's life, Andrew asked whether or not he could move events he had already put on the scale to accommodate his changing thoughts and opinions. When I asked what he meant, he responded by outlining that there are a number of much worse events that could happen in his life, and losing some playing time or his rugby career to injury was not as terrible as he had thought. I asked him where he would now put his injury on the scale and he moved it to "50% bad". Although he still believed that it was a bad situation, he acknowledged that he could experience worse events, including being paralyzed ("90% bad"), contracting an incurable disease ("85% bad"), and never playing rugby at any level again ("60% bad"). In essence, Andrew had gone from believing his injury situation was one of the worst aspects of his life ("85% bad") to having a more rational understanding of the circumstances he was experiencing ("50% bad").

Effective rational belief (E) phase

Within this phase, I worked with Andrew to promote a new, more adaptive rational belief. This change only occurred once he understood that the current beliefs he held were irrational and illogical in relation to other potential adversities he might experience in his life. I firstly asked Andrew if he could outline to me how he would change his belief that the injury was the worst thing that could happen to him to a more rational belief. Andrew struggled with this, as he had never considered an alternative way to think about these beliefs he held. Consequently, I worked with him by suggesting he could consider softening the tone of language used and using preferences as alternatives (Turner & Barker, 2013). Due to the directive nature of REBT, I suggested that Andrew might wish to consider a more rational belief like, "I really, really want to play rugby again, and . . . if I am not able to it will not be the end of the world and it will not reduce my worth as a person. It will be hard to bear but it will not be unbearable". Andrew acknowledged that this belief was perhaps more rational, but he also thought that this was underselling what he had achieved and what he could offer if he recovered from injury. Instead, he suggested the alternative belief could be, "Being injured is bad, but it is not the end of the world, and I know I can give everything to recover and try 100% to become a professional rugby player, and it may still not happen. I would like to recover and play again but I will be able to do other things with my life if I can't". When I asked Andrew to comment on why he wanted to include the aspect about giving everything to recover, he said it was because he felt it was something he could control. He now acknowledged that there were aspects of his situation, such as the injury itself, he could not control, but there were other aspects such as his motivation and determination throughout his recovery he could control and he wanted to be reminded of this in his rational belief. This new belief was one that Andrew now aligned himself to and kept reminding himself of throughout his recovery period.

Reinforcement

In this period, I worked with Andrew to reinforce the ABCDE and badness scale procedures we had used to challenge his beliefs and consequential behaviors by asking him what he felt he had learned from the process. Andrew outlined that he believed he was more knowledgeable about his current situation and the way his beliefs drive his behaviors, while also acknowledging his new beliefs around the injury process. The reinforcement session of the REBT process with Andrew took place 1-month after the final effective rational belief (E) phase had taken place. This timescale was chosen because it allowed Andrew to have some experience of reminding himself of his rational belief, while at the same time identifying instances during his recovery process where he had gone back to more irrational thinking. Although Andrew acknowledged the benefits of the process he had gone through, he identified that he had gone back to irrational thinking during particular events in his recovery period. These were primarily during tough rehabilitation sessions, where he had either been pushed to the limits of his capabilities, or had been involved in conversations with other players and coaches in the team asking when he was going to be back playing with the team. Andrew was, however, able to manage and deal with this maladaptive thinking and restructure his thoughts to be more positive and facilitative to his mental health. In essence, Andrew was using ABCDE in situ, self-regulating his own thoughts and beliefs based upon the conversations we had previously. This understanding allowed me to reiterate to Andrew that he had the capabilities to change any irrational beliefs he may have had, regardless of whether it was during a recovery from injury or not.

Humanistic counselling

While I used REBT as a technique to help Andrew understand his thoughts and beliefs in relation to his injury, the continuation of humanistic-based counselling with Andrew helped him to determine his own direction in the recovery process. This approach took place before, during, and after the introduction of REBT and continued until Andrew had fully recovered from his injury a number of months later. To me, it was fundamental that Andrew continued to be an active participant in the psychological recovery process and that through the adoption of REBT I was not just imposing skills and techniques I had at my disposal on him. The combined approach of REBT techniques and humanistic conversations, as outlined previously, provided Andrew the ability to respond well to particular demands and gave, I think, the most complete, person-centred approach in this situation. Our humanistic conversations, prior to his second injury, were around his reactions to his initial injury and how he was feeling psychologically and physiologically. Driven by Andrew himself, after the introduction of REBT, our conversations centred on his decision-making regarding what else he could do with his life to achieve self-fulfilment and actualization should he not be successful in his recovery from injury. This change in conversation by Andrew highlights the value that an integrative approach to practice can have for the client.

Outcome analysis

After Andrew had fully recovered from his injury, both psychologically and physically, and had started to train and compete with the team again, I asked him to reflect with me as to whether or not he believed his recovery process had been influenced by the work we had done. He offered the following reflection:

> Absolutely it has! I think there are a couple of reasons for that to be honest. Firstly, it gave me a better understanding of why I was behaving the way I was. I was falling out with people and getting really frustrated. When we did the ABCDE, I started to understand just how bad things were. It put it all in perspective – nothing is as bad as it ever seems. At the end of the day, I still have a family, I'm still healthy overall. That was what it made me realize. And I think starting to work through alternatives as well – knowing rugby wasn't everything or the only thing I could do. I just feel more relaxed about things. And even if I get injured again, I know it's not the "end of the world" as I thought before! I felt control . . . control of my thoughts and behaviours.

Andrew also felt that the process had been easy to follow, commenting that "at times" sport psychology can become "deep" if the conversation is focusing on difficult issues. He had found that the approach taken in response to his injury "was easier" because, due to the structure of REBT, it was "easy to understand and made it clear what was going on". He continued to come to the sessions we had arranged, owing to the fact that he felt they had value for his recovery.

As social validation, this form of evaluation is valuable in understanding, from Andrew's perspective, the recovery process he had gone through and the impact of the integrative approach on his injury rehabilitation and recovery. The work had helped Andrew understand that his irrational beliefs and consequential behaviors were controllable and gave him ways he could act in more adaptive ways.

In my own reflections on this work, I believe that Andrew was helped in his recovery by this intervention. When I first spoke to Andrew after his injury, I knew that he was experiencing anxiety and anger due to his body language and the way he spoke to me. A usually forceful character, Andrew had become withdrawn from others and spoke in a more timid manner. When I reflect upon how his attitude and body language changed throughout his recovery process, after every session he would comment on how much he valued the work I was doing with him and he also became more forthright with his opinions again. As our work together unfolded, he proceeded to become the Andrew I knew prior to his injury.

Critical reflections

Overall, the integrative use of REBT within a humanistic framework of sport psychology support was, for Andrew, a success as it helped support his psychological recovery from injury and increase his functioning. That said, some reflections on the strengths and limitations of the use of REBT as part of an injury recovery rehabilitation strategy may help to inform future applied practice.

Firstly, practitioners may need to consider the type and severity of the injury and how long the athlete is likely to be unable to train when using REBT as part of a recovery programme. When I worked with Andrew it was clear that after a period of time (approximately 2-months) the beneficial impact of the badness scale in reducing awfulizing to which he was prone would gradually decrease, resulting in him becoming more irrational in his beliefs again. Repeated sessions of REBT throughout longer-term injuries could be beneficial for athletes, ensuring that this type of "drift" might not be as pronounced.

One of the major benefits of REBT in the current context was that Andrew found the intervention easy to follow. It was, therefore, much easier for me, as the practitioner, to implement REBT because I did not continually have to explain the process to him. Rather, I could focus on helping him to change his beliefs via the intervention. When I first outlined what we were going to do and started to implement the intervention, he immediately identified why doing such an intervention may be beneficial, and we were able to quickly progress through the stages of intervention without him being unsure what we were doing and why we were doing it. For practitioners who place importance on their clients being able to collaborate in the work being done to inform its intended outcomes, the experience of working with Andrew suggests that REBT, as a technique-driven intervention, can be accommodating in this regard. Indeed, collaboration is a key part of what the REBT model emphasizes, and clients need to be active in the process.

One final consideration for future practice is the underpinning philosophical approach practitioners take with their work. Having an underpinning humanistic orientation to my practice, REBT and other technique-based interventions are not tools I would usually consider when choosing an intervention in my sport psychology practice. Through this case study, however, and other work I have carried out over the subsequent period, I have come to acknowledge and understand the value of having a skill set which is not solely and over-narrowly defined by the philosophical approach I take to the exclusion of all others, but that is also flexible enough to be concerned with the specific issues athletes present. In the case of Andrew, I may have been effective in helping his recovery from injury using just a humanistic approach. I believe, however, this would have taken a much longer period of time, with Andrew having to go through a more prolonged period of distress. Through broadening my approach, I was able to consider other alternatives to practice and offer a support programme, which gave Andrew short-term comfort and long-term benefit, helping him on his way to achieving self-actualization and recovery.

Conclusion

The current chapter outlined the case of Andrew, a professional rugby player who suffered significant knee injuries, and outlined how a combined integrative approach using REBT and humanistic counselling can be used to effectively support athletes with serious injuries (such as those Andrew encountered) and facilitate recovery. Although the process was successful in Andrew's case, in deciding whether to use REBT in other cases there is a need to consider the length of time athletes are likely to be out injured, but perhaps more fundamentally whether or not REBT represents a useful intervention on its own, or is best used in combination with other approaches (as in this instance), to provide psychological support for athletes with serious injuries.

References

Dryden, W. (2009). *How to think and intervene like an REBT therapist*. London: Routledge.

Ellis, A. (1957). Rational psychotherapy and individual psychology. *Journal of Individual Psychology, 13*, 38–44.

Ellis, A., Gordon, J., Neenan, M., & Palmer, S. (1997). *Stress counselling: A rational emotive behavior approach*. London: Cassell.

Rogers, C. R. (1959). A theory of therapy, personality, and interpersonal relationships, as developed in the client-centered framework. In S. Koch (Ed.), *Psychology, a study of a science. Vol. III: Formulations of the person and the social context*. New York, NY: McGraw-Hill.

Tripp, D. A., Stanish, W., Ebel-Lam, A., & Birchard, B. W. (2007). Fear of reinjury, negative affect, and catastrophizing predicting return to sport in recreational Athletes with anterior cruciate ligament injuries at 1 year postsurgery. *Rehabilitation Psychology, 52*(1), 74–81. doi:10.1037/0090-5550.52.1.74.

Turner, M. J., & Barker, J. B. (2013). Examining the efficacy of rational-emotive behavior therapy (REBT) on irrational beliefs and anxiety in elite youth cricketers. *Journal of Applied Sport Psychology, 25*, 131–147. doi:10.1080/10413200.2011.574311.

Turner, M. J., & Barker, J. B. (2014). Using Rational-Emotive Behavior Therapy with athletes. *The Sport Psychologist, 28*(1), 75–90. doi:10.1123/tsp.2013-0012.

Turner, M. J., Slater, M. J., & Barker, J. B. (2014). Not the end of the world: The effects of Rational-Emotive Behavior Therapy on the irrational beliefs of elite academy athletes. *Journal of Applied Sport Psychology, 26*(2), 144–156. doi:10.1080/10413200.2013.812159.

Editors' commentary on Chapter 15: "'It's the end of the world as we know it (and I feel fine)': the use of Rational Emotive Behavior Therapy (REBT) to increase function and reduce irrational beliefs of an injured athlete"

Robert, David, and Martin address a really important issue in their chapter. Injury will affect every athlete in their careers, to lesser and greater extents, and REBT can be a very effective approach to helping athletes rehabilitate, or in the worst cases, transition out of athletic performance. As highlighted in the chapter, awfulizing can hinder an athlete's efforts to successfully come through an injury. Research indicates that higher catastrophizing (a term often used instead of awfulizing) leads to greater pain, more distress, greater disability, poorer quality of life in response to injury, and is generally negatively related to all pain outcomes investigated such as intensity, distress, and functioning, whereas decreased catastrophizing leads to decreased pain, disability, and depressive symptoms (see Schnur, et al., 2010, for a review). Particularly relevant to athletes, catastrophizing is related to post-knee surgery pain (Pavlin, et al., 2005), and poorer pain adjustment and unrealistic thoughts about pain (Dixon, et al., 2004). Therefore, irrational beliefs may have an important part to play in the biopsychosocial understanding of pain.

The authors skilfully work with the athlete to dispute his "it is the end of the world" belief. Timing is vital here. We would not recommend disputing a client's awfulizing too soon after an injury, particularly if the injury is severe. In disputation, you are challenging the athlete, and in some cases, you are having a difficult conversation. Being too active-directive and challenging too soon can damage rapport. Morris et al. collaborate with the athlete, developing rapport before disputation, therefore when beliefs are disputed, teamwork (athlete-practitioner) becomes a vital component. When taken at its most fundamental level, even if the injury is career-ending, helping the athlete to see that this is not truly awful will be a difficult conversation and process, but if done right, will help the athlete to move on.

References

Dixon, K. E., Thorn, B. E., & Ward, L. C. (2004). An evaluation of sex differences in psychological and physiological responses to experimentally-induced pain: A path analytic description. *Pain, 112*, 188–196.

Pavlin, D. J., Sullivan, M. J. L., Freund, P. R., & Roesen, K. (2005). Catastrophizing: A risk factor for postsurgical pain. *The Clinical Journal of Pain, 21*(1), 83–90.

Schnur, J. B., Montgomery, G. H., & David, D. (2010). Irrational and rational beliefs and physical health. In D. David, A. Ellis & S. J. Lynn (Eds.), *Rational and irrational beliefs: Research, theory and clinical practice* (253–264). New York, NY: Oxford University Press.

16 Using Rational Emotive Behavior Therapy (REBT) to combat performance-debilitating unhealthy anxiety in an international level karateka

Clare Churchman

Introduction

I first became aware of REBT during my training as a clinical psychologist. To me the model offered a more complete formulation of people's emotional difficulties than other psychological approaches and offered clear points of intervention to help them achieve realistic aims. I undertook a specialist REBT placement as part of my doctoral program, completed the Primary Practicum in REBT at the Centre for REBT at the University of Birmingham in 2007 and followed up with the Advanced Practicum in REBT in 2008, again at the Centre for REBT. I have continued to use REBT regularly since then as my psychological approach of choice with clinical clients as well as athletes and I am currently working towards Associate Fellowship status. Being a clinically trained psychologist, my philosophy of practice with athletes is perhaps more holistic than it might otherwise have been. My usual focus when working with athletes is to understand the emotional distress that they are experiencing and to help them find ways to address and overcome it. In my opinion, improvements in performance will only be maintained when an individual is emotionally healthy. REBT provides an effective way to challenge debilitating irrational beliefs and promote psychological resilience in individuals working in high-pressure environments.

This chapter describes an REBT intervention with an international level karateka athlete, whilst also demonstrating that applied psychology in the real world can be messy and rarely textbook perfect. This is true in the clinic room but even more so in sporting contexts where psychologists attempt to conduct assessment and therapy with athletes around the complex demands of their sport. The chapter is written as a roadmap of therapeutic intervention, from initiation to ending stages, interspersed with reflections on the process by the athlete as service-receiver and myself as service-provider.

Context

When I met Tom he was a successful karateka athlete who had competed and medalled at national and international competitions in both kata and kumite since childhood. A few years earlier he had changed karate federations and had subsequently needed to learn new competition rules and fighting styles. He had found this psychologically challenging despite rising high in the ranks and being selected for the national squad. When Tom requested psychological intervention he was at the beginning of his competitive season and in the early stages of preparing for a major international competition, his largest and most important meet to date.

We arranged an initial meeting during which Tom briefly outlined the difficulties he was experiencing and I explained the basic theory of REBT and what he could expect if we worked together. This was followed up with an email and information sheets on the therapeutic approach so that Tom could make an informed decision on whether he wished to explore his difficulties in this way. I also suggested that he search for REBT on the Internet and gave him some websites to look at on the topic. After our initial meeting and reading of the material, Tom was in agreement to proceed with REBT sessions. After the sessions Tom later reflected, "I was eager to try some psychological intervention and prepared to believe that it would have a positive impact on me. I'd tried some stuff before but always doubted the process, 'it'll work for them but not me' etc., but this time it was important enough to want it to work and it did".

Tom and I agreed to meet regularly after a training session at his local training establishment. As both a Clinical and a Sport Psychologist I find the choice of where to meet athletes more difficult than with usual therapy clients. Although Sport Psychologists are often used to meeting athletes in non-traditional consulting spaces, many other therapists prefer designated controlled environments that are designed to maximize the client's ability to fully engage in the therapeutic process. Naturally there are advantages and disadvantages to both of these approaches and I think in sport, the practitioner should decide upon the choice of location carefully. Tom and I agreed the location as it was convenient for Tom in terms of time and access, there was sufficient private space for us to speak together confidentially and it was associated to the nature of Tom's engagement in therapy (i.e., anxiety about sport performance). The sporting nature of the location gave the opportunity for emotions to be explored *in vivo* whilst containing any emotional distress and separating it from other spaces in Tom's life such as those of home and family. However, the time of the session and nature of the space meant that he was often tired and that there was always the possibility of the session being interrupted by other users of the dojo. These factors could have affected Tom's ability to concentrate on and confront emotional issues through fatigue and concerns about privacy and confidentiality. Reflecting on this particular case, I think that the location was adequate and overall we were able to utilize it well, however, I could have pushed harder to set boundaries around the therapy from the start in order to ensure Tom's commitment to the therapeutic process. Although taking therapy *into* an athlete's space can increase opportunities to access psychological support, one particular disadvantage of doing so is that the athlete does not have to make the extra commitment of remembering the appointment, getting themselves there and entering into a more traditional setting which could help prepare and increase a person's readiness to engage in therapy.

We agreed to meet for ten 45-minute sessions, in the first instance, with a chance to review and add more sessions if needed after that. After we selected a time and location for our sessions it was also important to agree the boundaries of the therapy itself. I used a standard informed consent to therapy agreement which when signed clearly states that the client is agreeable to the psychological therapy I have offered; they are aware I provide that service within the limitations of my own professional expertise and governing standards set out by the Health and Care Professions Council (HCPC) and the British Psychological Society (BPS); they understand payment, cancellation and termination of therapy policies, the provision and limitations of confidentiality (including my use of supervision) and that informed consent is a process that may require further consideration during the delivery of the therapy service. For Tom, there was an added caveat around confidentiality due to the expectation that the work conducted would be written up as a case study.

Presenting issue

Tom self-referred for psychological work in order to deal with problematic anxiety that was negatively affecting his performances in competition as well as his enjoyment of the sport itself. He reported worrying more and more in the run up to competition about potential competitors, whether he would be able to beat them, whether he *ought to* be able to beat them, whether he would be able to achieve his goals and what people would think of him. This was disrupting his pre-competition routine and affecting his performance during a fight, leading to competition losses and feeling 'bad' about himself and his performance after competitions. He hoped to alleviate his anxiety so that he could perform to the best of his ability in competition throughout the year.

Needs analysis

Assessing suitability of REBT

Some practitioners use formal measures (usually questionnaires) to screen for the presence of irrational beliefs in their clients in order to assess suitability of REBT as a therapeutic approach; however, there are a number of conceptual problems with irrational belief scales (Terjesen, et al., 2009), for example, scales can include assessment of emotional distress, behavioral consequences, inferences or automatic thoughts as well as irrational beliefs (Robb & Warren, 1990). In addition, most people are unable to access irrational demands in the absence of their unhealthy emotion and their 'irrationality' would be missed when completing the questionnaire in a moment of calm or in the presence of an entirely different emotional experience, such as a healthy emotion (Jones, 2016). Therefore, in deciding whether REBT would be a suitable therapeutic approach, I followed the advice of Trower, et al. (2016, pg. 38–39) who recommend consideration of the following criteria:

1   "That the client is disturbed and/or behaving in a way that is dysfunctional to a degree that their quality of life (or in some circumstances, that of closely associated others) is seriously affected"

2   "That the emotional or behavioural problem is triggered by external psycho-social adversities or internal, physiological symptoms . . . rather than being the direct consequence of a physical illness or injury" and "that the core problem is specifically an emotional and/or behavioural disturbance"

3   "Whether the client is likely to be able to benefit", for example, whether the client has a learning disability or cognitive impairment that would preclude them from being able to fully explore their problem from a cognitive behavioural viewpoint

4   "Whether the client is ready for CBC [cognitive behavioural counseling]"; the authors suggest that clients should at least be in the contemplation stage of change (Prochaska & DiClemente, 1984)

5   Whether the client has another agenda that would interfere with the therapeutic process, for example, if due to on-going litigation they stand to achieve financial gain by remaining distressed

From his description, Tom's problem appeared to be emotionally based and, more specifically, appeared to be unhealthy anxiety, one of the eight dysfunctional emotional responses emphasized in REBT (first criterion) that was triggered in response to adversity perceived at the time of competition (second criterion). From speaking with him briefly at the time of his referral I had no reason to believe that he would struggle with the ideas and concepts of REBT (third criterion). His self-referral indicated motivation to explore his difficulties and challenge himself and he appeared psychologically robust in other areas of his life that could otherwise unsettle the therapeutic process (fourth criterion). There was no indication that Tom had an agenda that would affect the therapeutic process (fifth criterion).

Assessing the problem

REBT is an active-directive, change-focused brief therapy and as such therapists do not usually dwell on gathering lots of historical background information from clients, unlike therapists using other psychological approaches. REBT also posits that although emotional difficulties may have historical roots, clients are disturbed in the present because they still believe the irrational ideas with which they created their unhealthy emotional responses in the first place (Ellis, et al., 1997), therefore a focus on the present allows the client to see how they are actively reinforcing these beliefs. I used the early sessions to understand Tom's current situation and presenting difficulties but did not go into the details of his earlier life or long sporting career. Tom told me about his preferences within the sport (i.e., kata vs. kumite) and in which categories he fought. He outlined his training program, the competitions for the season and talked about his goals for them. These were often "to medal" and/or "do well". In addition to being seen as unnecessary practice in REBT, leaving the historical aspect out of early sessions enabled us to move faster in tackling Tom's main issue of anxiety. This was imperative as the competitive season was already underway and Tom had upcoming competitions with the national team to attend.

When assessing a client's problem with REBT I try to elicit the client's REBT-ABC (activating event, irrational beliefs and consequences) by following a semi-structured process such as that detailed by Trower et al. (2016) or by Dryden et al.'s (2010) REBT Competency Scale. However, even when using such structures it is important to remain flexible and non-dogmatic and remember that any understanding of a person's problem is just one explanation of many possible alternatives and is subject to change and amendment. REBT practitioners are encouraged to remember that assessment occurs constantly throughout the therapeutic process, with clinicians formulating and testing hypotheses within the principles of REBT (Ellis, et al., 1997).

After gaining an understanding of Tom's general presenting problem and goal we explored his experience of anxiety in more detail using the ABC as a guide. When assessing a client's emotional 'C' I rarely use standardized mood questionnaires for a number of reasons. On a practical basis these types of questionnaires are not based on REBT theory and the use of them would lead to confusion in the therapeutic approach, for example, mixing inferences (at A) and irrational beliefs (at B) with cognitive, behavioral and emotional consequences (at C); mixing aspects of the unhealthy emotion with its healthier, rational counterpart; and tending to look for a reduction in intensity of the emotion rather than a qualitative change in an emotional experience (e.g., less anxious rather than concerned). In addition they are often based on medical models of emotional distress and designed for psychiatric or clinical populations whereas the principles of REBT can be used to promote healthier psychological philosophies with clients who would not be considered to be experiencing problems worthy of a diagnosis. Instead of using formal measures I keep in mind the *relevant themes* associated with the various emotional responses (e.g., threat for anxiety, transgression of a rule for anger), as well as their *action tendencies* and *cognitive distortions*, and draw on this knowledge to determine which emotion the client is experiencing and whether it is healthy or unhealthy. I use the client's language wherever possible although it is often necessary to use REBT's emotional language when explaining the differences between healthy and unhealthy negative emotions. In this particular case I could understand early on from Tom's description of his problem that he was most likely experiencing unhealthy anxiety so I could enter the assessment process with a clear idea of what to look for.

When assessing anxiety, it is helpful to understand that it is a future oriented emotional response and therefore it is always best to elicit a client's anxiety about an upcoming event rather than have them describe a past experience of anxiety.

This helps the client connect to the emotion in the therapy session and therefore elicit the irrational beliefs. However, this can be difficult when working with competition related anxiety, particularly if competitions do not occur frequently during the course of psychological intervention. This was the case for Tom at the start of our sessions so we initially spent some time looking back at past competitions and recalling thoughts, feelings and behaviors that Tom believed had affected his performance. This kind of information gathering can be useful to help identify the client's perception of what has gone wrong and assists in the development of emotional insight, helping the therapist assess the degree of emotional responsibility held by the client. Then when the season started and he began to compete, Tom used a combination of thought diaries and his own competition notes to record thoughts, feelings and behaviors during a meet and our sessions focused on anxiety that he was feeling in reference to the competition that was coming up a few days later. These methods of identifying the C also highlighted a number of potential As. To explore these situations further in our sessions I used a combination of Socratic questioning, (e.g., "how do you respond when . . . happens?"), inference chaining (e.g., "if . . . then . . ."), Ellis's sentence completion ("and that would mean . . .") and 'Windy's Magic Question' ("Assuming the situation stays the same, what one thing could relieve your distress?", e.g., Dryden, 2001). Using these assessment strategies we were able to identify a number of specific situations (situational A) and inferences (critical A) associated with Tom's anxiety (C). These are detailed next.

When thinking about a meet coming up in the next week and who he would have to fight (situational A), Tom assumed "I'm not doing enough training!" and that he would therefore perform badly and likely be beaten (inference – critical A). Consequences associated with this A included feeling a sense of dread, underestimating his own skills and abilities whilst overestimating those of competitors, doubting his training regime, underestimating his ability to cope under pressure and anticipating the negative evaluation of others should he perform badly or make a mistake (anticipated shame). This thinking could also lead then to panic preparation rather than sticking to his original competition preparation plan.

At the meet itself there were a number of different triggers for an anxious response that were all associated with the perceived threat of performing badly, for example, when rating other competitors as stronger than himself; evaluating the day's performances as bad and believing that they would likely continue to be so; and evaluating pre-competition preparation as 'not enough' (inferences – critical As). Other triggers included Tom feeling anxious, nauseous and tense; thinking about his technique in an extremely focused and detailed way that disturbed flow and was quickly detrimental in a fight; attending excessively to a mistake; moving away from his fight strategy; getting drawn into his competitor's fight; and making rash moves that ultimately cost him points, sometimes got him disqualified and sapped him of energy. These were also the consequences when Tom found out that he was drawn against lower ranked fighters, opponents that he had beaten in previous competitions or who were rated as less competitive than himself (situational A). In these situations Tom perceived these competitors as "beatable" and that therefore he *ought* to win against them (inference – critical A).

If, when losing during a fight (situational A), Tom evaluated his performance as poor (inference – critical A), consequences included mentally resigning and giving up from the fight (possibly indicating a sense of loss and a feeling of depression), and overestimating negative judgment from others. Such a situation was often followed by feeling angry at himself for having given up or made mistakes and feeling ashamed in front of teammates and coaches about his "poor" performance.

Paradoxically, Tom noted that he did not often feel anxious when facing a final place fight. His inference here was that by reaching this stage he had already medalled and therefore had validated himself both in his own eyes and in those of others regardless of what happened in the final fight. Tom explained that "fighting to the best of my ability is more important than winning. If you're in the final you know you're going to get a medal, therefore you know you're doing well".

I then established whether there were any meta-emotional problems stemming from Tom's feelings of anxiety. Meta-emotional problems are where clients disturb themselves about their emotional problems (Dryden, 2002), for example, feeling ashamed about reacting in an anxious way. It is important to assess the presence of meta-emotional problems in order to decide which emotional problem to first target in therapy. Although working with the principle emotional problem would logically then remove the second, it is sometimes more appropriate to tackle the meta-emotional problem first, for example, when the presence of the meta-emotion interferes with the work you or the client are trying to do on the primary emotional problem or when the meta-emotion is clinically more important than the primary emotion (Dryden, 2002). Tom described feeling anxiety about his competition anxiety, although this time it was expressed in thoughts of being a coward for feeling anxious, doubts about himself and the way he lived his life, and reassurance seeking. This fed back into increased anxiety in situations such as competitions that were seen as chances to prove that he was not a coward.

A need for validation

Grieger and Boyd (1980) describe ego anxiety as a consequence of people believing that they must perform well and/or be approved of by others in order to accept themselves, and that it is awful when they do not perform well and/or are not approved of by others as they must be. Discomfort anxiety on the other hand occurs when people perceive their comfort to be threatened and believe that they should or must get what they want (or not get what they do not want) and that it is awful and unbearable when they do not get what they should or must. The exploration of Tom's As and Cs suggested that ego anxiety was prominent in his experience. A number of statements he had made throughout our sessions had highlighted this (e.g., "I haven't validated myself on the world stage"; "I want to feel like I've done well and have my coach tell me [that I've done well]. That can be as good as a win for me"; "There is an element of what people think . . . it validates you as a performer to win something big"). Such statements indicated the presence of one of the main irrational beliefs posited by REBT theory: "I must do well and win approval for my performances or else I rate as a rotten person" (Grieger & Boyd, 1980). It was becoming clear through the assessment that this belief was active in most areas of Tom's life and particularly affected his competition state.

Tom identified anxiety on competition day as the target problem for our detailed assessment, specifically feeling anxious in the build up to a fight against an opponent he perceived as stronger. As mentioned previously, anxiety is best assessed *in vivo* as most people are unaware of their demands when they are no longer feeling anxious. Indeed many clients find it difficult to access the demand even when they are really feeling the emotional problem, as this relies on the therapist being able to facilitate the right response at the right time. Within a session many people can explore their fears in a more balanced way and will often provide alternative rational inferences and beliefs to the ones they experienced at the time of the anxiety itself. As I was not going to the meet myself, the example would have to be explored in our session a few days later via notes and reflections that Tom would take on the day of competition. For this reason I spent some time preparing Tom in the session before the meet and ensuring that he was familiar with the As and Cs of the REBT model so that he could accurately record his experience on the day. In the session following the meet I encouraged Tom to reconnect to his anxious competition experience by encouraging him to recount the event in detail bringing in contextual cues that could support him to reconnect to the lived experience, for example, describing his competitor's physical appearance. Bringing emotion into the room is extremely important in REBT and it can be quite difficult for the practitioner to encourage this, often because the client has disconnected from the emotion by the time of the session but also because of a client's beliefs about how they should act in therapy and a practitioner's confidence in working with intense emotions during sessions. Once Tom was reconnected with his anxiety I used sentence completion and other similar probes (see, for example, Wessler & Wessler, 1980) to elicit his irrational beliefs about the critical A. The ABC was as follows (see Figure 16.1).

At this point of the process I elicited Tom's situational goal, that is, how he would prefer to respond to the situation. Setting a clear goal will help in the disputing phase to illustrate the futility of the client's irrational beliefs and consequences towards that goal and to help them come up with an alternate healthy but negative emotional state for their problematic situation. Tom's goal was to fight his own fight, stay focused on his own technique and strategy, not get distracted by his opponent's moves and be able to evaluate and analyze his performance with his coaches after the fight in a way that could be a useful learning tool rather than feeling anxious about their judgments, ashamed about performing poorly and low in mood for underachievement. Tom easily acknowledged that his current emotional C of anxiety was not conducive to his new goal, but that

---

Activating Event: "Prior to a fight and I'm thinking that I'm fighting poorly today, he's going to win, I'm going to get humiliated in this fight and let myself and my coaches down, they're going to be disappointed in me"

Irrational Beliefs	**Rational Beliefs**

Demand: "I don't want that to happen! I need them to be pleased with me; I need that validation from my coaches!"

Awfulizing: "It's so bad that it's awful when my coaches don't validate me"

Self-Depreciation: "My coaches being disappointed about this performance proves that I'm totally worthless, that I haven't achieved what I ought to have achieved by now . . . that's an awful thought too"

Unhelpful Consequences	**Helpful Consequences**

Emotional Consequence: Anxiety

Behavioral Consequence: Put pressure on myself, make more mistakes, get drawn into his strategy, tire myself out and perform even worse than I was doing to begin with

Cognitive Consequence: Overestimating how badly I'll perform and how disappointed my coaches will be

Physiological Consequence: Get tense during the fight, tire myself out

---

Figure 16.1 ABC form displaying Tom's situational and critical A, irrational beliefs and unhelpful consequences (permission to use table granted by P. Trower, 2016)

feeling *concerned* about his performance and what he and others would think afterwards would allow him to give it his best shot and not be hard on himself after the event. I asked him what the emotional, behavioral and cognitive elements of healthy concern could look like for him before we moved onto generating alternative rational beliefs that could then be disputed along with the irrational beliefs in the intervention phase. I led the development of rational beliefs, ensuring that the first part of each belief remained and asking Tom to suggest alternative endings. Tom was able to give theoretically consistent suggestions for the preference, anti-awfulizing and unconditional self-acceptance beliefs that did not require much adaptation before the disputation phase. I was lucky in that Tom understood the concepts and principles of the ABC model very quickly though this is not the case with all clients and more time on the teaching of REBT theory is often required.

Intervention

Change techniques can be broadly categorized as cognitive, imaginal and behavioral (see, for example, Wessler & Wessler, 1980). My natural tendency is to start with cognitive strategies such as disputing as this is something that can be attempted immediately and without much preparation, unlike behavioral techniques such as risk taking exercises and Albert Ellis's shame attacking. First, I ensured that Tom understood the B-C connection and then I began to teach disputation on each of the irrational beliefs indicated in his ABC example: "I don't want my coaches to be disappointed, therefore I *need* them to be pleased with me, I *need* that validation from others!" (demand); "It's so bad that it's awful when others don't validate me" (awfulizing); and "My coaches being

---

Activating Event: "Prior to a fight and I'm thinking that I'm fighting poorly today, he's going to win, I'm going to get humiliated in this fight and let myself and my coaches down, they're going to be disappointed in me"

Irrational Beliefs	Rational Beliefs
Demand: "I don't want that to happen! I need them to be pleased with me; I need that validation from my coaches!"	**Preference:** "I don't want that to happen! However, although I *want* them to be pleased with me, I don't *need* them to be pleased with me"
Awfulizing: "It's so bad that it's awful when my coaches don't validate me"	**Anti-Awfulizing:** "It won't feel great but it also won't be the end of the world and more importantly . . ."
Self-Depreciation: "My coaches being disappointed in this performance proves that I'm totally worthless, that I haven't achieved what I ought to have achieved by now . . . that's an awful thought too"	**Unconditional Self-Acceptance:** "My coaches being disappointed in this performance doesn't prove that I'm totally worthless. It only proves that I make mistakes the same as everyone else. My worth as a person doesn't depend on whether people think I fight well"

Unhelpful Consequences	Helpful Consequences
Emotional Consequence: Anxiety	**Emotional Consequence:** Feel concerned about the possibility I might get beaten here
Behavioral Consequence: Put pressure on myself, make more mistakes, get drawn into his strategy, tire myself out and perform even worse than I was doing to begin with	**Behavioral Consequence:** Make an effort to do my best, set myself some goals and try to pay attention to them, listen to my coaches' advice, try to stay in the game
Cognitive Consequence: Overestimating how badly I'll perform and how disappointed my coaches will be	**Cognitive Consequence:** Don't beat myself up if I make a mistake
Physiological Consequence: Get tense during the fight, tire myself out	**Physiological Consequence:** Ready but not tense

Goal: Fight my own fight, stay focused on my own technique, not get distracted by my opponent, feel ok if my performance is not top or if my coaches aren't happy with it. Use it as a chance to learn and develop

---

Figure 16.2 Tom's completed ABC form (permission to use table granted by P. Trower, 2016)

disappointed about this performance proves that I'm completely worthless" (self-depreciation).

Ellis believed that the demand is the key irrational belief and the other three irrational beliefs, awfulizing, depreciation and low frustration tolerance, are derivatives of the demand (Dryden, 2002), and so the demand is what I aim to dispute first. Using empirical, practical and logical disputes, Tom immediately understood the irrationality of demands and the rationality of desires and this for him was represented in an intellectual and an emotional shift with little need for further intervention. Teaching disputation is often not enough for clients, yet Tom was able to take it and immediately expand on this concept himself in the next competition, practicing statements such as "I *want* my coach to be happy with my performance but I don't *need* him to be happy in order to value myself as a person and a fighter" and "I might want my performances to always be great so people can respect me for them but I don't have to have what I want, no matter how bad I want it".

The next target was the self-depreciation belief, as I evaluated this belief as more powerful than the awfulizing belief. Again I used empirical, practical and logical disputation and exercises such as the "fruit basket" described in Wessler & Wessler (1980, pg. 125), the "pizza" (Jones, 2007); and the "Big I, little i" (Lazarus, 1977 cited in Ellis & Grieger, 1986). Again Tom understood the principles of conditional and unconditional self-acceptance immediately and quickly agreed that statements such as "even if I put in a bad performance and my coaches think badly of me, it doesn't prove that I'm worthless, just that I'm human, not superhuman!" and "sometimes I make mistakes just like everyone else!" were true, helpful and logical.

The awfulizing belief was the final irrational belief to be challenged and again for this we used empirical, logical and practical disputations as well as an imaginal technique of time projection (Lazarus, 1971), which involved imagining a bad performance, perceived negative judgment from others and reflecting on how long negative feelings about this situation would likely last. This allowed Tom to imagine a more realistic occurrence of the negative event. By the end of the disputation process Tom's complete ABC looked like this (see Figure 16.2).

Outcome analysis

Tom's response to the disputation process was immediately positive. Often clients find it hard to make the head – heart shift; they understand the model intellectually but struggle to *feel* it emotionally; however, Tom immediately connected to the model. The so called "tyranny of the shoulds" (Horney, 1950) or "musterbation", as Albert Ellis coined the phrase, was so clear to Tom that he was able to dispute it without issue and, even better, maintain his progress. The competitive season gave ample opportunity for Tom to practice his newly developed beliefs in the presence of potential threat of poor performance and disappointment and disapproval from others and he was able to dispute his irrational beliefs each week. Over the next few months Tom noticed a number of other sport related demands that he was putting on himself that he was able to dispute successfully. "I ought to be doing more training, so therefore I *should* be doing more training!" became "I ought to be doing more training but I don't have to do it just because I ought to. Realistically it isn't possible for me to do that right now so I'll just have to deal with what I'm able to put in". This enabled Tom to feel more in control, enjoy training more and focus on family and work without panicking about missed training sessions. Tom reported feeling relaxed and confident before and during competitive meets and was again enjoying the experience of competing. More importantly, Tom began to put in strong performances, and came back from almost every meet having medalled in one or more of his competitive bouts. Each successful performance instilled Tom's confidence in himself and his performances but also in the REBT model and techniques that he was using on a regular basis. Tom now received regular external validation, and still believed that it was great to have, but he did not *need* it like he had thought a few months earlier. A number of times Tom would tell me how he had caught himself making demands during a meet and how he had noticed it and challenged it.

Doubts about performance still appeared from time to time (e.g., "I don't want to go there and look like a mug") but once explored these were identified as appropriate and flexible *preferences* (e.g., "I don't want to go there and look like a mug . . . but there is no reason why I must not have what I don't want"), which were characterized by an appropriate concern response that involved advance planning, goal-setting and preparation. Goals for competitive performance became much more specific and process oriented (e.g., to commit to an attack) rather than outcome oriented (e.g., to win). Tom began to associate more closely with *concern* rather than *anxiety*, for example, feeling nervous but excited, telling me "I was on the right side of the diagram" (in relation to the ABC form we used in sessions similar to Figure 16.3). Tom found it helpful to maintain his own notebook of thoughts, challenges and goals to help him remember REBT principles, which he used regularly to great success.

Wider applications

As Tom became more skilled in his use of REBT, the more he was able to use these skills to explore other anxiety provoking situations. For example, Tom was able to apply the ABC model and disputation techniques to one of the previously mentioned situations: feeling anxious when facing an opponent that he believed he ought to be able to beat (for example, due to previously winning against this competitor, being ranked higher than them or perceiving himself as more experienced/fitter/stronger). Using the recently learned techniques, Tom was able to identify and challenge irrational beliefs with little support (see Figure 16.3).

We were also able to branch out from anxiety and explore ABCs linked to feelings of anger and guilt, for example, when competition organization was problematic and frustrating, or at being away from home and family on so many weekends during the competitive season. As Tom progressed through the season we also

Activating Event: "I'm better than this guy so I ought to beat him!"

Irrational Beliefs	Rational Beliefs
Demand: "I ought to beat this guy so I absolutely should!"	**Preference**: "I ought to beat this guy but there's absolutely no reason why I *have to* or *must* beat him just because I ought to. So many things can happen in a fight, it's not something that I can demand to happen!"
Awfulizing: "If I don't beat him it's going to feel so bad that it'll be totally awful"	**Anti-Awfulizing**: "If I don't beat him I'm going to feel pretty bad for a while but it won't be *100% awful*, it's temporary, it will pass, and it seriously won't be the worst feeling ever!"
Self-Depreciation: "Failing to beat him when I ought to and should will prove that I'm totally useless"	**Unconditional Self-Acceptance**: "Failing to beat him when I know that I can and that I ought to beat him won't prove anything other than the fact I'm a fallible human being"

Unhelpful Consequences	Helpful Consequences
Emotional Consequence: Anxiety	**Emotional Consequence**: In the zone
Behavioral Consequence: Not fighting in my style	**Behavioral Consequence**: Committed to the action
Cognitive Consequence: Expecting the worst	**Cognitive Consequence**: Not second guessing, instinctive
Physiological Consequence: Tense	**Physiological Consequence**: Relaxed but alert

Goal: Get in the zone and win!

Figure 16.3 Additional completed ABC form for anxiety

spent some sessions exploring his meta-emotional problem of anxiety about anxiety, and his thoughts that experiencing anxiety meant that he was a coward. We were able to use the knowledge gained about demands for validation in specific situations and generalize out into a much wider context of proving oneself in life and not just in sport (e.g., "I have to do well in order to prove myself and I need that validation to accept myself"). Tom was curious as to how he had developed this belief and since he had become practiced enough at REBT theory to use it independently we also spent one of our sessions in a more explorative way (see Figure 16.4). Placing the belief in the middle (the problem) we thought about predisposing life experiences that may have made the development of such a belief more likely, as well as more recent events that may have increased its current potency. After this we thought about how the irrational beliefs that had been the target of our intervention were perpetuating the problem, and finally some pointers for change. Although unusual in REBT practice, this session helped contextualize Tom's irrational beliefs about validation and aided him to generate successful disputation skills and healthy and rational alternative beliefs.

What made me vulnerable in the first place?

Experience of being bullied as a child, feeling scared, didn't like the feeling of anticipation, dread. Sensitive to seeing threat around me.

My dad was a high achiever, a hard man. He encouraged me to fight back but I didn't like it. Saw myself as a coward and I hated that.

I believe being a good fighter is important; fighters get more respect than those that do kata.

Recent Triggers

Got picked for national squad.

Don't know the rules or the style, it's all new, that's a disadvantage.

Pressure at home, doing well would pacify the situation?

Now I need to get picked next year as well.

The Problem

Unhelpful beliefs – I want to do well and I *have to* do well in order to prove myself, for people to respect, admire, validate me…I *need* that external validation to accept myself. It's awful not to be approved of as I must be. I can't stand it…

When the demands are met, i.e. believe I can win, have been getting validation etc., there's no anxiety. Anxiety happens when in a situation that threatens the demands above and there's a chance that the demands won't be met – I feel anxious, focus on other competitors, feel muscle tension, performance goes down and validation goes with it. Unhelpful belief gets stronger.

Next ABC chain down – am I a coward for feeling anxious? I don't want to be a coward, I *shouldn't* be a coward! I *need to* prove that I'm not a coward! (Vicious cycle that acts as an anxiety reinforcing loop)

How to challenge it?

Need to challenge the demands to *have to do well* and that external validation is not just desired but *needed*. Keep them desires, *I want to do well. I want others to notice that and respect me but I don't need it in order to accept myself*… change the anxiety to healthy concern.

Figure 16.4 Explorative formulation of need for validation

Critical reflections

Overall, I consider this piece of work to be successful in a number of ways; subjectively the client felt better within himself, was concerned about performance where necessary but not anxious like before and objectively he put in strong performances and medalled at most competitions during the season. His fast understanding of the REBT approach together with a motivation to tackle the problem head on and support his practice with his own use of self-help books, videos and podcasts enabled Tom to quickly put REBT concepts into practice. The exploration of the possible origin of his irrational demands also gave Tom a better understanding of their development and a reason to challenge them further from his adult perspective. Although not necessarily part of REBT theory, historical contexts can be useful in showing clients the development of their beliefs through childhood and empowering them as adults to choose a different perspective on life. Tom's feedback on REBT was very positive too; he has since been able to use REBT in his own practice as a coach. He provided the following feedback: "I use REBT often and coach my own fighters on the ideas I have learned about from the sessions. For me it makes perfect sense and has worked very well. Occasionally I was unable to call upon it and then suffered anxiety, but I think this was down to lack of planning around the day and having too many variables there, which we discussed. Controlling everything I could – music, food, timing, etc. reduced the pressure and having my book of written goals was vital, with my REBT statements in. Without it, even though I could recall the goal and theory, my belief in the content was not as strong. Got to have the book!"

In critique of my own work as a practitioner, in practical terms I think I should have attended at least one meet with Tom in the assessment phase. Although it can be anxiety provoking as well as distracting for an athlete to have their psychologist on hand asking about what they are thinking in any given moment, being present in the emotional experience can help the practitioner observe outwardly visible consequences without being too intrusive. This would be particularly helpful if the athlete is struggling to identify their emotional experience and would also help to gain specificity in the ABC. Another important aspect of REBT that I sometimes overlook is the setting of homework assignments. As mentioned previously, Tom undertook his own homework in between sessions by identifying and challenging his beliefs on an almost weekly basis, either when in competition or in training camps, or sparring with other squad members who would also be opponents in competition. When he reported back how his own self-directed learning had taken place, he occasionally indicated that he had challenged his inferences rather than his beliefs. Although psycho-education took place within the session, we perhaps could have come up with agreed tasks that would have consolidated the difference between inferences at A and irrational beliefs at B.

My most significant reflections of this work are on the understanding of anxiety from an REBT perspective as there were a number of different avenues that could have been taken with Tom and could be taken with athletes experiencing anxiety in general. Tom was particularly in tune with his emotional experience and its associated thoughts, which made the assessment and intervention process easier. However, with another client it might have been difficult for me to get past "I want to win, so I have to win!" This would have led me to help Tom to dispute why he did not *have to* win, which is not always an easy strategy (albeit theoretically correct) for practitioners to take in the world of sport where winning usually entails monetary gain as well as recognition. Most importantly, it most likely would have led to disputing a discomfort anxiety (e.g., "I can't stand not winning!") rather than exploring further and uncovering the ego anxiety that was behind it (e.g., "I want to win, so I have to win, because not winning would prove that I am worthless").

Another reflection is that much of REBT theory suggests that the preference (and therefore demand) construct is one-dimensional; however, Trower and Jones (2015) posit the distinction of two different preference-demands: the "want-must" and the "ought-must" defined respectively as our wishes and desires, and our obligations or duties. Examples relevant to sport might be: "I must win because I 'want-must' be successful in everything I do" and "I must not lose because I 'ought-must' never let others down". The client's unhealthy consequences should alert the practitioner to the presence of one or other belief; an unmet want-must may lead to anxiety, anger or depression, whereas an unmet ought-must may lead to anxiety, guilt or shame. In the case of anxiety, a want-must belief may be more prominent in an athlete seeking approval from others, whereas an ought-must belief may be demonstrated by an athlete *avoiding disapproval* (Trower, 2016). In my work with Tom I did not explore this distinction as well as I could have, focusing predominantly on his approval seeking behavior and want-must belief to do well, gain approval and therefore be validated because without this validation he would be worthless and nothing (compared to being a morally bad person if he were to gain *disapproval*). On reflection my instinct suggests that he probably experienced both beliefs during the course of our sessions.

In REBT theory the experience of anxiety is ultimately the consequence of a demand *to be certain* and ABCs of this could be formulated at a number of levels, for example, "I need to know for sure that I will win this fight", "I need to know for sure that others will approve of my performance (or that I won't be disapproved of)" or, in the case of discomfort anxiety, "I need to know that this awful experience will not last forever". In my experience, deciding at which level to formulate requires consideration of the client's needs, their progress in REBT so far and their ability to understand potentially more abstract principles. In this particular case Tom was able to understand the step from *needing to win* to *needing approval and validation from others* but we did not go further in exploring the next level of abstraction, which to me would have been from "I need to know for sure that I'll win" to "I need to know for sure that I'll have approval".

Summary

This chapter has detailed a course of REBT sessions with an international level athlete experiencing performance related anxiety due to an irrational demanding philosophy for external validation. Through familiarization and practice of the REBT ABC model, Tom was able to identify his unhelpful demands leading to anxiety and successfully challenge them, along with self-depreciation and awfulizing beliefs, experiencing helpful concern in performance situations. Both subjective and objective change was noted after REBT intervention and was maintained over the course of the competitive season via Tom's dedication and motivation to the therapeutic process.

References

Dryden, W. (2001). *Reason to change: A rational emotive behavior therapy (REBT) workbook.* New York, NY: Brunner Routledge.

Dryden, W. (2002). *Fundamentals of rational emotive behaviour therapy: A training handbook*. Whurr Publishers Ltd.

Dryden, W., Beal, D., Jones, J., & Trower, P. (2010). The REBT competency scale for clinical and research applications. *Journal of Rational-Emotive Cognitive-Behavioural Therapy*, 28, 165–216

Ellis, A., Gordon, J., Neenan, M., & Palmer, S. (1997). *Stress counselling: a rational emotive behaviour approach*. New York, NY: Continuum.

Grieger, R., & Boyd, J. (1980). *Rational emotive therapy: A skills based approach*. New York, NY: Van Nostrand Reinhold Company.

Horney, K. (1950). *Neurosis and human growth*. New York, NY: Norton.

Jones, J. (2007). Personal communication.

Jones, J. (2016). Personal communication.

Lazarus, A. A. (1971). *Behaviour therapy and beyond*. New York, NY: McGraw-Hill.

Lazarus, A. A. (1977). Toward an egoless state of being. In A. Ellis and R. Grieger (Eds.) (1986), *Handbook of rational-emotive therapy*. New York, NY: McGraw-Hill.

Prochaska, J., & DiClemente, C. (1984). *The trans-theoretical approach: Crossing the traditional boundaries*. Homewood, IL: Dow Jones Irwen.

Robb, H.B., III., & Warren, R. (1990). Irrational belief tests: new insights, new directions. *Journal of Cognitive Psychotherapy: An International Quarterly*, 4(3), 303–311.

Terjesen, M. D., Salhany, J., & Sciutto, M. J. (2009). A psychometric review of measures of irrational beliefs: implications for psychotherapy. *Journal of Rational-Emotive Cognitive-Behavioural Therapy*, 27, 83–96.

Trower, P. (2016). Personal communication.

Trower, P. E., & Jones, J. (2015). Demanded wants and oughts: An overlooked distinction in REBT? *Journal of Rational-Emotive Cognitive-Behavioural Therapy*, 33, 95–113.

Trower, P., Jones, J., & Dryden, W. (2016). *Cognitive behavioural counselling in action* (3rd ed.). London: Sage.

Wessler, R. A., & Wessler, R. L. (1980). *The principles and practice of rational-emotive therapy*. San Francisco: Jossey-Bass.

Editors' commentary on Chapter 16: "Using Rational Emotive Behavior Therapy (REBT) to combat performance-debilitating unhealthy anxiety in an international level karateka"

As the final chapter in the book, and perhaps the springboard for the reader to explore REBT texts in more depth, it seems appropriate that Clare has provided a comprehensive overview of the many theoretical and technical issues that face practitioners. Many aspects of this chapter are worthy of additional comment, although one that might have the widest relevance is that of meta-emotional problems. One thing that unites the vast majority of the individuals with whom we have used

REBT is that their presenting problems are layered, and that the task of assessment might be compared to peeling an onion. The primary problem is often accompanied by a 'problem about the problem' (e.g., feeling depressed about on-going anxiety), hence the term 'meta-emotional problem'. It is helpful if the practitioner is alive to this possibility and carefully assesses for the presence of meta-emotional problems, since not doing so can hamper the progress of interventions. Consider an athlete with longstanding competition anxiety. In simplified terms, her 'primary' ABC might look like this:

A – I might not perform well (inference) in the forthcoming competition (situation)
B – I must perform well (demand) and I can't stand the idea of doing badly (LFT)
C – Anxiety (emotion) and an unhelpful outcome focus (cognition)

If a meta-emotional problem about the anxiety is also present, this can be formulated using the same model simply by re-stating the primary C as the new A:

A – Anxiety (emotion) and an unhelpful outcome focus (cognition)
B – I should not be anxious (demand) and it proves how weak I am (self-depreciation)
C – Depression (emotion) and reduced motivation to train (behavior)

It is helpful to formulate in this way both to demonstrate the generalizability of the model and as a means of promoting individual choice and ownership over the direction of therapy. The focus of the intervention can be a collaborative decision, although as Clare demonstrates in this chapter, sometimes there is intuitive logic about in which order problems might be addressed (Dryden & Branch, 2008). In the previous example, intuition might suggest that it will be hard for the athlete to make progress on her anxiety whilst simultaneously condemning herself for feeling anxious, and therefore, addressing the meta-emotional problem (depression about anxiety) might be the more helpful option.

Reference

Dryden, W., & Branch, R. (2008). *Fundamentals of Rational Emotive Behaviour Therapy: A training handbook*. Chichester: Wiley-Blackwell.

Index

Note: Pages in *italics* indicate figures; pages in **bold** indicate tables.